Dr Catherine Blackledge was born in 1968. Following a science degree and PhD, she worked as a science and medical journalist. This is her first book.

The Story of V

Opening Pandora's Box

Catherine Blackledge

PHOENIX

A PHOENIX PAPERBACK

First published in Great Britain in 2003
by Weidenfeld & Nicolson
This paperback edition published in 2004
by Phoenix,
an imprint of Orion Books Ltd,
Orion House, 5 Upper St Martin's Lane,
London WC2H 9EA

A CIP catalogue record for this book
is available from the British Library.

ISBN 0 75381 776 4

Diagrams by Raymond Turvey (Turveybooks Ltd)

Typeset by Selwood Systems, Midsomer Norton

Printed in Great Britain by
Clays Ltd, St Ives plc

For Baby Anne
and her family
of chicken farmers and weavers

CONTENTS

ILLUSTRATIONS

Colour

The vagina giving birth – from *The Yoni: Sacred Symbol of Female Creative Power* by Rufus C. Camphausen, Inner Traditions, Vermont, 1996.

The yoni as yantra – from *Yantra: The Tantric Symbol of Cosmic Unity* by Madhu Khanna, Thames & Hudson Ltd, London, 1979.

'The Origin of the World', Gustave Courbet, 1866 – Bridgeman Art Library/Musee d'Orsay, Paris.

Vulvas from *The Yoni: Sacred Symbol of Female Creative Power* by Rufus C. Camphausen, Inner Traditions, Vermont, 1996 (five) and by Jill Posener (three) from *Femalia* by Joani Blank, Down There Press, San Francisco, 1993. Reproduced with permission.

Female bonobos © Frans Lanting.

Black & White

1.1 – from *The Witch on the Wall: Medieval Erotic Sculpture in the British Isles* by Jørgen Andersen, Rosenkilde & Bagger, 1977.

1.2 – from *Images of Lust: Sexual Carvings on Medieval Churches* by Anthony Weir and James Jerman, Routledge, 1986.

1.3 – from *The Great Mother: An Analysis of the Archetype* by Erich Neumann, translated by Ralph Mannheim, Princeton University Press, 1963. Staatliche Museum Preussischer Kulturbesitz, Antikenmuseum, Berlin; Museum fur Volkerkunde, Berlin; British Museum.

1.4 – The Castello Sforcesco, Milano. Photo Bartorelli.

1.5 – from *Images of Lust: Sexual Carvings on Medieval Churches* by Anthony Weir and James Jerman, Routledge, 1986, Fortean Picture Library; *The Witch on the Wall: Medieval Erotic Sculpture in the British Isles* by Jørgen Andersen, Rosenkilde & Bagger, 1977, National Monuments Record, London; *The Yoni: Sacred Symbol of Female Creative Power* by Rufus C. Camphausen, Inner Traditions, Vermont, 1996.

1.6 – Terence Medean/Fortean Picture Library.

1.7 – Bridgeman Art Library/Kunsthistorisches Museum, Vienna; Bridgeman Art Library/Musée des Antiquités Nationales, St-Germain-en-Laye, France.

1.8 – from *The Great Mother* by Erich Neumann; British Museum. Bridgeman Art Library/Ashmolean Museum, Oxford.

2.1 – redrawn from *The Language of the Goddess* by Marija Gimbutas, London: Thames and Hudson, 2001.

2.2 – from *Making Sex: Body and Gender from Greeks to Freud* by Thomas Laqueur, Harvard University Press, 1990.

2.3 – from *Eve's Secrets: A New Theory of Female Sexuality* by Josephine Lowndes Sevely, Random House, 1987.

2.4 – from *Making Sex: Body and Gender from Greeks to Freud* by Thomas Laqueur, Harvard University Press, 1990; The Mind Has No Sex: Women in the Origins of Modern Science by Londa Schiebinger, Harvard University Press, 1989.

2.5 – from *Making Sex: Body and Gender from the Greeks to Freud* by Thomas Laqueur, Harvard University Press, 1990.

3.1 – from 'Communications from the Mammal Society', *New Scientist*, © Stephen Glickman.

3.2 – from *Sexual Selection and Animal Genitalia* by William G. Eberhard; Harvard University Press, 1985; *Female Control: Sexual Selection by Cryptic Female Choice* by William G. Eberhard, Princeton University Press, 1996.

3.3 – redrawn from *Female Control: Sexual Selection by Cryptic Female Choice* by William G. Eberhard, Princeton University Press, 1996.

3.4 – from *Sexual Selection and Animal Genitalia* by William G. Eberhard; Harvard University Press, 1985.

4.1 – from *Eve's Secrets: A New Theory of Female Sexuality* by Josephine Lowndes Sevely, Random House, 1987; 'New Treatise Concerning the Generative Organs of Women' by Reinier de Graaf, annotated translation

7.4 – redrawn from 'The Female Orgasm: Pelvic Contractions' in *Archives of Sexual Behaviour,* Bohlen Joseph G. et al., *11* (5); (1982), 367.

7.5 – redrawn from Slob A. K. et al., 'Physiological Changes During Copulation in Male and Female Stumptail Macaques' in *Physiology and Behaviour, 38* (1986), 891–5.

7.6 – from *Primate Sexuality: Comparative Studies of the Prosimians, Monkeys, Apes and Human Beings* by Alan F. Dixson, Oxford University Press, 1998.

Ella habla por en medio en las piernas.

She speaks from between her legs.

INTRODUCTION

This book is about views of the vagina. Unorthodox views, colourful views, blinkered views and revolutionary views. Inside these pages, you'll find vaginal perspectives from a vast array of sources. There are views of the vagina from science, from history, from mythology and folklore, literature and language, and anthropology and art. My aim is to provide as full and frank a picture as possible of female genitalia. A wide-angle vaginal view, if you will. And my hope is that, because of this book, you won't ever look at the vagina in quite the same way again.

How do you feel about female genitalia? What does the vagina mean to you? For many, the vagina is the seat of female sexual pleasure, the site of the creation of humankind and the channel for its birth. For both women and men it is also a potent arouser of sexuality. Yet these are not the only views of the vagina. For some, the vagina signifies sacred sexuality. It is an object of worship, recognised as the font of life, an icon of fertility. In stark contrast, the vagina appears elsewhere as an emasculating, castrating fearsome toothed organ – the *vagina dentata.* Meanwhile, many, if not all, cultures see this portion of female anatomy as something which, in public, women must cover up at all costs. The word 'vagina' is one that is avoided in the majority of conversations, and from the top shelves of convenience stores doctored female genital images peer down. So many ways of perceiving the vagina, so which one do you plump for?

Before I started researching and writing this book, I too had my own conception of the vagina. And, I must admit, it was a somewhat limited viewpoint. I had a vagina between my legs, it was about sex, about pleasure, about bleeding and about pissing. It could also, unfortunately, be about pain. And, in the future perhaps, it would be about childbirth. Those were the facts about my female genitals. But, regarding how I felt emotionally about my vagina, I really couldn't say. If asked I would probably have said: 'Fine, good, it's a good, pleasurable part of me.' However, if I felt so positive, why did I sometimes blush when I said the word vagina? Was there shame or embarrassment mixed in there too?

One problem for me in knowing how to view my vagina was that the western culture I grew up within gave me confusing messages. Possessing a vagina means that I have the unique power to bring new life into the world, yet from birth I was treated differently from people who don't own one. And typically, being treated differently meant not being treated as well as the vagina-less person. Having a vagina meant I could be expected to work all my life for less money than if I was minus female genitalia. I could expect to be treated as a second-class citizen, downgraded constantly because of my cunt. I also recognised that if I'd been born into another society, the implications of having a vagina would have been far more restricting and threatening, potentially fatal.

Considering these emotions surrounding my vagina, and despite the pleasure it provided, how could I feel good about or proud to sport female genitalia, when their possession appeared to hamper irrevocably my progress as a person? The truth is, I wasn't happy with what I had between my legs. Or, more precisely, I wasn't satisfied with my perception of female genitalia, what I knew about the vagina. I hoped there was something more, some alternative way of viewing my vagina. This is, I feel, where the desire and idea to write a book about the vagina came from. So I set off on my own personal odyssey – to discover if there are other means of understanding female genitalia, and to see if I could gain a more balanced vaginal perspective. Could I change the way I felt about female genitalia? The result is this book, and the journey was both treasure hunt and treasure trove.

As someone who has been immured in the world of science since my youth, an important first port of call was to consider how the disciplines of science, medicine and anatomy today see women and their genitalia. This was an eye-opener. Controversy and confusion reigned, with the situation compounded by an astounding lack of recent decent research. Arguments were raging over whether females have a prostate, and if they do, what is its function. On the topic of the clitoris, opinion was divided over both the true structure of the clitoris and its role in sexual pleasure and reproduction. Some studies clearly showed how sensitive the interior of the vagina is, while other authors continued to state confidently (albeit erroneously) that the vaginal interior is insensitive. And when it came to orgasm, and the function of the female variety, fanciful theories flourished, but there were no satisfactory answers.

This basic lack of understanding of female genitalia – in terms of structure, function and pleasure – bothered me. Why, if female genitalia embody arguably the most important job on this planet – creating, supporting and giving birth to offspring – was there so little clear, accurate and consistent information available? Why was funding so hard to come by when the words vagina, vulva or even reproductive canal or tract were in the title of your research or grant proposal? This was the twenty-first century after all. And yet, in the midst of this medical mess of outdated and biased beliefs, I started to hear the sound of an alternative story, one that was unconventional and still in its infancy. To my surprise and delight, as I began to look below the surface media-friendly face of science, I realised that something astonishing was happening in the field of reproductive biology. No less than a vaginal revolution was brewing.

Female choice is the theme of this scientific revolution, and the piece of dogma that is being overturned is the idea of the vagina as a passive vessel – acting simply as a channel for the passage of sperm in one direction and offspring in the other. For centuries, the notion of female genitalia as a passive vessel with no controlling part to play in reproduction is the one that has been in ascendance. This, in part, explains why so little time and money has been expended in the past on figuring out the actual structure and function of female genitalia. Yet the idea of the vagina as a passive vessel is possibly one of the greatest scientific misconceptions of all.

What more and more research is revealing is a fascinating picture of female genitalia as an extremely powerful and complex organ of choice and control, capable of wielding an extraordinary level of influence over the outcome of sexual reproduction. Staggeringly, studies are beginning to show that in many, if not all, cases it is the female, courtesy of her intelligent genitalia, who decides whether or not a male will have a chance to become a father. This new way of thinking does, of course, have serious implications for technologies that purport to mimic the processes involved in sexual reproduction. This is because most assisted reproductive technologies are based on the assumption that female genitalia represent a passive vessel.

With the importance of female genitalia in terms of sexual reproduction in mind, this book also takes a tour of many different species' vaginas. There's a lot to look at. Just a quick glance reveals that vaginal variety across species is stunning. I was unprepared for the sheer beauty and diversity in design, for the realisation that female genitalia are an awe-inspiring marvel of elaborate and intricate internal engineering. For some reason, with nothing else to tell me anything different, I had assumed there was somehow a vanilla, 'one size fits all' vagina. There is no such thing, as you will see. Females store sperm, they eject sperm, they destroy sperm and they carefully and precisely select the most genetically compatible sperm for them with their amazing genitalia. This exploration of other species' genitalia includes penises as well as vaginas, for, of course, in order to appreciate the vagina in all its full glory, an understanding of its common partner in pleasure is essential – and vice versa. The sex lives of rabbits, of bonobos, of birds and bees, and many other species of animal are all here to illustrate how vagina and penis come together in delightfully inventive ways.

Having examined the ins and outs of other species' genitalia and sexual behaviour, this book reappraises those apparently sticky questions, such as: 'Is the clitoris a penile remnant?', which have been mired in controversy for years. And, having taken the approach of considering other vaginal styles, it supplies many answers too. You'll discover that men as well as women have a clitoris, that nose and genitals are intimately linked for a very good reason and that the nose has a clitoris too. Moving inside, and the role of the vagina's internal ecosystem as both sperm bodyguard, bouncer and sorter is uncovered, as is that of the female prostate and the infamous fact of female ejaculation. Even female orgasm and female sexual pleasure get an evolutionary explanation.

My quest to find a more fulfilling view of the vagina led me, surprisingly, to reconsider the nature of scientific research. Science is usually taken to be an objective, rather than a subjective, discipline. That is, it claims to be able to inform its audience about an object or idea independently – without a person or society's emotions or perceptions influencing it. And yet, everywhere I looked, the subjective nature of scientific research was in evidence. For example, until recently, the females of many species were said to be monogamous, preferring to mate with only one male. This theory has now been shown to be wrong – females of the majority of species are polyandrous, choosing to mate with multiple males. In fact, the idea of the monogamous female was a scientific notion driven by ideology not evidence. The ideology in this case was the outdated idea that females did not and could not experience sexual desire and pleasure like males could and did. The lesson is that science can be as subjective as any other discipline, and that in order to understand scientific theories you have to look at the culture that creates them.

The perils of getting stuck with just one perspective – and how that affects scientific reasoning – were emphasised again for me when I decided to look at the history of how western science, medicine and anatomy has viewed the vagina. This historical viewpoint at first revealed a very one-sided approach to visualising the vagina. Put simply, ancient and arbitrary doctrine dictated that man was the measure of woman, with his penis the yardstick by which to grade her genitalia. The result of this dogged and dodgy logic was that Renaissance anatomists found themselves proclaiming that the vagina was an unevolved, unfurled penis, ovaries were testicles, the uterus was a scrotum and the clitoris was a penis too. And they did this despite striking evidence to the contrary, because they had to stay in step with what the authorities of the day told them to say. So much for science being objective.

Adopting a historical vantage point on the vagina also uncovered some astonishing facts. Some men of anatomy were brave enough to speak out, to voice their views about the vagina devoid of prior dogma. Their pioneering words and images exploring the structure and function of female genitalia are depicted here. One of the shocking points to emerge from this historical frame of reference was that it seems more was understood about the structure of the clitoris in 1672 than when I was born in 1968. Why did the information published in 1672 remain virtually unknown nearly three hundred years later? Why had this outstanding work not been built upon and communicated widely? The answers, as you'll see, lie with how female genitalia came to be understood incorrectly as a passive vessel, contributing nothing to sexual reproduction. Western religion, and the morals of the day, also had a major role to play in this matter.

Religion – a society's belief system – is always a contentious subject and in looking at how different religions have regarded female genitalia in the past, I found the most polarised views possible. On one side was the west, with its attitude of the vagina as the gateway to hell, the source of all trouble and strife in the world, and the potential downfall of men. Here the vagina was an object to be feared, ridiculed and loathed. Belief systems originating in India and China, however, taught that female genitalia were the symbolic origin of the world, the source of all new life and the route via which longevity and eternal life could be attained. Here the vagina was an icon to be worshipped, loved and honoured. The divine vagina. And, in case I couldn't believe the words, extremely vocal vaginal art – painted, sculpted and engraved – confirmed that this is how many people in vastly different cultures have conceived of female genitalia across thousands of years.

Casting my net wider in my search for alternative vaginal vistas, I investigated language, literature, mythology, art and anthropology. A myriad aspects appeared. The languages of cultures outside the western world talk of female genitalia in glowing, sensual, pleasurable terms. I stumbled with excitement upon an understanding of the origin of the word 'cunt'. Literature, mythology and anthropology expanded my mind, making me think again about the importance that different people place on female genitalia. The vivid vaginal art, myths and folklore of many societies made me laugh out loud, and cry. These include the voracious 'vagina girls' from New Mexico, the genital chanting and songs from Hawaii, the clitoris cat's cradle game, the various vibrant descriptions of differently contoured clitorises, the audacious Baubo belles and the shameless Sheela-na-Gig girls. Looking further back in time to prehistory, I found that the vagina was venerated, looked up to as a symbol of fertility, and a means of averting evil. It seems there were other ways of looking at the vagina. I had found something of worth, something to speak out about, from between my legs.

This, then, is my story of the vagina. It is, aptly enough, in no way a straight story. And it cannot be the complete story of the vagina. *The Story of V* will change again over time, I'm sure. My desire was simply to try to tell this untold story from as many perspectives as possible, using as many voices as possible – and to as many people as possible. From a scientific perspective, I hope this book will make known the crucial role that female genitalia have to play in sexual pleasure and reproduction. From an emotional standpoint, I hope the different views represented here illustrate the value of the vagina and the female of the species for as many individuals as possible – women and men alike. Things that are not known and not valued are easy to dismiss and destroy – as the history of attitudes towards female genitalia shows all too clearly. My desire is that by revealing female genitalia in terms of structure, function, smell, sexual pleasure and reproduction, orgasm, art, language and mythology, the vagina will become and remain valued and known – in all its fascinating, arousing, compelling and beautiful aspects.

One important choice I made when writing this book was to include images of female genitalia – both in black and white (throughout the book) and in colour (the central pages). My desire here was to show the vivid and striking variety of vaginas – uncut and unedited. I also wanted to provide what I believe is a much-needed counterpoint to all-too-common and easily accessed pornographic images. Women and men should know what a vagina au naturel looks like. However, if you are reading the American or Japanese editions of this book you will notice that the central images are not in colour, but are in black and white. For Japanese readers, the reason for this is that it is illegal in Japan to publish colour photographs of genitalia. For American readers there is no legality issue, rather it is a cultural one. It was impossible to find an American publisher willing to produce the book without replacing the colour vaginal photographs with black and white ones. It seems the colour photos must be omitted if large bookstores in the United States of America were to stock and sell the book.

Both of these attitudes sadden and shock me. Why are colour images of vaginas so feared? Why is it easier to publish doctored and degrading vaginal images than ones celebrating female genitalia in their natural glory? It seems the underlying feeling in these countries is still that the place where we all come from must be veiled in some way from view. My only hope is that this attitude will change in time. I believe it will, and I also recognise that this fear of showing colour images of the vagina underlines the power and significance of female genitalia.

An act of synchronicity connects the beginning and end of this book. The act is, not surprisingly, a vaginal one, and one that has been carried out by women for millennia. As the first chapter of this book relates, the most common vaginal gesture in history is that of a woman raising her skirt to deliberately display her genitalia. The gesture is a bold, proud, potent one and has been used with devastating effect, as you'll see. This genital act can also be a defiant one too, as I discovered. After finishing the first draft of this book, I went to my local charity shop to splash out on a new skirt. The shop was crowded, and as I left the changing room, I bumped into a man naked from the waist up. 'That's nothing,' said the woman at the counter, 'You'll never guess what I saw last week.' I knew instantly. Her story was of an older woman, possibly a refugee, accused of stealing from the shop. Backed into a corner, with nowhere to turn, the woman did the only thing she could to regain a sense of pride and her place in the world. She raised her skirt to reveal her naked vagina. It seems that she had not forgotten the power of the vagina, and she was not ashamed.

I wouldn't have been able to carry out my own unveiling of the vagina if I hadn't had an enormous amount of support – from my family, my friends, peers and colleagues, including those at Weidenfeld & Nicolson, and from people who haven't even met me. I'd like to acknowledge all those people in so many different fields of research who have listened to me, talked to me, advised and quizzed me, and given so generously of their time and their knowledge. Not only have I been amazed at what there was to find out about the vagina, I've been happy to discover just how helpful people are, and I've found succour in the most surprising and strange places, so thanks, Buffy, Spike and Joss. My biggest thanks, though, go with all my heart to my family for their physical, financial and emotional support: Mum, Dad, Grandma, Helen and Gerard, Andrew, Paul, Janette and Jaime, Charlotte, Dominic, Benedict, and Steve and Maisy. And finally, thank you to Mum and Dad for picking me up (literally) when I needed it, and loving me no matter what; to Janette for always being there for me – you've taught me so much about relationships; and to Steve, for coming back for me and showing me something new. I love you Steve and I'll remember.

1

THE ORIGIN OF THE WORLD

There is a Catalan saying: '*La mar es posa bona si veu el cony d'una dona*' – 'The sea calms down if it sees a woman's cunt'. This Catalan belief in the power of the vagina is, in fact, the source of the good luck custom of fishermen's wives displaying their genitals to the sea before their men put out on the water. The flipside of this faith is, logically enough, that a woman can cause storms if she urinates in the waves. Moreover, according to folklore, it's not just the oceans that are soothed by the sight of a woman's vagina. A flash of female genitalia has the power to calm other forces of nature too. For example, women in the southern Indian province of Madras were known to subdue dangerous storms by exposing themselves. And Pliny, the first-century historian of the ancient world, writes in his work *Natural History* of how hailstorms, whirlwinds and lightning are all quieted and dispelled by a face-off with a naked woman.

The remarkable ability to mollify the elements is far from being the only capacity that folklore and ancient history ascribe to the act of a woman revealing her vagina. For many, female genitalia also present a potent apotropaic package. That is, the sight of a woman deliberately exposing her naked vulva is deemed to be capable of preventing evil from occurring. Driving out devils, averting vicious spirits, frightening carnivores and scaring opposing warriors and threatening deities away – all these heroic and dangerous deeds are reputed to form part of a woman's genital might. As a consequence, tales of women's vaginal derring-do are found in various cultures. Take Pliny and his fellow ancient historian and philosopher Plutarch (*c.* 46–*c.* 120 Common Era CE). Both these men described how great heroes and gods will flee in the face of female genitalia. Elsewhere, the report of a sixteenth-century traveller in North Africa records the belief that lions will turn tail and run from this sexual sight. At funerals, women were hired as mourners, with the express aim of exorcising demons via vaginal display. Russian folklore relates how when a bear appears out of the woods, it can be put to flight by a young woman raising her skirt at it. It seems that in the face of adversity, the best option open to a woman is to lift her skirt. For a man, it would be to make sure you're standing next to one of the sisters.

This view of the vagina may seem startling, disturbing even. Vaginas can calm the elements and drive out devils? It's certainly the case that this is a way of looking at female genitalia that is atypical in most cultures today. In the western world of the twenty-first century, the idea of women showing their genitals tends to be inextricably bound up with sex, pornography or images of women in accommodating positions rather than ones of power and influence. For many, the idea of a woman revealing her vagina is seen as offensive, and seldom positive, let alone something to be welcomed or to hide behind. For women themselves, the idea of deliberately displaying their vagina in public is more likely to provoke emotions of shame and embarrassment than feelings of respect and authority. Adding to the modern-day negative associations surrounding the naked vulva is the fact that a number of cultures put great effort into ensuring female genitalia are rarely viewed, and never publicly. At present, the most potent concept associated with the naked vagina is probably that of childbirth – the moment when a woman's vagina stretches wide and, miraculously, provides a baby with a safe gateway into the world. This parturition picture, it could be said, is also the one 'acceptable' public face of female genitalia (see colour plate section). The one vaginal image people are comfortable observing, without too much shame or embarrassment.

Yet it's apparent that women around the world have been lifting their skirts to full effect for centuries. From Italy – where folklore from the Abruzzo region tells of the power of a woman raising her skirt to display her genitals – to India, where the gesture was also understood to dispel evil influences, tales of deliberate female genital exposure abound in history, folklore and literature. One eighteenth-century engraving by Charles Eisen for an edition of the book *Fables* by Jean de La Fontaine depicts the ability of the exposed vagina to dispel evil forces beautifully (see Figure 1.1). In this striking image, a young woman stands, confident and unafraid, confronting the devil. Her left

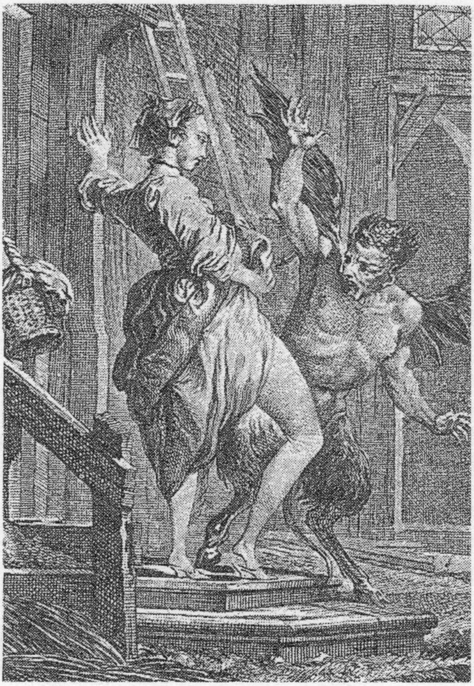

Figure 1.1 The devil defeated by vaginal display.

hand rests lightly on a wall, while her right raises her skirt high, displaying her sexual centre for Satan to see. In the face of her naked womanhood, the devil reels back in fear. In this way, the story relates, the young woman defeats the devil and saves her village, which Old Nick had been attacking. A couple of centuries earlier, the French writer Rabelais had his old woman of Papefiguiere rout the devil in the same manner, and reproductions of this vivid confrontation between the vagina and the devil can be found on seventeenth-century drinking mugs. A delicious sight to sup from, I'm sure.

The belief in the power of the exposed vagina to repel foes or expel demons is also, it seems, an enduring and widespread one. Significantly, accounts of women revealing their vaginas in order to achieve a particular effect are not rooted in any one historical period or any one culture. Instead, they span millennia, from the ancient past through to the present day (as my story in the introduction shows), and cross continents too. In his essay 'Bravery of Women' Plutarch recalls a vulva-displaying incident where a large group of women lifting their gowns together changed the outcome of a war. He describes how, in a certain battle between the Persians and the Medes, the Persian men, losing heart against the strong advancing Median forces, turned tail and attempted to flee from them. However, their way was blocked by a group of their own women, calling them cowards. These Persian women proceeded to raise their skirts, exposing their nakedness to their fellow men. Shamed by this vaginal display, the Persian men returned to face their enemies, eventually defeating them.

Fast forward nineteen hundred years or so, and the western press describes similar incidents. In the *Irish Times* of 23 September 1977, one Walter Mahon-Smith contributed the following item:

> In a townland near where I lived, a deadly feud had continued for generations between the families of two small farmers. One day, before the First World War, when the men of one of the families, armed with pitchforks and heavy blackthorn sticks, attacked the home of their enemy, the woman of the house came to the door of her cottage, and in full sight of all (including my father and myself, who happened to be passing by) lifted her skirt and underclothes high above her head, displaying her naked genitals. The enemy of her and her family fled in terror.

Outside the western world, anthropological data collected during the last century regarding the people of the Marquesas Islands reveals a similar reverential attitude to female genitalia, albeit with a slight twist. This Polynesian culture credits female genitalia with supernatural influences and these vaginal forces, Marquesans say, are strong enough to frighten gods or to drive out evil possessing spirits. Hence exorcisms carried out in this part of the world consist of a naked woman sitting on the chest of the possessed. For this society, the belief that women have extra mysterious powers courtesy of their unique sexual anatomy extends elsewhere. For instance, Marquesans also consider that a woman can curse an object or person by naming them after her genitalia. I haven't yet tried this one myself.

So according to many individuals and communities, the vagina is an extremely influential organ – and one possibly to be feared if you're on the receiving end of a vulval flash. However, there is another aspect to the gesture of female genital display. Some genital practices highlight how the protection provided by the displayed vagina is not only about preventing harm. Just as importantly, vaginal protection can encompass a more nurturing, nourishing influence. Indeed, historical evidence suggests that female genital display can also be about promoting fertility, such as causing plants or the earth to flourish. Up to the twentieth century, in many western countries, belief in this vaginal ability can be seen in the custom of peasant women exposing their genitals to the growing flax, while saying: 'Please grow as high as my genitals are now.' And as strange as it may seem, the fairy tale of Snow White, or Biancaneve, is suggested to have arisen from an ancient Italian ritual designed to enhance the fecundity of the earth itself. A beautiful, noble girl would be sent down a mine which was running low in iron ore in order to expose Mother Earth to her vital female essence or energy. Biancaneve, so the theory goes, came from the Dolomites region of the Cordevole river north of Belluno in Italy, an area which was known for its magnesium-rich iron mines.

The fertility effect of the displayed vagina can work in more subtle ways too. In ancient Egypt, women exposed their vaginas to their fields in order to bring about a double whammy effect, if you will. First off, the gesture was designed to drive evil spirits from the land, but the consequence of this apotropaic action was desired too. With no evil spirits around, the women would increase the yield of their crops. Hence the act of deliberate vaginal display is both evil-averting and fecundity-enhancing, as the former function promotes the latter. This double aim is also thought to lie at the heart of the custom recorded by Pliny, who noted how a woman can rid a field of pests by walking around it before sunrise with her genitals exposed. Giving thanks for a bountiful harvest and asking for the same fruitfulness next year may well lie at the heart of one of the concluding parts to Marquesan harvest festival celebrations – the *ko'ika to'e haka*, the clitoris dance. Significantly, this traditional dance features young women in wrap-around skirts which they raise to expose their vaginas and clitorises and the ritual tattoos emblazoned around their genitalia.

The Greeks call it *ana-suromai*

So where does it come from, this proud, potent female gesture that crosses time, continents and cultures? What could be the source and significance of this evil-averting, fertility-enhancing genital act which appears so alien and outrageous to many twenty-first-century eyes? One of the first and most explicit descriptions comes from one of the world's earliest known civilisations – that of ancient Egypt. The act of a woman deliberately displaying her vagina was, in fact, a common motif within the rituals, celebrations and beliefs of ancient Egypt, as historians of the day recorded. One of these chroniclers was the famous Greek explorer and historian Herodotus, who travelled extensively through Egypt in the fifth century Before the Common Era (BCE). As this Greek man saw it, the ancient Egyptians' bizarre world was a reversal of his own – one where, as he put it, 'women go in the marketplace, transact affairs and occupy themselves with business, while the husbands stay home and weave'. And within what seemed to him to be a topsy-turvy environment in terms of gender roles, female genital display was an integral part of religious beliefs. Perhaps because the gesture was so common, perhaps because it was so shocking to him, or perhaps because he needed to find some way of explaining the Egyptian custom to his Greek peers, Herodotus gave the revealing act a name – *ana-suromai*. Derived from a Greek word meaning literally 'to raise one's clothes', *ana-suromai* is also often referred to as *anasyrma* or *anasyrmos*.

The Egyptian event that Herodotus recorded an eye-witness account of was the annual festival of Bubastis, the biggest and most popular of all ancient Egypt's festivals, the Glastonbury or Kumbh Mela of the day. The deity involved in these celebrations was the cat goddess Bast or Bastet, one of the more popular deities in ancient Egypt's pantheon of gods and goddesses. Said to rule pleasure, dancing, music and joy, Bast's main place of worship was the temple at Bubastis ('house of Bast', now Zagazig) on the Nile. Here, every year, noted Herodotus in his *History* (written in 445 BCE), hundreds of thousands of revellers gathered by boat to celebrate the feline goddess in a riotous religious carnival.

Now, when they sail on the river to the festival of Bubastis, men and women together crowd into each barge. Some of the women carry castanets and make much noise, while other women play flutes; both men and women sing and clap their hands. Whenever they pass close to a town, they bring the barge in nearer to the river bank, and then ... some of the women dance, while others stand up in the boat and expose their genitals ... They also shout out abuse and yell mocking jests and jokes at the village women standing along the river's edge. They do this at every town along the river. On arrival at Bubastis they make a festival with many sacrifices, and more wine is said to be drunk at this feast than during all the rest of the year. According to the reports of the inhabitants of Bubastis, as many as seven hundred thousand men and women (including children) assemble together here.

Cats are, curiously, still irretrievably associated with female genitalia and all things female. In Britain, 'pusse' first surfaced in 1662 as a vaginal descriptor; now the term has become 'pussy'. In Italy, the words for a female cat, chatte and gatta, both signify the vagina. Cats in many cultures also have associations with sex, female sexuality and, sometimes, prostitution. Women are feline, men never. Various cultures recognise and respect cats as having mystical powers, as a witch's companion or familiar, for instance, while some, in particular in Japan, believe cats bring good fortune. Japanese brothels also use the cat as a sign to indicate the nature of the establishment – a place where the vagina can be viewed and more. Despite the intervening centuries, cats and the vagina are still linked, just as vulval display was with Egypt's feline pleasure goddess, Bast.

Herodotus wasn't the only Greek man abroad to marvel at the striking visual display of *ana-suromai.* Diodorus Siculus of Sicily was another awestruck witness. This celebrated historian, who wrote a history of the world in forty books, travelled to Egypt in 60 BCE, some four hundred years after Herodotus reported on the skirt-raising celebrations of the Bubastis festival. Diodorus' report comes from Memphis, Egypt's oldest capital city, which was named after the virgin moon goddess Men-Nefer. In Memphis, the site of sacred female genital display was the Serapeum temple, home to a live bull which was tended and worshipped as a sacred animal, known as the Apis. For the Egyptians, the Apis, the great horned creature, was the incarnation of the supreme god Ptah, a deity of creative power. As a mark of Ptah's importance, when one bull died, it was replaced with another live animal. And it was this changeover of sacred bulls that provided the catalyst for ritual acts of *ana-suromai*. According to Diodorus: 'For the first forty days after the installation of a new Apis, women are permitted into the temple to see the bull face to face. They come and stand before him, tucking up their gowns.'

The focus of this particular vaginal rite is suggested to have been to strengthen the virility of the Apis bull. This fecundity-augmenting idea fits with an increased understanding of the core concern of ancient Egyptian society – that of promoting fertility, be it of the land or the people. Many of the Egyptians' sacred rites and the belief systems they followed are now understood as flowing from their fetish for fertility, and are increasingly read as a means to achieving and enhancing fertility. Could it be that the act of *ana-suromai* – be it that of the ancient Egyptians or twentieth-century westerners – stems from an original desire to swell the generative powers of the earth and its people?

The mythology of raising the skirt

The mythologies of different cultures represent a particularly important place to look for clues as to the origin and meaning of women raising their skirts to reveal their genitalia. As stories or traditions which claim to enshrine a fundamental truth about the world and human life, and which are regarded by their own particular culture as authoritative, a society's myths can be seen as statements about vital issues of life, although their truth is not necessarily literal, historical or scientific. Indeed, it has been said that it is impossible to understand the people of a particular society without having an understanding of their mythology. Significantly, myths exist in all societies, present as well as past, expressing beliefs, shaping behaviour and justifying institutions, customs and values. Similarities and parallels between myths from different societies often exist, not all of which are readily or completely explainable by the influence of one culture on another. In such cases of congruence, it's suggested that these myths embody common patterns of thought about what the fundamental issues of life are.

A belief in the power of female genitalia and the gesture of raising the skirt to display the vagina is found in various cultures' mythologies. It appears that this is a view of the vagina, a way of looking at and understanding female genitalia and women, that many societies did not want to forget. Moreover, as with stories from folklore and history, two types of vagina-exhibiting legends emerge: ones which focus on the evil-averting effects of public vaginal display and ones which centre on its fertility-enhancing ones. The first type of *ana-suromai* stories come from the mythologies of Greece and Ireland, both countries with a strong legend-telling tradition. These are of the evil-averting variety and focus on the militant apotropaic might that women can wield by exposing their genitalia collectively. Together, these legends say, women have the ability to shame and defeat an advancing enemy with what is between their legs. These myths mirror Plutarch's recollection of how in ancient history the Persian women faced down their men.

The Greek myth of Bellerophon also recalls the widespread belief in the power of the vagina to influence the oceans. Bellerophon is famous as the male hero who tames the winged horse, Pegasus and following his acquisition of Pegasus, Bellerophon appears to be invincible. He manages to do what all others have failed in doing – killing the Chimaera, the ferocious fire-breathing she-monster with a lion's head, goat's body and serpent's tail. He then conquers, amongst others, the Amazons, the fierce race of women who were said to live along the shore of the Black Sea. However, this great warrior is himself defeated as he returns to the Lycian city of Xanthos, to face his enemy the King of Lycia. On approaching Xanthos, Bellerophon calls on the god Poseidon to flood the Xanthian plain. Poseidon hears his prayer and starts to send wave after wave rolling in against the city. As Bellerophon rides up to the city on Pegasus, the Xanthian men plead with him to stop the inundation of their land, but to no avail. At this point, the women of Xanthos come wading forwards to meet their enemy. Hoisting their skirts to their waists, the crowd of women charge at him, exposing themselves. The result of this genital display? The waves recede, the winged horse Pegasus is frightened and Bellerophon retreats in shame, vanquished by vulvas.

A very early Gaelic legend about the Irish sun god Cúchulain also tells both of the potency of the *ana-suromai* gesture and how, when used collectively, it gains in force. The event occurs as a result of the youthful Cúchulain ('Hound of Culain') deciding to do battle against his own Ulster countrymen. Many try to dissuade him from this disastrous plan, but no one is successful. Then Ireland's women decide to act. Led by the chieftainness Scannlach ('The Wanton'), one hundred and fifty women group together to block his path. A version of this ancient legend, written circa 1186–92, records:

> and they all exposed their nakedness
> and their boldness to him.
> The boy lowered his gaze away from them
> and laid his face
> against the chariot,
> so that he might not see the nakedness
> nor the boldness of the women.

Out of Africa

Echoes of these Greek and Gaelic myths and the emotions they elicit are found in the twentieth-century customs of a number of societies, in particular in Africa. *Anlu* is a traditional practice of the Kom people of West Cameroon who, significantly perhaps, still trace their descent matrilineally, i.e., a person's position in society is dependent on the vagina they emerged from. *Anlu* is in essence a disciplinary technique used by women involving ritual genital display and dance. Offences warranting the practice of *anlu* (the word is derived from the root – *lu*, meaning to drive away) include abuse of old or pregnant women or parents; incest; seizing a person's genitals during a fight; and insulting a parent by using profanities such as: 'Your vagina is rotten.' Importantly, *anlu* is practised by Kom women collectively against a perpetrator.

The following description of *anlu* is by a Kom male:

> *Anlu* is started off by a woman who doubles up in an awful position and gives out a high-pitched shrill, breaking it by beating on the lips with four fingers. Any woman recognising the sound does the same and leaves whatever she is doing and runs in the direction of the first sound. The crowd quickly swells and soon there is a wild dance to the tune of impromptu stanzas informing the people of what offence has been committed, spelling it out in such a manner as to raise emotions and cause action. The history of the offender is brought out in a telling gossip. Appeal is made to the dead ancestors of the offender, to join

in with the *anlu*. Then the team leaves for the bush to return at the appointed time, usually before actual dawn, donned in vines, bits of men's clothing and with painted faces, to carry out the full ritual. All wear and carry the garden-egg type of fruit which is supposed to cause 'drying up' in any person who is hit with it. The women pour into the compound of the offender singing and dancing ... No person looks human in that wild crowd, nor do their actions suggest sane thinking. Vulgar parts of the body are exhibited as the chant rises in weird depth...

The final act of *anlu* is that, when repentant, the offender is taken by the women to a stream and ritually purified. Those who do not recant their crimes are ostracised by the community until they do. The Kom ritual of *anlu* is significant in that it shows that rather than being ashamed of their genitals or the insults thrown at them, these African women use their naked vaginas to shame, turning the tables deftly. The use of fruit associated with a 'drying up' effect also hints at a fertility aspect to the custom. What is more, modern-day acts of *anlu* have been used to defend the fertility of the Kom's land. In 1958, in an amazing display of collective female force, seven thousand women rose up to protest against government regulations changing for the worse the way women farmed their land. The women won.

Anthropological research highlights how collective vaginal displays are used to reaffirm African women's pride in their gender and genitals, as well as to shame others. Up until the second half of the twentieth century, the Bakweri women of West Cameroon employed collective direct action against any male who insulted a female's genitals. In a traditional ritual, all the women of the village would surround the offending male, demanding immediate repudiation and material recompense. If this was not forthcoming, the women would begin to dance, singing suggestive sexual songs, making genital gestures and displaying their vaginas. '*Titi ikoli*,' one song goes, 'is not a thing for insults, beautiful, beautiful.' The Bakweri explain the expression *titi ikoli* in various ways. It can mean 'beautiful' as well as 'something valuable and above price'. However, it also 'refers to an insult'. Plus there is the association of female genitals, and women's secrets and the revealing of these. By itself *ikoli* means a thousand, while *titi* is a juvenile word for 'vulva'.

Making derogatory remarks about female genitalia is punishable by vaginal display en masse elsewhere in Africa. For the neighbouring Cameroonian people, the Balong, this practice exists because it is said that if a man insults his wife's genitals 'it is like insulting all women, and all the women will be angry'. Added to this is the understanding that just one vaginal insult could have a negative effect on all of the women of the village, including newborns. What this effect is is unclear, although it is possible that it is related to a woman's ability to bear healthy babies. Therefore if any man throwing genital slights refuses to compensate the village women, 'they will take all their clothes off. They will shame him and sing songs.' In more recent years, court procedures have replaced the women's direct vulval sanctions. Indeed, court records from 1956 state the general principle that 'it is unlawful to insult the lower part of women'. Imagine if using the word 'cunt' in an insulting way was illegal in the west. This idea seems just as heretical as that of women taking pride in their genitalia, and everything they represent, and yet both do exist. For some, defending the good name of female genitalia is important.

In fact, it appears that vaginal display in response to slights and snubs was a relatively common shaming gesture in many African societies well into the twentieth century, possibly a quick and effective way of saying: 'Respect, remember where you come from.' Research highlights how Azande women would 'tear off their grass covering from over the genitals and rush naked after the intruder, shouting obscene insults at him and making licentious gestures', while the Kikuyu deliberately displayed 'the private parts towards the thing or person cursed', and Pokot women were known to mortify a miscreant publicly by singing and dancing 'around him and putting their naked vulvas in his face'. At the end of the eighteenth century, male European explorers in southern Africa described how Khoisan women would expose their genitalia to them. What these men did not know, though, was that this was a recognised Khoisan way of insulting and shaming voyeurs.

The act has resonance out of Africa too. Across the globe in Papua New Guinea, an Ilahita Arapesh woman can mock and shame a man by flashing her vagina at him in public. For the Ilahita's linguistic cousins, the Mountain Arapesh, the most shameful thing that can happen to a man is to have a woman's vulva put to his mouth. This association with shame derives from this people's mythology. One myth describes how collectively a group of women punish a male rapist by stamping on him, piercing his penis with sago needles, and slapping his face with their aprons. The woman who was raped then forces the male's mouth to her vulva, thus shaming him. It is also said that for a gypsy man, the greatest shame he can suffer is to have a woman pull her skirts over his head. This female act designates the male unclean, and signifies social death for him.

The cunt as catalyst

Returning to mythology, the second type of myth encompassing the motif of skirt-lifting lightens things up a little, for provoking laughter and life, rather than shame, is the focus of these great legends. This time the civilisations up for inspection are Egypt and Japan, as well as Greece again. In Egyptian mythology, the female displayer is Hathor, the goddess of joy, love, sexuality, childbirth and nourishment, and the daughter of the sun god Ra. The story of Hathor's vaginal display also involves Hathor's partner, Horus, and the long-running conflict between Horus and his uncle Seth over who will assume kingship of Egypt. During the course of one of their particularly heated disputes, the warring men insult the present ruler, Ra. Angered, Ra storms out of the court and refuses to participate in any further proceedings, thus bringing them to a halt. It is at this point that Hathor intervenes. Her method of calming her father? She exposes her genitalia to him, which causes him to laugh. Put at ease by her display of womanhood, Ra then returns to court, enabling the wheels of government to begin to turn again. A translation of a papyrus from 1160 BCE recalling the myth reads: 'Hathor . . . came and entered before her father, the Master of the Universe, and she uncovered her nakedness in his face, so that he was forced to laugh thereat.'

While Hathor's method of appeasing her parent is certainly novel, the act of genital exposure is apparently a highly effective catalyst in dispelling a sombre mood or static state. This idea of the cunt as catalyst, is also reflected in the two other myths in this category. In both the following famous legends, a woman, by revealing her vagina, surprises a goddess out of her sadness. Laughter is again key, and dance is too. In these Greek and Japanese myths, though, a point that is only hinted at in Hathor's story – that of her act allowing the 'system' to operate again – is now highlighted. These stories, which contain vital truths about life, stress that the act of revealing publicly the hidden core of womanhood initiates a process of change that operates on a world scale, as well as on an individual level. That is, creating laughter in an individual is one consequence; the other is ensuring that the earth remains a fertile place after the violent actions of men have plunged it into darkness and sterility. As a result, both myths also act as metaphors for human and plant cycles of birth, death, rebirth and resurrection, and the ever-changing seasons. In both cases the revealed vagina acts as a reminder of female fertility and a means by which negative and destructive energies are dispelled, recalling the still-held global belief in the evil-averting and fertility-enhancing influence of a woman deliberately displaying her genitalia.

The first legend centres on Amaterasu-o-mi-Kami, in Japanese mythology the Shinto sun goddess, 'the heavenly shining one' or 'Heaven Radiant Great Divinity', the bringer of life and light. She is also the most important deity in Japan's pantheon of gods and goddesses. Indeed, all empresses and emperors of Japan, including the present-day emperor, trace their imperial lineage back to Amaterasu. According to the myth of Amaterasu, which was first written down in the year 712 and is still famous in Japan, the sun goddess is angry and indignant at the increasingly violent actions of her brother, Susanowo, the storm god, known as 'the impetuous male'. After Susanowo wrecks Amaterasu's heavenly fields, voids excrement in her palace and, while in the sacred weaving hall, strikes Amaterasu's vagina with a spindle-shaft, piercing it, the sun goddess is so enraged and despairing at his behaviour that she decides to withdraw from the world, shutting herself up in a cave.

In doing this, Amaterasu plunges heaven and earth into darkness. Constant night reigns, calamities of all kinds ensue and earth's fertile nature begins to fade. Extremely concerned at the future of a world without light, warmth and food, the eight hundred Shinto deities gather to discuss the best possible way to appease the sun goddess, but not even the god of wisdom can think of a way to bring her out of the cave. Enter the goddess Ama-no-Uzume-no-Mikoto, the 'dread female of heaven'. Ama-no-Uzume starts to dance on an upturned bucket or basket, lifting her skirt and exposing her sacred genitals ('heavenly gate' in Japanese) to the assembled deities. Her revealing dance causes the watching gods and goddesses to laugh and applaud noisily, and as a result heaven and earth start to shake. Curious as to what could have caused this commotion, Amaterasu cautiously comes out of hiding, and in doing so brings the sun's rays and fertility back to the earth. The potency of Ama-no-Uzume's exposed vagina is also revealed in the Shinto story of the meeting of Ama-no-Uzume and another Shinto deity – Sarutahiko, a phallic god, before whom all demons shrink with fear. However, when Sarutahiko is confronted by the goddess' genitalia, it is the phallic god who loses all his strength and 'wilts away like a dead flower'.

The corresponding Greek myth is well known and concerns Demeter, the Earth-Mother or Corn-Mother, goddess of fertility and governor of the cycle of the seasons and the growing of grain. Demeter is in utter despair and sadness at the loss of her daughter, Kore (also known as Persephone), who has been abducted into the underworld by the god Pluto (Hades). In her grief, she leaves heaven and wanders desolate on the earth in search of her child. As she mourns, refusing to eat or drink, the earth loses its energy source and starts to become barren and infertile. Eventually Demeter arrives at Eleusis, some fifteen miles northwest of Athens. There, disguised as an old woman, she takes a job as a nurse. But she is still lost in grief, and continues to refuse to nourish herself, causing the crops to shrivel, and famine ensues. While at Eleusis, Demeter is visited by an older woman called Baubo, who, on seeing the goddess' sorrow, tries to comfort her. Her words have no effect, but then Baubo chooses to lift her gown, pointing out her naked vagina to Demeter. On seeing this bold display of womanhood, the goddess laughs and, shocked out of her suffering, accepts some sustenance. With this restorative act, life on earth begins to return to normal. In this way, Baubo's actions are instrumental in restoring the world to balance, harmony and fertility.

From *ana-suromai* to 'the open'

These legends provide a very dramatic reminder that the common modern view of what the vagina represents is not the only one to have existed. At some point in human history, female genitalia were considered potent enough to be used as the catalyst for bringing the earth and all life back from the brink of destruction. A very powerful image and idea indeed. Considering the significance of these myths to their respective societies, it is maybe not surprising to discover them being re-enacted throughout history, becoming part of a culture's rituals and customs. For example, Herodotus in his *History*, Book II, mentions an important ritual involving the baring of Hathor, and, as we shall see below, the myths of both Demeter and Baubo and Amaterasu and Ama-no-Uzume are associated with ancient rituals. Such re-enactments of the original act of the goddess or god are, typically, carried out to remember publicly the significance of the gesture. Rituals or rites are also, in some cases, performed in an attempt to resurrect the primal power associated with the deity.

What is perhaps unexpected is that, in some cases, the rituals and symbols linked to the act of *ana-suromai* have resonance not just in ancient societies, but in modern ones too. In Japan, Kagura, 'that which pleases the gods', is an old Shinto ritual which is held annually to commemorate the ancient myth of Amaterasu and Ama-no-Uzume, and how light was made to shine once more into the darkness. Still enacted today during the annual Kagura festival, this once sacred ritual has become a modern one. However, it is now, in essence, a striptease, as a dancing priestess playing the part of Ama-no-Uzume displays her vagina in front of the faithful temple visitors (the audience).

Echoes of the Amaterasu myth and the sacred ritual are also found in another Japanese tradition – the modern art of *tokudashi*. Performances of *tokudashi* – revealing the vagina – are given every night in the red-light districts of Tokyo and Kyoto, as well as elsewhere in Japan. Also known colloquially as 'the open', a *tokudashi* show emphasises the light-bringing aspect of the vagina with a strange twist – the audience are given tiny torches by the performer just before she displays herself.

A number of writers have been entranced enough by the act of *tokudashi* to include it in their work. The following description is from *Behind the Mask* by Ian Buruma.

> The girls shuffle over to the edge of the stage, crouch and, leaning back as far as they can, slowly open their legs just a few inches from the flushed faces in the front row. The audience ... leans forward to get a better view of this mesmerising sight, this magical organ, revealed in all its mysterious glory.

> The women ... slowly move around, crablike, from person to person, softly encouraging the spectators to take a closer look. To aid the men in their explorations, they hand out magnifying glasses and small hand-torches, which pass from hand to hand. All the attention is focused on that one spot of the female anatomy; instead of being the humiliated objects of masculine desire, these women seem in complete control, like matriarchal goddesses.

The impact on the nation's consciousness of the myth of the sun goddess Amaterasu can also be seen in contemporary Japanese cinema. The movie *Weather Girl* – the story of how lifting her skirt on national television acts as a catalyst for change for weather woman Keiko – was one of the major Japanese cinematic success stories of the 1990s in terms of both prizes and popularity.

In ancient Greece, ritual *ana-suromai* was a part of a number of ancient religious festivals – all associated with the goddess of fertility Demeter, her daughter Kore, and Baubo. These festivities included the famous Eleusinian Mysteries and the Thesmophoria, as well as other Greek mystery religion celebrations, such as the springtime festival of the Floralia (the Flourishing One), celebrated in April. It's known that the Thesmophoria was a small three-day women-only festival celebrated each October at the time of autumn grain sowing, while the annual autumnal festival of Eleusis is said to have lasted for over eight days and involved thousands of celebrants – men as well as women. Details of various written accounts point to rebirth and fertility as the central themes of these cult celebrations, with the ritual genital display a re-enactment of the mythological meeting between Demeter and Baubo. Moreover, according to Herodotus, the rites performed at the Thesmophoria were similar to the mystery rituals he had observed in Egypt.

Descriptions of what took place at these ancient fertility festivals in honour of Demeter paint a picture of celebrations filled with lifted skirts, dancing and ribald language and steeped in vaginal gestures and fertility symbols – a heady, fecund mix, indeed. Shocking sexual jokes were uttered – their function, academics suggest, is two-fold, being both apotropaic and fertility-enhancing, just as the act of deliberate female genital display can be. As sows were a symbol of female fertility, female pigs, often pregnant, were the most common sacrificial offering. Both archaeological and written evidence has revealed their symbolic use, with small terracotta models of pigs (dated to between 5300 and 4500 BCE), as well as pig bones, being uncovered at temple sites associated with Demeter, Kore and Baubo.

Participants at the Syracusan Thesmophoria festival and at the Eleusis celebrations also carried *mylloi*, cakes made of honey and sesame and shaped like vulvas. Such vulval loaves – split ovals decorated with lace and sugar – still form part of Catholic festivities in some parts of Italy and France. Known as *miches* or *michettes* in the Auvergne region of France, this vaginal *pain bénit* ('holy bread') is baked now in another woman's honour. Instead of rising in recognition of corn and fertility goddess Demeter, these vulval loaves are eaten to celebrate the Purification of the Virgin, that is, the Virgin Mary, the Christian religion's top-ranking woman.

Vaginal imagery is found elsewhere in the ancient Greek rituals. At Eleusis, the third element of being initiated into the mysteries of women was known as the Deiknymena (the Displaying). This was the displaying of the *hiera*, the holy relics, and was seen as the most profound or sacred part of the ceremonies. Texts suggest that these divine objects included fertility symbols such as pomegranates, fig branches, a snake, and a representation of the vulva (*kteis*). The precise nature of some of these holy icons remains sadly unknown, as their descriptions are somewhat vague. Christian writer Clement of Alexandria (*c.* 150–215 CE) chose to state merely that the *hiera* included 'unutterable symbols' of the earth goddess Thetis. The mind reels: what was so unutterable?

The writings of many early Christians on these ceremonies in honour of goddesses provide a clue, and they also give a unique, and entertaining, insight into how the Christian church viewed female genitalia and women (and alternative religions). Christian chroniclers commonly described the ritual female genital display and use of sexual language, jokes and objects by women as obscene and scandalous. Most seem to have been shocked, and talk of the rites in terms of shame, not pride. The early Christian writer Arnobius said of the rite of *ana-suromai*:

> She takes that part of the body by which the female sex gives birth and on account of which woman is called 'the bearer' [*genetrix*] ... Then in the midst of the other things that are customarily done to assuage grief and bring it to an

end, she exposes herself, and showing her organs lays bare all the parts veiled by shame. The goddess' gaze falls on the pubis and feasts on the sight of this extraordinary sort of consolation.

Later, the eleventh-century historian Psellus added his own spin. His judgements and others on this re-enactment of Baubo's actions are, of course, why a woman today would be described as bawdy and shameful, or a bawd (*baude*) or broad, if she did the same, making herself visible and open to all. Psellus chose to describe the sacred events in the following way: 'She pulled up her gown revealing her thighs and pudenda [*gynaikefos kteis*]. Thus they gave her a name which covered her with shame. In this disgraceful manner the initiation ceremonies came to an end.'

The art of *ana-suromai*

Considering the wealth of ways in which the belief in the potency of women displaying their genitalia has been passed down over the centuries – via mythology, tradition and ritual dance, as well as orally and in ancient historical texts – it is not surprising to find the act of *ana-suromai* has been stunningly depicted in many cultures' ancient art treasures too. The art of *ana-suromai* can be found on archaic sculptures, statuettes, amulets and figurines, and carved on seals and jewellery. Some of the oldest skirt-lifting images date from 1400 BCE, and are found on cylinder seals from Syria. These show women either splay-legged displaying their genitals, or lifting their robes to reveal their vagina – gestures that have been interpreted as having sacral significance. Elsewhere, a gold bracelet found in Reinheim, Saarland, Germany, bears, at one end, the image of an owl-goddess exhibiting herself, and dates to around 400 BCE. Many such artefacts are Egyptian, dating from the Ptolemaic period (323–30 BCE) or the second and third centuries CE.

One of the most striking aspects of these archaic images is the women's sense of pride and joy in their genitalia. There is no shame on show here, just a display of unabashed dignity. One delightful character – a small terracotta squatter – adds to the pleasure by placing her right hand on her vulva, touching herself as she gazes straight forward (see Figure 1.2). The effect is stunning. If you want to see her,

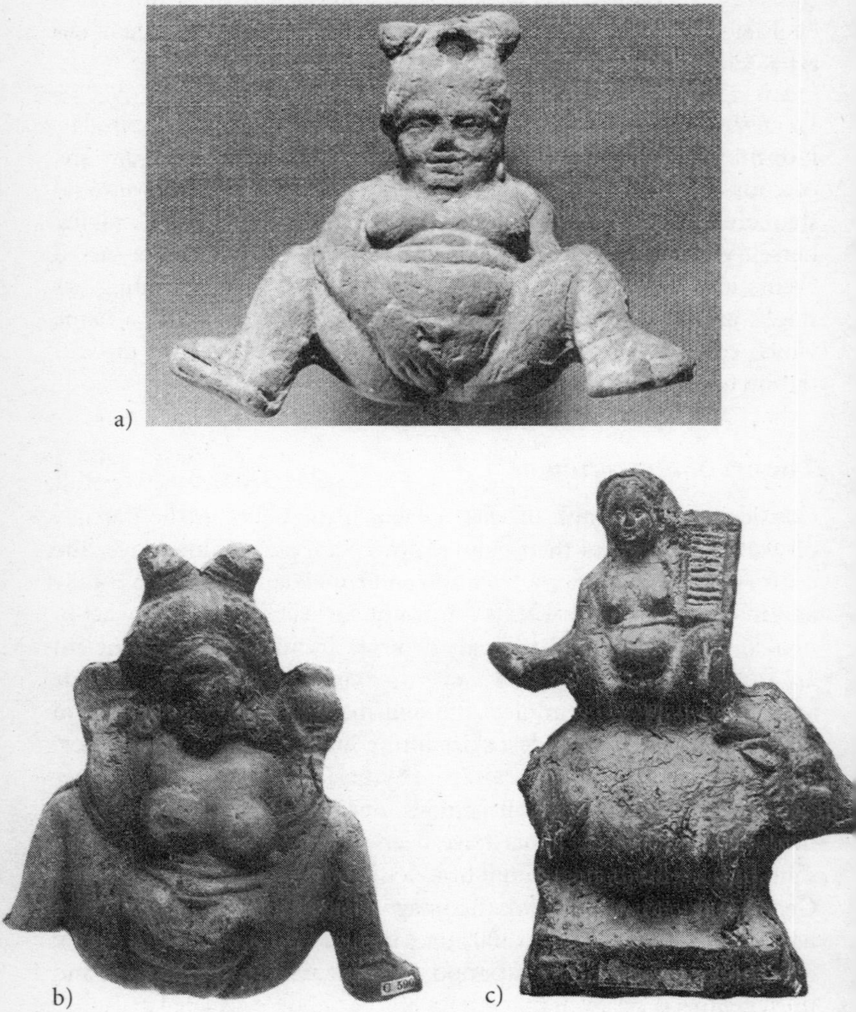

Figure 1.2 Terracotta squatters: a) with direct gaze this vagina displayer touches herself; b) the British Museum's voluptuous vagina displayer has a *polos* or crown on her head and holds a vessel in her hand; and c) this vagina displayer from southern Italy rides a sow while revealing her vagina.

she is in the Copenhagen Museum. A sister squatter is on view in the British Museum. Two others – terracotta statues from Alexandria, Egypt (second/third century CE) – show women standing proud, in full-length gowns, complete with decorated and detailed headdresses. Facing forwards, eyes direct, they gracefully raise their fancy frocks to reveal their naked vaginas to all.

The identity of these figurines is perplexingly uncertain. Are they queens, goddesses, important women of the day? Some say they are representations of Baubo or her acolytes. As many of these statuettes are Egyptian, others point to Hathor or the closely connected goddess Isis, 'the female principle of Nature', who was revered as the inventor of agriculture. Isis was also later worshipped by both the Greeks and Romans. Certainly there are many characteristics of these figurines that link them to fertility or creator goddesses such as Demeter, Hathor or Isis. One statuette dating from the Ptolemaic period not only has her skirt raised high, hands resting on her wide-open legs, and her perfectly carved vulva on display; she is also sitting astride an overturned harvest basket. Moreover, delicate sculptural details point to the high regard this woman was held in – she is wearing a long-stranded necklace and has carefully coiffed hair and a *polos* or crown on her head. Whoever she is, she is powerful, and it shows. The British Museum's terracotta squatter also sports a distinctive headdress, and has a vessel held high in her left hand.

Elsewhere, pigs again come into play within the art of vaginal display. One of the more famous female exhibitionists rides resplendent on the back of a large, possibly pregnant sow (see Figure 1.2). Found in southern Italy in the early nineteenth century, this terracotta Baubo, if it is she, sits with legs apart, her right hand raising her right leg slightly, as if to give a better view. In her left hand she holds what looks like a ladder, although it is difficult to be certain. Does the presence of a pig link this vagina-displaying woman to Baubo and Demeter? As has been noted, pigs are a symbol of female fertility, and similar terracotta sculptures of pigs, as well as the skeletal remains of sow sacrifices, have been found at temples associated with Demeter and Baubo. Perhaps the pig does provide the link and the identity of the mysterious vagina-displaying female.

There are other connections between Baubo, pigs and female genitalia. Look at language, for instance. Baubo also means cavity (in

Greek this is *koilia*, which is also a word for a female's genitals), while the Greek word for pig, *khoiros*, was also a commonplace term for female genitalia, particularly the vagina. Plus in Latin, *porcus* was the nursery name used by women, in particular nurses, to describe girls' vulvas or little girls themselves (from *porca*, the Latin for 'sow'). This link probably explains why one of the worst Italian expletives is '*porco dio*' – that is, 'pig god', or perhaps that should be 'vulva god'. Intriguingly, the association between Baubo and the sow has also remained resonant throughout history. The nineteenth-century German writer Goethe made use of this bond in Faust, when he wrote: 'The venerable Baubo now, Comes riding on her farrow-sow.' Meanwhile, across the globe, the Venezuelan love goddess, Marie Leonza, is said to ride on a tapir (a snout-nosed pig-like South American mammal), brandishing a human pelvis and, Medusa-like, turning men into stone.

The Baubo belles

One of the most amazing art collections incorporating female genital display also provides perhaps the most direct evidence linking these images with the myth and cult of Baubo and Demeter. In 1896, in Priene in Turkey, German archaeologists unearthed a group of seven small terracotta females from a site that was known to be an important temple dedicated to Demeter. The statuettes, which range in size between 7.5 and 20.3 cm, all date from the fifth century BCE. They were christened 'Baubos' for two reasons – the temple they were found at, and what they are all revealing. The attributes of these standing female figures are both extraordinary and extremely striking. They are also unique in Greek art.

The viewer's focus is firmly fixed on their genitalia, for what the artist has done is to make the face, abdomen and genitals become one. These are, quite simply, vagina or vulva women. However, these stunning naked women are not unadorned; some have elaborate headdresses, others ribbons or hair arranged in an extravagant topknot – the so-called *lampadion* ('little torch') style, typical of the Hellenistic period. One female holds a torch in her hand, another a lyre, others baskets of fruit – in one a bunch of grapes is visible. Together they create a rich, fertile, fecund assembly (see Figure 1.3). They are the

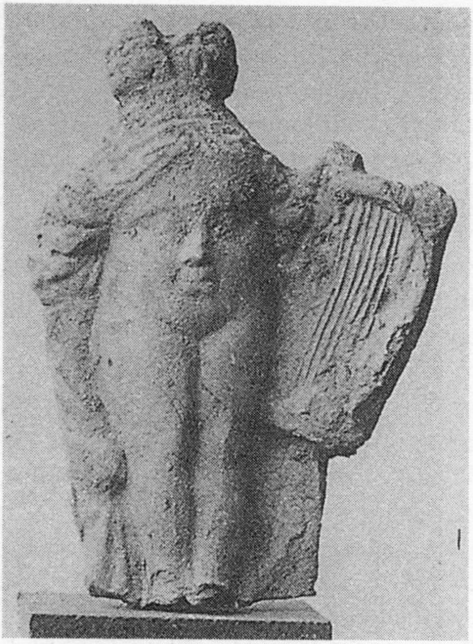

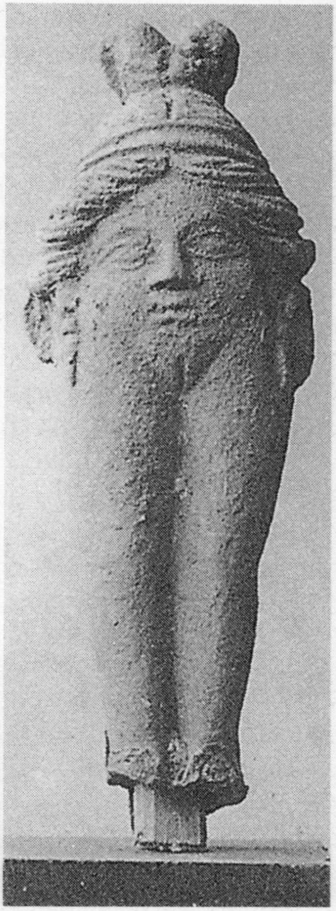

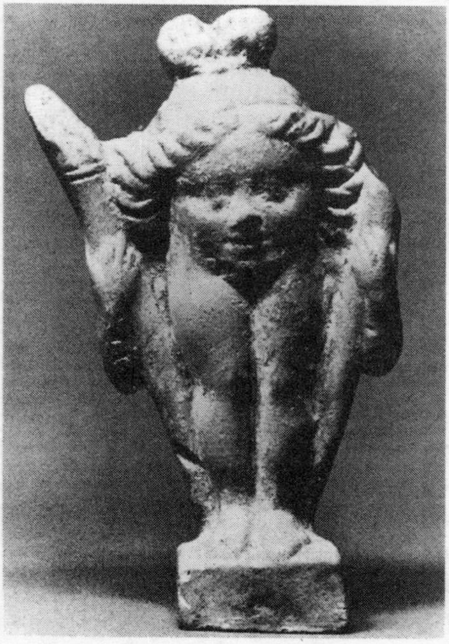

Figure 1.3 The Baubo belles: the vagina personified and adorned (fifth century BCE).

vagina personified. The Baubo belles, icons of fertility.

Many of the examples of the artwork of *ana-suromai* come from Egypt, what is now Turkey, and Greece. However, Japan has its skirt-lifting treasures too. The Japanese Shinto-Buddhist goddess Kannon or Kwannon is sometimes depicted hitching her skirt to reveal her genitalia, and a statue of her in the Kanshoji temple at Tatebayashi shows her doing just that. Dating from the eighteenth century, this figurine is still venerated today – with worshippers coming to touch the sacred *yoni* and anoint it with red ochre, in order to receive its blessing. (In China, this deity is known as Kuan-Yin, or the Yoni of Yonis, *yoni* being a Sanskrit word for the vagina.) Another Japanese yoni-displaying goddess is Benzai-ten, the goddess of art, music, poetry and physical love, and one of the most popular deities in Japan. A wooden statue of her on Enoshima Island, near Kamakura, dates from *c.* 1200. She is also the patron of sex workers.

The skirt-lifting sculptures and figurines so far described are, in the main, associated with a desire to enhance fertility – be it of plants or people – an idea that is suggested by the sites the statuettes were discovered at, and their carving characteristics. Some *ana-suromai* artwork, however, seems to express the evil-averting nuance of the genital myths. That is, the ability of a woman to drive out the devil or evil spirits by raising her skirt to reveal her vagina. Two terracottas, in particular, underline the act of *ana-suromai* as a potent and potentially apotropaic one. These sculptures are Hellenistic, dating from the first or second century CE, and both depict a vulva-revealing woman together with the symbol of the evil eye (read now as the ability to inflict harm with just a glance). In the first image, the vagina-revealing crowned woman rides astride the oval evil eye motif. In the second, she simply squats, showing a dark-painted pubis, green gown hitched high on her thighs, necklace adorning her chest, with a magnificent crown incorporating the evil eye on her head. In her hand she holds a red situla, a musical instrument that is associated with rituals to the goddess Isis. The effect of combining the symbol of the vagina with that of the evil eye – both images traditionally drawn as concentric ovals with a hole or pupil in the centre – is striking and memorable, and has led some scholars to suggest a connection, albeit twisted, between the two iconic images. This, however, is another story.

Nearly one thousand years separates these Mediterranean

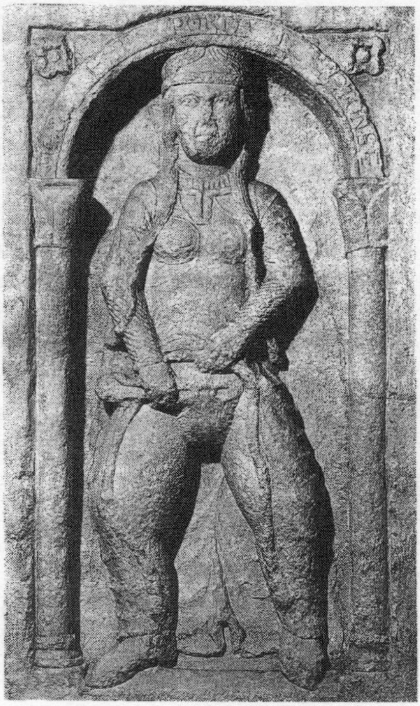

Figure 1.4 The medieval Porta Tosa skirt-raiser stands proud, protecting her city.

sculptures from Italian figures of women lifting their gowns discovered in Como and Milan. The Milanese maiden dates to the twelfth century and formerly stood above the medieval Porta Tosa gateway into the city (it is now in the museum). This impressive sculpture shows a standing woman in a full-length gown (see Figure 1.4). In her right hand she holds a dagger placed above her exposed genitalia, plush with pubic hair. Her left hand raises her dress to just above the top of her *mons veneris* (mound of Venus), as she stares proudly forward. Above her head there is an archway inscribed with the word 'Porta' – door. Her original role, as she stood above a key entranceway to the city, is now thought to have been one of protecting and guarding the city against evil influences. Why else would she stand there, so proud, beautiful and ferocious? And unknowingly, this woman also provides a gateway to one of the most perplexing puzzles in medieval sculpture – the significance of the Sheela-na-Gig girls.

The Sheela-na-Gig girls

Medieval Europe is the surprising source of one of the richest arrays of sculpted female genital display. Some of these carved-in-stone female figures stand proud with their genitalia on show. Some squat, hunkering down on their haunches. Others splay their legs or place them akimbo. Many reach back, with one or both their hands passing around their thighs from behind and reappearing between their legs, fingers inserted in their vagina or pulling apart their labia to give a better view. Some female figures use their hands to point to their displayed and often massively enlarged vulvas, some with raised labial rims, while others touch themselves with a finger. Some have pubic hair. One sculpture stands just over 30 cm tall, yet her large slit of a vulva measures nearly one fifth of her total height. Another figure sports large breasts and the most extremely generous genitalia, which fill out the entire space between her legs. This pillow-like pudendum – the most ample of all of these images – comes complete with a well-marked clitoris, and an oval vaginal opening (see Figure 1.5).

As well as the standers, squatters and splayers, there are the acrobats, females lifting their feet to their ears, the better, it seems, to reveal their almond-shaped or circular open cunts. A twist on the acrobats are the two-tailed mermaids, clasping their fish tails to their ears in place of legs, but still showing off their genitalia. While some of the women appear to be bald, others have elaborate hairstyles, or are veiled or wear headdresses. And of course the classic act of *anasuromai* – raising their skirts to reveal their naked womanhood – is depicted too. The one thing these varied female sculptures have in common? The emphasis on their displayed and nude genitalia.

These seemingly shameless female exhibitionists are the Sheela-na-Gig girls. Showing off their carefully chiselled genitals in the most outrageously explicit manner, they look down from hundreds of medieval buildings across a well-defined geographical area of Europe – England, Ireland, Wales, western France, northern Spain and Scotland. Significantly, their architectural location is confined to a particular type of structure – places of worship and power, which, in the period they date from (1080–1250), translates as Christian churches and castles. The majority adorning churches or cathedrals are carved on to stone corbels – the stone blocks which jut out like beam ends

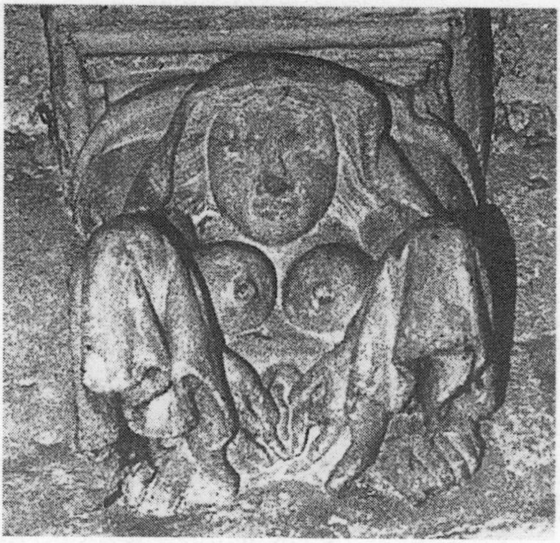

a)

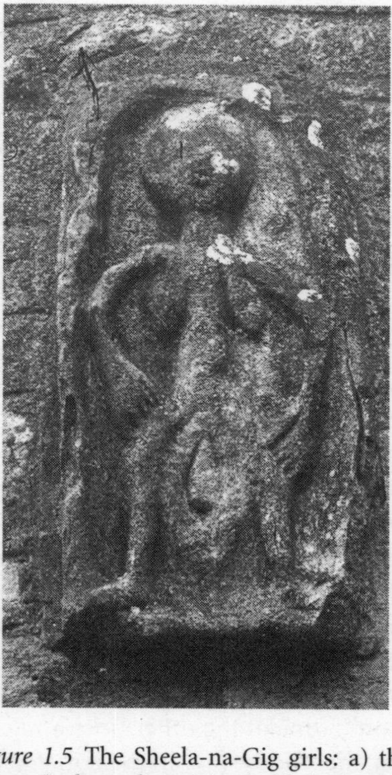

b)

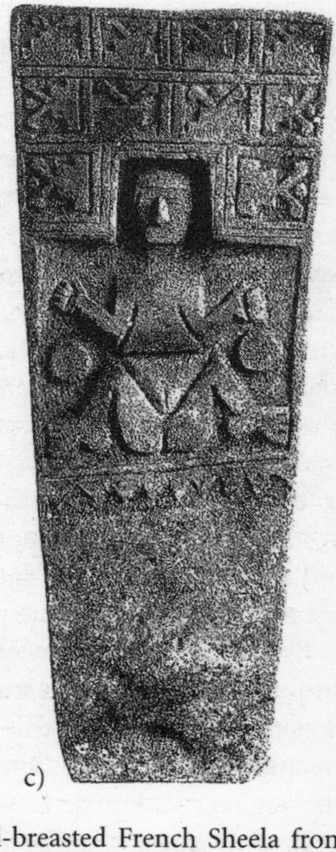

c)

Figure 1.5 The Sheela-na-Gig girls: a) the full-breasted French Sheela from Sainte-Radegonde, Poitiers holds her vaginal lips apart; b) the Sheela on Oaksey Church, Wiltshire has the largest genitalia of all her sisters; and c) across the globe in Ecuador, a squatting vaginal displayer on a stone stele.

from exterior walls – although some appear on flat slabs of stone or stand above the church's arched entrance on the keystone (the central stone).

It is astonishing that so many of these fabulous Christian vaginal icons survive. In seventeenth-century England, many were ordered to be hidden, destroyed, buried or burned. Many are defaced, their apparently offending lower halves hacked or smashed away or the carefully carved vaginal clefts crudely filled in with cement. One of the most famous English Sheela-na-Gigs is from the Church of St Mary and St David in the village of Kilpeck in Herefordshire. This Sheela is fortunate to have survived through to the twenty-first century. During the nineteenth century, a vicar of Kilpeck, ostensibly disgusted with his surroundings, ordered the defacing of those images which upset his sensibilities. The famous flaunting Kilpeck Sheela-na-Gig somehow survived this act of vandalism, as did a sister acrobat.

The source of the sobriquet Sheela-na-Gig (also written as Sheilagh-na-Gig or Sheelagh-na-Gig) is unclear. Some scholars say the name means 'woman of the castle'. Written in Irish as *Síle na gCioch*, the first element of the name, *Síle*, according to Dineen's Irish-English dictionary, refers to the female figures as stone fetishes, designed to confer fertility. Another Irish explanation gives a suggestion for the second half of the title, pointing to the phrase *Síle in-a giob* – which means 'Sheela on her hunkers or haunches', i.e. Sheela squatting. Other research reveals 'gig' or 'giggie' to be related to the dance, the Irish jig, which itself comes from the French word *gigue*, which was in pre-Christian times an orgiastic dance. The 1785 *Classical Dictionary of the Vulgar Tongue* states that to 'goats gigg' implies 'making the beast with two backs; copulation'. Moreover, etymologists note that in the seventeenth and eighteenth centuries, 'gig' was another word for wanton, metamorphosing (as words do) by the nineteenth and twentieth centuries into meaning rectum, as used in the phrase 'up your giggie'. The same phrase today is, of course, 'up your arse'.

By the mid twentieth century, though, 'gig' had come to be a term for female genitalia (this was also the time that the title Sheela-na-Gig began to stick). Using this etymological explanation, Sheela-na-Gig means something like 'vagina woman', or, taking *Síle* into account, 'the vagina of a female fertility icon'. Some of the other titles applied, such as Hags of the Castle, Julia the Giddy (an Irish term for an immodest woman) and The Whore, appear to reflect the feelings of the bequeather. Others, like Cathleen Owen or Sheila O'Dwyer, are thought to refer to local legends and particular women. Another theory, though, points to a much older origin for the term. In Sumer, the ancient name for southern Iraq, historians record that the women of the temple at Erech were known as the *nugig*, the pure or spotless.

The rationale for the sculpting of the Sheela-na-Gig girls is also uncertain. Their ubiquity solely on important places of worship and power points to their significance. After all, why would a medieval village waste money on carving images on their church if they had no meaning, or a wealthy landowner commission senseless castle designs? The view of the vagina that the Sheela-na-Gig girls give must be communicating a vital message, but what? Answers vary. Because of their precise geographical spread and the strength of Celtic beliefs in these countries, some historians claim them as representations of the Celtic religion's great goddesses. Other scholars see them merely as a means of horrifying parishioners with depictions of the sins of the flesh, of Eve, and of womankind. As female pigs with exposed genitalia are also part of the vaginal display repertoire on churches, some researchers have suggested a link to the myth of Baubo and Demeter.

Some of these pig sculptures, like the Spanish sow at Uncastillo, Navarra, appear to have human genitalia; others, like the pigs at Jubia, La Coruna, and Cervatos, Santander, simply exhibit exposed genitals; while the sows adorning the churches at Alloué, Vienne, and Vielle-Tursan, Landes, have extremely large vulvas. However, whether this particular porcine theme to the Sheela-na-Gigs was designed to echo the centuries-old association between Baubo's fertility-promoting act of *ana-suromai* and the fertility symbolism of pigs remains undetermined. The occasional habit of placing additional items with the women only seems to add to their mystery. Circular discs held under the arm have been read as bread rolls, a letter T as indicating *terra* (earth), while the clasping of daggers, sickle or moon-shaped objects, and the carved letters ELUI, merely confound matters more.

Evil-averting, fertility-enhancing

Two other possibilities as to the significance of the Sheela-na-Gigs are lent weight by folkloric practices and the precise positioning of some of the figures. Up until the last century (and indeed, for some people today), Sheelas were seen as fertility figures – if a woman rubbed or touched them, then her fecundity would be enhanced. Certainly many of the stone carvings have vulvas that have been rubbed smooth or worn away with the constant touching over centuries. Even eye contact was apparently enough: the tradition surrounding a Sheela at St Michael's Church, Oxford, required that all brides look at the figure on the way to their wedding. But enhancing fertility may not have been the only aim in mind when staring at or stroking these stone images. It's also suggested that the Sheelas served an apotropaic function – namely scaring the devil and driving evil spirits away from the holy sanctuary of the church, or, in the case of castle Sheelas, protecting inhabitants against those with wicked intent. Indeed, the Sheela of Carrick Castle, County Kildare, Ireland, was, according to local residents, the 'evil eye' stone of the castle – designed to drive away unwanted visitors or avert ill fortune.

The location of the majority of the sculpted Sheelas is certainly suggestive of them having protective power. In churches they are commonly carved into the keystone or quoin – the central stone at the top of an arch or entrance – perfectly placed to repel evil. Such positioning fits with the millennia-old global custom of placing protective images or tutelary objects above doors and gateways – areas traditionally seen as points at which potentially evil influences might find entry to a dwelling or town. On castles, many, such as the Sheela of Caherelly Castle, County Limerick, are to be found on walls guarding the road. This Irish Sheela appears a particularly formidable figure, and is placed as part of the defences of the old medieval town, overlooking the bridge and the approach to the town.

The idea of placing an image of a woman exposing her vagina on sites in need of beneficial influence is found elsewhere in the world, as we've seen with the twelfth-century Italian maiden from Milan, positioned as she is above a key entrance to the city. But it's not just a European tradition. In Cerro Jaboncillo, Ecuador, a stone stele of a woman squatting, vagina exposed, similar to the Sheela-na-Gig figures, stands guard at a critical junction where three roads meet (see Figure 1.5). This motif is also found in Indonesia, this time carved into doors, and again the aim is apotropaic. Vaginas that protect appears to be a common and widespread concept. And as the

Sheela-na-Gig girls show, skirt-raising is only part of the story. Sometimes there are no skirts at all, just a vulva in your sight. It seems that for many cultures throughout history, that view is potent enough to avert evil or confer fertility.

Images of Venus

As we've seen, the mythologies of various cultures, and the artistry, rituals and iconography associated with them, provide an explanation for the belief in the power of female genitalia to protect and enhance fertility; but these ancient myths and legends do not provide the whole answer for this widespread and enduring vaginal belief. What about before the skirt-lifting myths were first told? What prompted early civilisations to weave these legends, stories that contain messages so fundamental to life that they must be passed on in narrative form to future generations? Considering this, where to next in the search for the source and significance of the belief in the power of the vagina?

Venus is the next stop – the goddess, not the planet. In the western world, Venus (or Aphrodite, as she was known to the Greeks) is one of the better-known goddesses of Roman mythology. And it was Venus' popularity, plus her position as the goddess of love and beauty, that combined to make hers the monicker of choice when, in the second half of the nineteenth century, archaeologists began to uncover a wealth of Stone Age depictions of the naked female form. Some were sculpted palm-sized figures, fitting compactly into a person's hand and appearing remarkably portable. Other Venuses are larger and carved into rockfaces. All were unambiguously female, flaunting their fecund curves of breast, buttock and belly, underpinned by the arc and cleft of vagina. One figurine's vulva is so cleverly carved that her labia minora, her inner lips, seem swollen as if aroused. Vertical grooves trace the cleft of the vaginal opening of other figures, while some exhibit a more revealing attitude – with oval or almond-shaped vaginal vestibules – as if their labia are parted.

So far, over two hundred 'Venus figurines', as they have come to be called, have been found across a huge geographical area, ranging from as far east as the steppes of Siberia through to the caves of France in the west, and down to the dangling boot of Italy in the south. These prehistoric portrayals of the female form also span an incredibly long expanse of time, covering some twenty thousand years – a period of Stone Age history which is known as the early portion of the Upper Palaeolithic (30,000–10,000 BCE). The oldest figurine found to date is the 'dancing Venus of Galgenberg'. Carved from green serpentine stone, with a delicately bored vaginal opening between her legs, she was discovered in 1988 near Krems, in Austria, and has been dated to between 29,200 and 31,190 years old. The greatest number of Venuses, however, date from around 27,000–20,000 BCE. Significantly, in comparison to the hundreds of female figurines found, only a handful of depictions of the male form have been discovered, and there is a vast age difference between the two sexes. The few male figures found date from around 5000 BCE. For around twenty-two thousand years it seems men just didn't carry much weight in the Upper Palaeolithic art scene.

This focus on the female and the lack of attention to the male is a great quandary for many researchers, and has generated much heated debate. A large part of such discussions have centred on the genitalia, not surprisingly, as the vagina is often the focus of these figures. Probably the most famous of the Venus women is the Venus of Willendorf, found in Willendorf, Austria, in 1908 and dated to between 26,000 and 20,000 BCE (the Gravettian period of the Upper Palaeolithic). Worked in limestone, this figurine is just 11 cm high, but remarkably rich in detail. Indeed, according to one archaeologist, she has 'the most carefully and exquisitely carved realistic vulva in the entire European Upper Palaeolithic' (see Figure 1.6). Certainly her labia and vaginal cleft are clearly delineated, with a hint of clitoris visible too.

The prize for the Venus figurine with the most exaggerated vulva should, perhaps, go to a fantastic carving made out of limonite and found in Monpazier, in the Dordogne, southern France. Dating from between 23,000 and 21,000 BCE, this female displays a deliciously curved oval vulva, slit down the centre. Some say she is pregnant, her vulva swollen as if in pre-parturition, and point to her voluptuous breasts, rounded abdomen and exaggerated buttocks. Whether pregnant or not, the way in which the artist sculpted her external genitalia is striking and symbolic, iconic even. Indeed, this particular approach to depicting external female genitalia is an incredibly popular and persistent design. This concentric ovals vaginal style is found over and

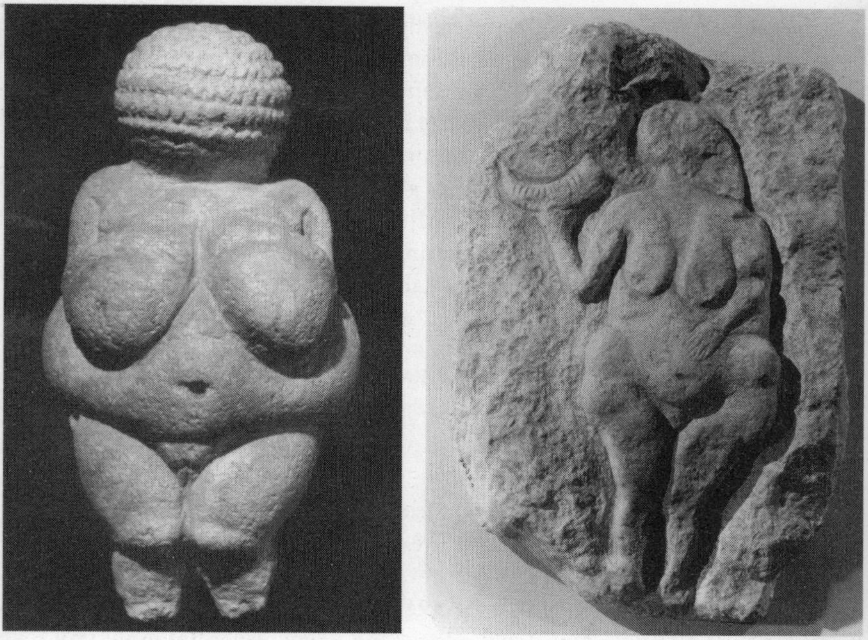

a) b)

Figure 1.6 Images of Venus: a) the Venus of Willendorf with her delicately carved vulva; and b) the Venus of Laussel holds her horn of plenty and directs the viewer's gaze to her vagina.

over in prehistoric art, even appearing on pottery and cylinder seals produced more than twenty thousand years later, as we will shortly see.

Another Palaeolithic Venus is curiously precise and explicit in making her vagina the centre of attention. Carved into a hard limestone block in a cave shelter at Laussel, in the Dordogne, this Venus, at 46 cm high, is larger than most others. Dubbed the Venus of Laussel, she dates from around 24,000 BCE. With her left hand, this curvaceous, obviously adult female pointedly directs the viewer's gaze straight to her vagina (see Figure 1.6). In her other hand she holds what looks like a horn; however, it may also represent the crescent moon or the curved horns of a woman's Fallopian tubes. The meaning of the thirteen grooves engraved on this ambiguous object remain to be deciphered conclusively. One suggestion is that they signify the moon's cyclicity – the fact that thirteen moons occur in every year. Another is that they point to a female's menstrual cyclicity, which mirrors that of the moon. A third idea is that they flag up ovulation, as day thirteen of a woman's menstrual cycle is commonly when she ovulates – a peak point of fertility. However, whether a reminder of the cyclical fertility of the earth or of that of women themselves, the Venus of Laussel appears a potent symbol of fecundity, with the emphasis firmly on her genitals. Two other carved female reliefs were also found at this site, creating what many researchers see as a fertility shrine.

The first Venus figurine to be found, the Vibraye Venus, reveals two alternative ways that Upper Palaeolithic sculptors made the vagina and female fertility the focus. First of all this ivory-formed female is bereft of face, arms or feet. The stress is again on the female sexual centre, hence her alternative title, the Venus Impudique, the shameless Venus. This Venus, like her sisters from Laussel, Willendorf and elsewhere, was coloured with red ochre when found. In the case of the Vibraye Venus, this pigment decorated just her genital area. The use of red ochre by Palaeolithic people is, in many cases, thought to refer to the female menstrual cycle. One particularly unambiguous reference – a female figure with twenty-eight red dots between her legs – was found in 1980 in the Ignateva Cave in the southern Urals, Russia. Red ochre has also been found staining small clefts, cavities and fissures in a number of prehistoric cave sites. These natural stone formations, which are suggestive in themselves of the shape of the vulva, then appear to be smeared with the flow of menstrual blood, conjuring an even more powerful vaginal image. The reverence in which women and their life-giving, bleeding genitalia were held is palpable from these stained cleft rock forms.

Vulvas, vulvas, vulvas

The fascination of female genitalia for Palaeolithic artists was expressed in other modes, as well as the Venus figurines, as the prevalence of etched-on-rock vulvas from this period reveals. These extraordinary rock-incised, and in some cases painted, vulva images have been found emblazoned on caves, bone, stones and shelters in various Stone Age sites, in France, Spain and Russia among other places. The carvings of vulvas are also, in the main, older than the sculpted Venus figures, and typically date from the Aurignacian period of the Upper Palaeolithic (27,000–30,000 BCE). Not surprisingly, as the artistry occurs over a vast geographical span and thousands of years, the size, shape and style of the vulvas depicted often differ. Some are striking in how realistically they describe how a woman's external genitalia look – either face on, thighs together; or full frontal, legs parted.

The thirty-thousand-year-old cluster of vulva engravings from the caves at La Ferrassie, France, trace a more oval template (see Figure 1.7), while painted vulvas on the walls of Spanish caves at Tito Bustillo and Castillo are described as bell-shaped. Some designs, like those at Castillo, are associated with plant images. Others illustrate a woman's pubic triangle as just that – triangular with a median cleft. One of the most recently discovered Palaeolithic cave complexes, at Chauvet, in the Ardèche, south-east France, features such a vulval design – a large black downwards-pointing triangle situated deep inside the ancient site. This is also believed to be one of the oldest vulva images yet discovered, possibly dating to 31,000 BCE. Fast-forward twenty-three thousand years or so, and ancient artists are carving strikingly similar vaginal designs, as artists continue to do today (see Figure 1.7).

The different ways in which Palaeolithic artists represented the vulva has led to accusations of archaeologists going vulva hunting – viewing every V-shape, oval, U-design or triangle as a representation of female genitalia, much as towers, pointed objects and straight lines are typically construed as phallic. However, despite the vulva-hunting jibes thrown at some prehistoric artistry, there are a vast number of Palaeolithic vulval images which are acknowledged unequivocally as archaic representations of female genitalia. For some it is their style, or the ritual over-marks, that point to their genitalic nature; for others it is their undisputed similarity to the real thing.

The Bédeilhac vulva is one of the latter. Sculpted on the ground, in clay, it is a remarkably realistic likeness of a woman's external genitalia, with – in the appropriate position – a small stalactite for a clitoris. Another Palaeolithic style is also a giveaway for vaginal authenticity. In some imagery, the vulva does not stand alone; rather it appears in context with other aspects of female form. Examples of this particular vogue adorn either side of the entrance to a cavern in La Magdeleine, France. Half sculpted, half naturally formed out of the rock face, the

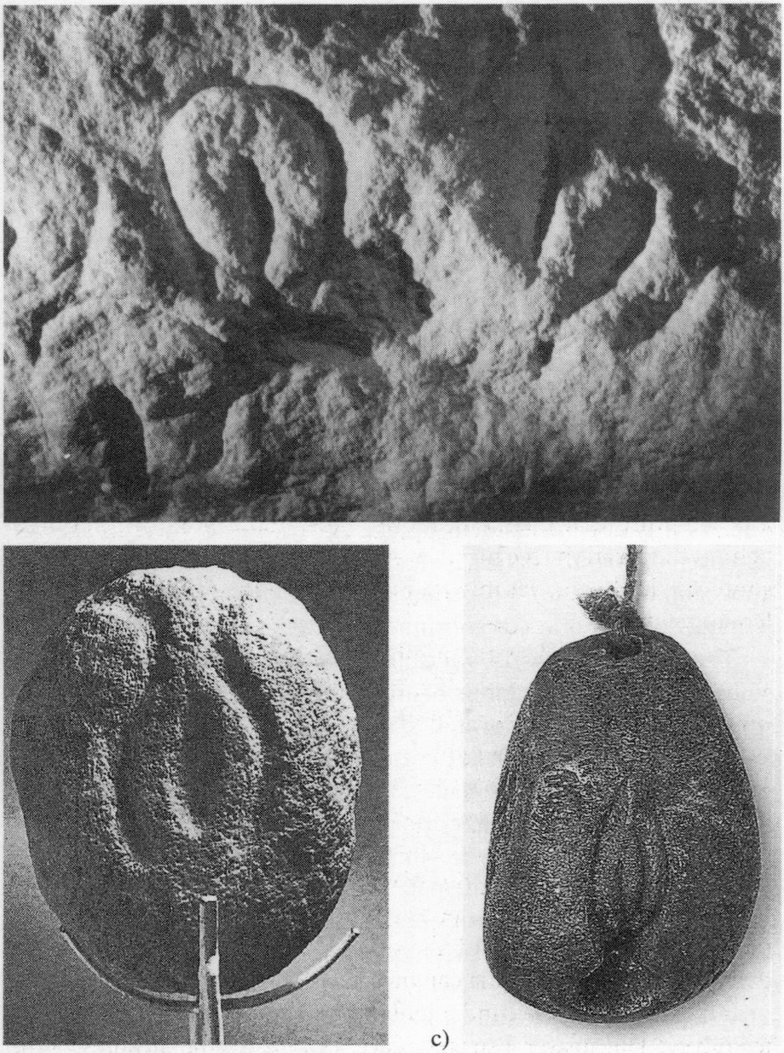

a)

b)

c)

Figure 1.7 Enduring vaginal design: a) La Ferrassie, in the Dordogne is home to thirty-thousand-year-old vulval stone carvings; b) fifty-four of these sandstone scuptures were found at Lepinski Vir placed in triangular shrines at the head of vulva-shaped altars (6,000 BCE); and c) worn by the Bashi people of Kivu, eastern Zaire, this is a vaginal amulet of carved bone.

figures stretch about a metre in length. Depicted in a reclining, supine position, they raise one arm to rest their heads, but it is the deeply incised sexual triangle that catches the eye. A clear-cut illustration of vulval imagery.

One of the most beautiful and memorable of all examples of Paleolithic artistry is carved into the walls of a cave at Angles-sur-L'Anglin, Vienne, France. Here, some 17,000 to 14,000 years ago, another prehistoric artist worked with the natural curves of the rock surface to create a monumental and lasting work of art – a trinity of vulvas. However, take a step back from the genitalia and there is more to see. Traced lightly around the deeply engraved vaginas, and appearing to rise out of the rock face, three female forms can be discerned. These three graces, goddesses even, are of particular interest for a variety of reasons: their threefold nature; their two-tone sculptural style and their unusually large dimensions – the first figure from breasts to legs measures 120cm. This frieze of the essence of female form times three is a sculpture that seems to convey more than most the emotions behind the creation (see http://www.archaeometry.org/id02.htm. It is simplistic in design, yet intense in effect, and the focus is irrefutably female genitalia.

This, to my mind, is the vagina as icon, sacred, inviolable, worshipped. The site and source from which all human life springs. The font of all new life. The origin of the world. Such vulval prehistoric images represent, it is thought, humankind's first use of symbolism. They are also the oldest view of the vagina: this primal perspective depicts female genitalia as a symbol of fertility, of the power of creation, of hope for the future, and of a belief that despite disease and death, new life will always come forth – from the female. Moreover, it is in these ancient images, potent emblems of fertility and rebirth, that I believe the origin of the age-old faith in the power of the deliberately exposed vagina can be found.

But what about the fundamental message the myths were aiming to convey? The answer, I suggest, is very similar to the meaning of the prehistoric images. First off they say: 'Female genitalia are the font of all new life. They are the symbolic origin of the world. The vagina is where we all come from, it is humankind's common source.' However, the genital myths contain a warning too. They add: 'Don't forget where you come from, what is important. To revile, defile or abuse the vagina or women is to turn against life itself. And no good can come of that – just destruction of the earth and her bounty.' Together, this is the message, some would say the moral, the skirt-lifting, vagina-revealing myths and folklore wish to communicate. Coincidentally and intriguingly, this vital theme works on a scientific level too, as we shall see later.

Venerating the vagina

Many people may feel uncomfortable with the idea that prehistoric depictions of female genitalia reflect a belief in the vagina as a symbol of fertility but this theory is one that is gaining increasing support. This is in large part due to the fact that academic consensus is shifting towards viewing vaginal Palaeolithic art as the work of a people whose prime focus was fertility. Fertility is now recognised as the focal point of the beliefs of other ancient societies, such as ancient Egypt, and many scholars argue that such fruitfulness – whether of land or loin – would also be of primary importance to prehistoric people. In fact, it's hard to find convincing arguments against this. Fertility, or more correctly, trying to control fertility – by enhancing, suppressing or biasing it – has been the major concern of all known human societies, and still is today. So, in a world where fertility was prized above all else, it seems a reasonable suggestion that the visible source of all new life – the vagina – would be seen as vital to ensuring the continuation of life, and would be expected to play a powerful role in any fertility rites.

The fact that the male or his penis does not appear in a prominent way in works of art until much later in prehistoric times is explained by the lack of direct evidence at this time linking man to the birth of offspring. Although today it's common knowledge that despite not conceiving, gestating or giving birth to a child, man still represents a crucial portion of the reproduction equation, this information is not innate. Humankind is not born knowing these facts of life, and so it's recognised that at some point in time the belief that women were solely responsible for bringing new life into the world would have existed. In such a scenario, female genitalia would assume additional significance. Veneration of the vagina and women in all likelihood occurred, hence the growing acceptance of vaginal prehistoric images as symbols of fertility.

Early theories of how conception occurs highlight how the understanding of the sexes' roles in reproduction has changed over time. The Greek poet Homer (*c.* 800 BCE) reveals how the male had yet to be given a starring role in conception, with his description of how mares get pregnant via fertilisation by the wind. A later western theory proposed that the air was filled with microscopically small ethereal 'animalculae' which, by chance, wind or draught, found their way into the female, causing pregnancy. Indeed, impregnation of the female by the elements, be it the wind or the rain, is a common theory of conception, which still has resonance in some religions and cultures today. The Christian church's view of the Virgin Mary's conception is, of course, that she was 'visited' by the ethereal Holy Spirit. In contrast, Trobriand Islanders talk of how Bolutukwa, mother of their legendary hero, Tudava, conceived when drops of water entered her virginal vagina. Her name reflects this – *Bo* means female, and *litukwa* dripping water.

The myths of many cultures also reveal the ancient belief in the female being solely responsible for bringing life into the world. The earliest known recorded creation myth comes from Sumer, where, in a tablet giving a list of Sumerian deities, it is the goddess Nammu, written with the ideogram for 'sea', who is described as 'the mother who gave birth to heaven and earth'. Sumerian mythology also records how man was created from clay by this great mother goddess. Elsewhere, early Egyptian mythology spoke of how 'In the beginning there was Isis, Oldest of the Old. She was the goddess from whom all becoming arose.' The Pelasgian creation myth states how in the beginning, Eurynome, goddess of all things, rose naked from Chaos, and dancing set creation in motion. Orphics said that the black-winged goddess of the night was courted by the wind and subsequently laid a silver egg, from which Eros hatched. In eastern Africa, it is a virgin woman called Ekao who falls to earth from the sky and bears the first child.

For the Kagaba Indians of Colombia, belief in woman as the source of all is summed up by the following song:

> The Mother of Songs, the mother of our whole seed, bore us in the beginning. She is the mother of all races of men and the mother of all tribes. She is the mother of the thunder, the mother of the rivers, the mother of trees and of all kinds of things. She is the mother of songs and dances. She is the mother of the

older brother stones. She is the mother of the grain and the mother of all things. She is the mother of the younger brother Frenchmen and of the strangers. She is the mother of the dance paraphernalia and of all temples, and the only mother we have. She is the mother of the animals, the only one, and the mother of the Milky Way.

However, despite the recognition that, in prehistoric times, man's role in reproduction was less clear than woman's, and in spite of the increasing acceptance of the vagina as a primeval fertility symbol, it should be said that there can be no absolute answer as to the precise significance of this ancient vaginal art. The images cover a vast period of time and a wide geographical spread, so their meaning will, in all likelihood, have varied. Thirty thousand years on, we can only surmise, and our suppositions are of course coloured by the culture we come from, as well as the facts to hand. For example, the notion put forward by many mid-twentieth-century male minds that the vulva artistry and Venus sculptures were prehistoric pornography was both a product of its time (stemming from a culture which viewed the revealed naked vagina as more pornographic than powerful), and the result of an incorrect idea that Palaeolithic woman stayed at home while her partner went out to search for meat. It's now known that hunter-gatherer societies were and are remarkably egalitarian in structure, and it is increasingly accepted that women may in fact have had the more powerful position in such societies in Stone Age life. One result of this new understanding of ancient cultures is the dismissal by the majority of researchers of the view of prehistoric vaginal art as pornography. The fact that some researchers are broad-minded enough to perceive that female genital display and the female form can serve purposes other than pornographic ones is another factor in the rejection of this theory.

Written in stone

Whether the idea of female genitalia as archaic symbols of fertility will stand the test of time remains to be seen. It is, as all ideas, a creation of both fact and cultural fancy, as subjective as the next suggestion. However, in contrast to the pornography notion, the theory that these views of the vagina focus on enhancing fertility is rooted more firmly in an increased understanding of the roles of women and men in ancient times, and what was most important in their lives. There is also other evidence in support of this argument. Significantly, stone carvings connecting the vulva with fecundity are not confined to prehistoric artists. Other, more modern societies appear to have put their faith in the power of such vulval images.

In Bolivia, on a mountain pass below the eastern Cordilleras mountain range, is a site sacred to South America's Chimane Indians. This remote spot provides sculptural evidence supporting a link between stone-carved female genitalia and fertility. Here, in the 1950s, a grouping of stone blocks decorated with deeply carved vulvas was discovered, the largest measuring 37 × 40 cm and incised to a depth of 10 cm. Seen as a sanctuary by the Chimane, this site was also a source of rock salt, and a place where rituals and ceremonies were performed, as, for the Chimane, salt is related to fertility and human procreation. The Bolivian vulva boulders have not been dated; however, they do bear a startling resemblance in form and technique to the Palaeolithic vulva carvings discovered across Europe.

Stone vulva carvings from Mexico also point to an enduring association between female genitalia and fertility – be it plant or human. Engraved on rocks in Baja California are plants, surrounded by carved oval vulvas. Ethnographic evidence couples these carvings with human fertility rites and the concept of 'Mother Nature'. A short distance north, in California, it was naturally vulva-shaped rock formations that were venerated by native people. In San Diego County, five natural stone *yonis* are to be found at Jamul, with another cluster occurring at Canebrake Creek. Some have painted labia, representing menstruation, just as prehistoric vulva rock formations have been found to have. According to archaeological and ethnographic evidence, the Californian stones were places of worship for the indigenous Kumeyaay tribe and the related Northern Diegueno. These Native American people chose to build their villages near these stone vaginal forms, symbols of their Earth Mother. And while the precise function of the thirty-thousand-year-old European vulva stones is lost in time, testimony from a Kumeyaay medicine man in 1900 relates the use of the Californian stones in fertility rites, describing how the *yoni* stones were visited by young women who had not yet become pregnant.

Natural vulva-shaped rock formations are worshipped elsewhere in the modern world. In Japan, parents encourage their children to play near such genital rock forms, like those in Kyushu, as they are believed to bestow good luck and health on all in their vicinity. In Thailand, on the island of Koh Samui, two natural vulval rock formations in the cliffs continue to be places of prayer and pilgrimage, with local people leaving flowers there in the early morning. The best known of the female forms is called Hin Yaay, the Grandmother Stone. Japan, America, Mexico, Bolivia and prehistoric Europe – taken together these vulval designs in stone provide, I believe, very weighty evidence in favour of female genitalia as the primal icon of fertility.

These age-old ideas are probably what lie behind a belief in *yoni* magic – the ability of the vagina to protect people or influence events. Amulets inscribed with vaginal imagery – typically two concentric ovals, some complete with vaginal cleft or clitoral mound, or embossed pubic triangles – are used around the world in a bid to confer protection and fertility on the owner. Contemporary examples of ivory, bone and silver come from Ethiopia, the Netherlands and Zaire (see Figure 1.7). Some vaginal amulets and charms are also worn as pendants. Moreover, in Hawaiian mythology, it is the 'travelling vagina' of the goddess of dance Kapo that can magically protect. Detached from her body, Kapo's vagina is dispatched to distract the hog god Kamapua'a from further assault on Kapo's sister, the volcano goddess, Pele. These protective actions earnt Kapo the epithet *Kapo-kohe-lele*, 'Kapo of the travelling vulva'. This is the stand-alone vagina in action.

The divine vagina

There is a third aspect to the ancient view of the vagina as a fertility emblem – capable of protecting against evil and enhancing fecundity. This view is possibly the most controversial – probably because it steps into areas many people see as sacrosanct. The sacred cow in question is religion, and the final facet is viewing the vagina as divine. The idea of the vagina being conceived of as an object of worship, the vagina as godhead, if you will, may seem preposterous, blasphemous even, to some. However, a belief in female genitalia as the symbolic origin of the world, the font of life, is expressed in various religions and belief systems, both ancient and modern. Perhaps it's not surprising that this view exists. After all, female genitalia embody key godly qualities. They possess creative power, they are the very visible gateway into this world, so why not the vagina as the personification of the life force in the world?

Reverence towards the vagina remains deeply resonant today in various belief systems originating in the eastern hemisphere, including those stemming from India, such as Hinduism, Buddhism and Tantra, and from China too (Taoism). In fact, Shakta, one of the three most important mainstream forms of Hinduism, is centred on the belief that the creative power of the universe is embodied in female genitalia. Within this religion, the goddess Shakti (or Sakti), the principal deity, represents the energy of the universe and creation. Shakti also symbolises female genitalia and is considered to be the power source of every deity and every living thing. In the belief system of Tantra, a similar refrain is heard. According to holy Tantric scripture: 'The manifested nature, the universal cosmic energy is symbolised by the *yoni* [vagina], the female organ engulfing the lingam [penis]. The *yoni* represents that energy which gives birth to the world, the womb of everything manifested.' Then there are the Buddhist texts, such as the *Subhasita Samgraha*, which states explicitly that 'Buddhahood resides in the female organ.' (One beautiful Japanese terracotta shows the Buddha meditating in front of a vagina twice as big as the deity.)

In Taoist thought, this idea of female genitalia as the origin of all life in the universe is expressed in the following words from the *Tao te Ching*:

> The Valley Spirit never dies.
> It is named the Mysterious Feminine.
> And the doorway of the Mysterious Feminine
> Is the base from which Heaven and Earth sprang.
> It is there within us all the while.
> Draw upon it as you will, it never runs dry.

The view of the vagina as the symbolic source of the universe is also expressed in language. The Sanskrit word for female genitalia is *yoni*, a term that also encompasses the meanings 'womb', 'origin' and 'source'.

Take a look in an English dictionary, and you'll see that even there the definition of *yoni* is multi-layered. The first meaning describes the word as: 'the female genitalia, which are regarded as a divine symbol of sexual pleasure, matrix of generation and the visible form of Shakti'. However, the second meaning states that the term also indicates 'an image of female genitalia as an object of worship'. India's famous sexual texts, such as the *Kama Sutra* (compiled by Mallinaga Vatsyayana around the fourth century), talk of perceiving the *yoni* as being 'a sacred area, a pad of pleasure, an occult region worthy of reverence, and a symbol of the cosmic mysteries'. Meanwhile, an early Hindu text advises that it is those who worship the vagina, 'this altar of love', who will have their desires granted.

This reverent and religious way of looking at the vagina has, of course, resulted in various mythologies and rituals. Every day in India, pilgrims visit the Kamakhya Pitha temple and cave complex near Gauhati, in Assam, in order to pay their respects at a sacred site that they regard as *axis mundi* – the centre of the universe. The *axis mundi* is the Yonimandala, a natural *yoni*-shaped cleft rock in the cave which 'menstruates' once a year, when red-coloured water wells up out of it. At other times of the year, the *yoni* is kept moist by a natural underground spring. According to Hindu mythology, the Yonimandala represents the place where the *yoni* of the goddess Sakti fell, after her dismembered corpse plunged to earth. A temple was thus erected in her *yoni*'s honour.

The annual 'menstruation' is interpreted by worshippers as nature's confirmation of the importance of venerating the vagina, and as evidence that the earth is a goddess. The bleeding of the sacred stone is, however, understood to be a result of the welling-up of the underground spring at the onset of the monsoon season, and the red coloration attributed to the presence of iron oxide. Natural rock formations and caves reminiscent of the *yoni* are also worshipped elsewhere in India, as female genitalia are seen as a sacred symbol of the goddess. Two of India's most important Hindu goddesses, Durga and Kali, are honoured as embodiments of the vagina's powers of birth and death, creation and destruction. Even the Indian version of paradise – the island Jambu – is vagina-shaped.

The fact that vagina worship still has a place in public consciousness today means that images depicting the act of displaying the vagina (akin to those of medieval Europe's Sheela-na-Gig sculptures) are seen as sacred. The squatting, *yoni*-exposed figurines gracing many Indian temples are viewed as goddesses, their vaginas often shining from the constant touchings of devotees' fingers wishing to invoke the goddess' largesse. In India, Laija Gauri, the 'shameless goddess', is the *yoni* queen. Significantly, though, shameless in this context has the meaning of 'perfectly modest'. This goddess is free of guilt and inhibition, her vagina is displayed in glory, not shame. This is, of course, in stark contrast to the west, where the common reaction to Sheela-na-Gig figures has been to brand them as obscene. A vastly different perspective.

The creative triangle

One of the most common cross-cultural vaginal symbols underlines the view of female genitalia as sacred and creative. This symbol is the downwards-pointing triangle, the form that a female's pubic hair traces and also, if you could see it, the shape of the interior structure of the uterus. As prehistoric artists and others show, this triangle has always been associated with female genitalia. Indeed, from the Neolithic period onwards, goddess figurines from many cultures around the globe sport sexual triangles (see Figure 1.8). In Egypt, the entrance to the queen's chamber in the pyramid of Cheops is indicated by a downwards-pointing triangle, while the early cuneiform character for woman is an inverted triangle with a median line. In the gypsy community the oldest hieroglyphic for woman was a triangle. Delta, the fourth letter of the Greek alphabet, is the root of the Greek word for womb, *delphys*, and was used to refer to the shape of female pubic hair. It is also, when capitalised, drawn as a triangle, and according to the *Suda* lexicon (*c.* 1000 CE), the delta was the letter of the vulva. The deltas of rivers, are, of course, their mouth, which, when viewed from the air trace a downwards-pointing triangle. It is thought that the delta of the Tigris and Euphrates at Qurna, Iraq, is the site of the Garden of Eden.

For many people, however, the three-sided vaginal design has even greater significance. Greek mathematician Pythagorus, and his followers, the Pythagoreans, who conceived of the universe as a manifestation of mathematical relationships, considered the triangle

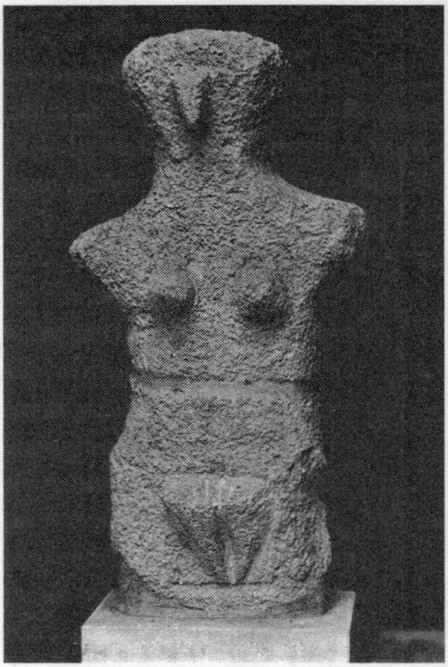

b)

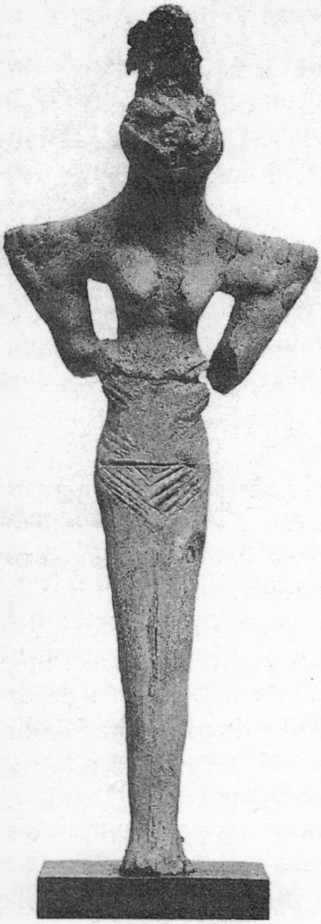

a)

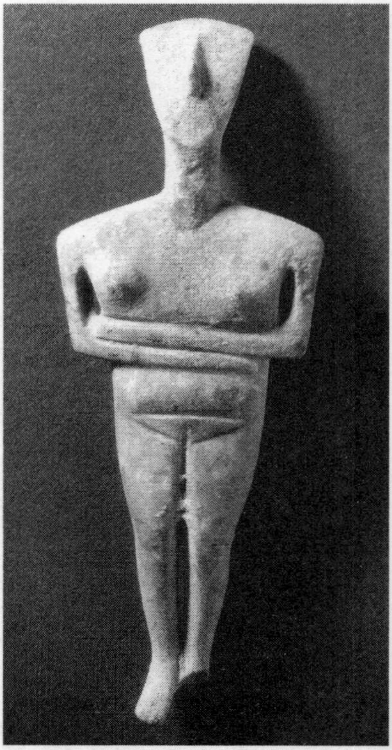

c)

Figure 1.8 The divine triangle: a) this terracotta Babylonian goddess appears like Tiamat the dragon woman (Ur, 4000–3500 BCE); b) this Greek goddess' deeply-clefted triangular vulva is massively enlarged (Aegean Islands, *c.* 2500 BCE); and, c) simplistic and elegant, this marble Cycladic goddess figurine is from Naxos (*c.* 3000–2000 BCE).

sacred. This reverence was not only because of the triangle's perfect shape, but also because the Pythagoreans read the three-sided form as a symbol of universal fertility, of the generative power of the world, of energy per se and the source of all being. Curiously, these ideas still have resonance, for in the modern language of logic theory, the symbol V signifies the whole universe, all that in one way or another exists. Today, in India, the downwards-pointing triangle, when painted red, becomes the ultimate symbol, or *yantra* (the visual equivalent of a mantra) of femaleness and generation. Hence the altars of Hindu temples often sport red-stained triangles, and Indian family-planning billboards cautioning couples to have no more than two children feature two red inverted triangles.

For Tantrics, the downwards-facing triangle is the emblem of femaleness, Shakti, female energy, and creative-genetrix feminine power. It also symbolises the supreme goddess and is recognised as the primary symbol of life. And as space cannot be bounded by less than three lines, the triangle is seen as the primal symbol – 'the first symbolic form to emerge from the cataclysmic chaos preceding creation'. In Tantric Buddhism, it is known as the *trikona* (triangle, or *yoni*), and is understood as the 'source of the dharma [the Hindu essential principle of the cosmos]', or the 'gate of all that is born'. Many yantras depict interlocking or overlapping triangles. To my mind, one of the most beautiful yantras is that of the supreme goddess (see colour plate section).

It seems that triangles and vaginas also had sacral significance for more ancient civilisations. These images are an astonishingly common feature of megalithic stones and tombs – some in surprising ways. For example, the Neolithic stones of Crucuno, near Carnac in France, incorporate the triangle/vagina in their design through their particularly precise architecture. During the autumnal equinox, the rays of the sun create a spectacular downwards-pointing triangle on a central stone. Many megalithic tombs have a large triangular stone at the entrance, or standing deep within the burial mound, often complete with vulval engravings. Triangular amulets of stone, clay or bone have also been found in ancient graves and caves, as have carefully placed goddess figurines with their beautifully inscribed triangular vulvas. So why did these people choose to bury their dead surrounded by symbols of female genitalia? Was the vagina viewed as an icon of regeneration or rebirth, as well as of creative power? Was this a bid to boost the deceased's chance of being reborn?

Vaginal resurrection

Rebirth is, of course, a central concept of many religions, and for a number of faiths, ideas of regeneration do appear to be intimately connected with female genitalia, with the vagina seen as the gateway between one world and the next, both the physical and the spiritual. There is some logic to this. If you entered this world via the vagina, why not attempt to be reborn through it too? Such a theory is evident in the Polynesian myth of the hero Maui, who crawls into the vagina of the first female on earth, Hine-nui-te-po, in an attempt to return to her womb and win immortality. Followers of Tantra also contend that since all humans are born via the vagina, female genitalia should thus be honoured as the gateway to life. Indeed, one part of Tantric ritual, *yonipûjâ* (adoration of the *yoni*), involves meditating on the *yoni*'s significance as the gateway to life. Tantrics also envisage the vagina as the entrance to the past as well as the future.

The idea that rebirth, like birth, would come from a woman's womb is perhaps why many Neolithic burial sites are uterine or vaginal in interior design, often with vulva-like openings. From above ground they swell outwards, as a woman's womb does in pregnancy, and indeed, the word 'tomb' derives from the Latin word *tumulus*, meaning swelling or pregnancy. Dolmens, stone formations that commonly consist of two vertical stones topped by a large horizontal slab, are commonly associated with female genitalia, fertility and rebirth. In Ireland, marriage contracts were arranged at the foot of these Neolithic 'hotstones', and, when pregnant, women threw clothes through the stone opening to ensure an easy birth. In India, pilgrims crawl through the vaginal apertures of dolmens in an imitation of divine rebirth, while in Malekula, Melanesia, the word for a dolmen means 'to come out from, or to be born'.

In Japan's Shinto religion, one sacred structure symbolises female genitalia, the Great Mother and the gateway between this world and another. This is the Torii arch, a distinguishing feature of Shinto shrines. Some arches, such as the shrine to the sun goddess, and the goddess of cereals, stand in woodland, while others stand in the sea.

On the feast day of the dead, one Japanese ritual involves sailing small boats filled with food and messages for the dead through the Torii arch. Chinese mythology also stresses the importance of the 'pearly gate' of the goddess of the Sea, through which all pass at birth and death.

Associations between the vagina and rebirth resonate elsewhere. Shells, in particular cowries, are a common Japanese symbol of the vagina. In some provinces of Japan, for instance, the word for vagina is *kai* – shell. Significantly, though, this vaginal symbol is also connected to ideas of birth and rebirth. According to Japanese tradition, holding a cowrie shell in your hands when giving birth is beneficial, hence the name *koyasuigai*, 'easy birth shell'. Another ancient belief holds that painting your body with a smear of powdered shell can procure rebirth. Shells still form the basis of love charms and talismans in Japan today, and are believed to confer protection on the holder. In ancient Egypt, a culture obsessed with the idea of rebirth, cowrie shells decorated sarcophagi. Why? Is this about ideas of rebirth too, connected via the shell as a vaginal symbol? Is this why finding cowrie shells among the grave goods of Stone Age burial sites is not uncommon?

Meanwhile, why the connection between shells and the vagina? Some suggest that it's because of the involute, folded, contoured appearance of shells, which bear a marked resemblance to the folds and curves of external female genitalia. Looking at a unique Neolithic Japanese figurine from the Jomon culture, which has an enormous cowrie shell sculpture as a vulva, this association seems rather clear. This yoking of shells and vaginas has found favour in many cultures. In ancient Greece, *kogchey*, a cockle seashell, was also a word for female genitalia, as was the more general word, *kteis*. In fact, *kteis* remained a widely accepted term for the vulva until into the fifteenth century, and it is suggested that Allessandro Botticelli's famous painting of the Birth of Venus – which places the goddess of love emerging from the sea standing on a scallop shell – plays with this idea. In English, 'shell' can be traced via the German word *scalp* to the Old Norse word *skalpr*, meaning 'sheath' (in Latin, *vagina*).

According to Pliny, the Latin name for the cowrie shell is *concha venerea* ('the shell of Venus'), or *porcellana*. The latter porcine name apparently derives from the appearance of the shell – said to be curved like a pig's back on one side and shaped like a sow's vulva on the other. This connection between pigs, shells and vulvas is also the source of the word porcelain. Some say the delicate, almost translucent ceramic material has a shell-like appearance; others pronounce it labial. Perhaps this is why the sixteenth-century sex text, the *Ananga Ranga*, describes one particular vaginal style as that of the Shakhini, or conch-woman, and conch soup is still considered a potent aphrodisiac in many countries.

From the sacred to the profane

But to come back to veneration of the vagina. Eastern belief systems, stemming from India, China and Japan, contain aspects of vaginal theology. Is there anywhere else? Surprisingly, and controversially, there is a place for vagina worship in the religion of Islam. The site is none other than the Kaaba, the cube-shaped building at Mecca which for Muslims is the most sacred shrine and to which all Muslims turn when praying. The black stone embedded here (believed to be a meteorite) is seen as the heart of Islam, the holy of holies. However, according to the ninth-century Arabian philosopher al-Kindi, it is Al'Lat, the ancient Arabian moon goddess, who in one of her three aspects (crescent moon – the virgin; full moon – the mother; waning moon – the wise old woman) was worshipped at the Kaaba – before Allah ever was. And the black stone, which is framed by a silver band in the shape of the vagina, is a symbol of Al'Lat's *yoni* (Al'Lat is, grammatically, the feminine form of Allah). As an aside, Al'Lat is not the only ancient deity to be venerated in the form of a black stone. Both the Greek goddess Artemis and the Phrygian goddess Cybele or Kubaba (as she was earlier known) were also worshipped in this way. Cybele, 'the Creatrix of All Things', was said to have fallen from the skies as a meteorite.

What about vagina veneration in the west? Are there any vulval symbols remaining to look at? At first glance, there does not seem to be much of a legacy left. The major western religion, Christianity, is famously renowned for being sex-negative and sexist. For centuries the men of the Christian church pushed the notion that sex was not for pleasure, but solely for procreation. Indeed, in their eyes, intercourse for pleasure was contrary to natural law and hence sinful.

The result of this line of reasoning was some very binding sex laws. In England in the twelfth and thirteenth centuries, the church declared sex illegal on Sundays, Wednesdays and Fridays, as well as for forty days before Easter and Christmas.

Preached hand-in-hand with the idea of sex being sinful is the thesis that the Christian god could only be in the image of a male; hence women have always been second-class citizens in Christianity, and added to these was the notion of the early Christian fathers that it was woman and her wicked sexual ways that were to blame for humankind's original fall from grace. One of these men, Tertullian, did not mince his words when he described Eve. 'You are the devil's gateway ... you who softened up with your cajoling words the man against whom the devil could not prevail by force.' Later, Christian authorities of the Middle Ages likened women's genitalia to the 'yawning mouth of hell'. It sounds like they were scared.

Not surprisingly then, when it comes to female genitalia, the emphasis in the western world post the advent of Christianity has mainly been on hiding or veiling the vagina, rather than revealing or celebrating it. For centuries, women could only take an active role in Christian life if they renounced their genitalia – and took a vow of celibacy. And when not ignoring the vagina, the Christian alternative appears to have been prompting women to feel shame about their genitalia and put a fig leaf over them, rather than feel pride in what was between their legs. The writers of the Old Testament chose to turn around the centuries-old female act of raising the skirt to display the vagina and use it for their own purposes. Instead of shaming others with this act, biblical words were used to push women into being ashamed by it – ashamed of their own genitalia and ashamed of their sexuality. In the Old Testament (Jerusalem 13: 26–27), Yahweh yells at Jerusalem that unless she repent of her criminal ways:

> I will also pull your skirts up as high as your face
> and let your shame be seen.
> Oh! Your adulteries, your shrieks of pleasure,
> your vile prostitution!

Elsewhere (Nahum 3:5) the prophet Nahum addresses Nineveh, warning in a vitriolic, virulent outburst:

I am here! Look to yourself! It is Yahweh Saboath who speaks.
I mean to lift up your skirts as high as your face
and show your nakedness to nations,
your shame to kingdoms.

One of the most influential theologians of the early Christian church, St Augustine (354–430), made his view of the vagina clear with his infamous comment that we are all born *inter faeces et urinam*, 'between shit and piss'. Resonances of this belief are found in language – one German word for vagina is, bluntly, *Damm*, the dam between faeces and urine, an unclean place. There are other, less direct ways that language has been used to attach shame to female genitalia. *Aidoion* is an archaic Greek word for both female and male genitalia (although more commonly female), that is generally translated as implying shame and fear. However, there is another story here. *Aidoion* also implies reverence and awe, and when first used did not contain a shaming overtone. The duality of the word is also reflected in the word it derives from – *aideomai*, which can mean to be ashamed, but also means to stand in awe, or to fear or regard with reverence, recalling perhaps the age-old emotions surrounding the exposed vagina. Significantly, *aidoios*, which is derived from the same root, was an adjective frequently used for women that meant deserving of respect, and also meant awe before that which is sacred and powerful. It seems that over the centuries, the ways in which authorities chose to use words for female genitalia meant that their meaning shifted from a complex potent mixture to focus solely on shame.

The vagina in art and architecture

Despite the generally hostile environment to vaginas and vaginal iconology in the Christian western world, some religious symbolism still exists. A common vaginal motif found in European works of art and architecture is the almond or mandorla (from the Italian for almond). Almonds and female genitalia are linked first and foremost via their shape. However, according to classical mythology, almonds are said to have sprung from the vagina of the goddess of nature and mother of all living things Cybele, who was worshipped from 6000 BCE through to the fourth century CE. Together these two associations probably explain why almonds were considered a fertility charm in Roman times, with newly-weds being showered with them.

In Christian art, in particular medieval paintings and sculptures, it is an almond-shaped area of light – a mandorla – that is often used to surround the Virgin Mary and her child. A more contemporary use of this vaginal halo is the famous one-hundred-foot-high tapestry that forms the altar centrepiece adorning Coventry Cathedral in Britain. It is essentially a gigantic mandorla out of which 'Christ in Glory' arises. As a vaginal halo, the mandorla is often found framing other important religious icons. An early-fifteenth-century painting, 'The Triumph of Venus', shows the goddess standing naked in a vaginal-shaped setting. Rays of light radiate out from the labia-like edges to illuminate the surrounding group of men (apparently famous from different periods as great lovers). Moreover, the strongest beams of light shoot directly from her vagina. Early stone statues of the Buddha are also often found enclosed in mandorlas, as are Tantric images of goddesses.

The almond-shaped oval, or mandorla, is seen as sacred in other ways too. For early Christians, it was a symbol of worship, and was known as the *vesica*, or *vesica piscis*. In this Christian context, this holy symbol is said to have represented the vagina of the Virgin Mary, while as a symbol of the vagina in general, it was, and still is, used in magic rituals. Curiously enough, the *vesica piscis* also reveals how veneration of the vagina exists in the strangest of places – even forming the basis of one of the most important buildings in Britain. Research shows that the shape of the *vesica piscis*, the symbol of the vagina, underpins the geometry of part of Windsor Castle. For at the heart of St George's Chapel are two intersecting *vesicas*, which set the blueprint for the rest of this beautiful medieval building. But why *vesicas*, and why here?

The answer lies in the mysterious Order of the Garter – England's highest order or society of knights – which was founded by Edward III in the fourteenth century. These knights, known as the Knights of the Garter, have a famous motto: 'Honi soit qui mal y pense' – 'Shame on you if you see evil in this'. And the 'this' in question? It appears that it is none other than the vagina. Indeed, a text by the Italian medieval scholar Mondonus Belvaleti, states explicitly in an essay on the chivalrous Order of the Garter that it 'took its beginning from the female sex'. The spiritual home of the Order of the Garter is St George's Chapel at Windsor, which is covered with symbols representing female genitalia. It seems viewing the vagina as a sacred orifice has left a far stronger legacy in the west than you might immediately suppose.

Some academics also point to the traditional cruciform design of most Christian places of worship as being based on the architecture of female genitalia. While other researchers choose to dismiss this seemingly heretical idea out of hand, there are certainly some similarities and some credence to the theory. On passing through a church's curved doors, one enters a vestibule, just as the vaginal vestibule lies behind a woman's labia. The main body of the church, which leads directly to the altar, the site of transformation, echoes the central vaginal aisle leading straight to the uterus, which magically transforms egg and sperm into new life. To either side of the altar (uterus) are two passageways (Fallopian tubes) which lead to the vestries (ovaries). The idea that places of worship were modelled originally on female genitalia is also lent weight by the fact that many Neolithic tombs and prehistoric sites of sacral importance, such as the incredible curving stone temples of Malta and Gozo (4500–2500 BC), appear designed to represent the body of the goddess, or her genitalia.

Finally, many researchers point to the western world's ultimate emblem of love – the heart – as none other than a vaginal icon. It's certainly the case that if you look at female genitalia when they are aroused, when the outer labia are plumped up and parting of their own volition, the form the visible vagina outlines is unmistakably heart-shaped (see colour plate section). Can you think of a part of the human body that traces a more heart-like figure? Hearts themselves are definitely not heart-shaped. Perhaps the western world's obsession with the heart as a symbol of love really is a relic of our vagina-worshipping past. Or how about the favourite lucky charm – the horseshoe. Does this stem from the U- or bell-shaped carvings found on prehistoric figurines, including that of the Venus of Willendorf's genitals, and copied over centuries? Who knows? There can be no absolute answer, but it's an intriguing possibility.

A vaginal awakening

While hints of vaginal iconography do still exist in the west, the general sex-negative mood of western culture suggests that flagrant, flaunting, proud art depicting female genital display is far more likely to be censored or covered up than commended. It's certainly the case that when painted images of the female nude appeared in the west, the morals of the day dictated that hands or drapes must be placed modestly and discreetly over the 'offending vaginal cleft', and horror of horrors, no one must depict women sporting pubic hair. The astounding 1866 painting by pioneering French Realism artist Gustave Courbet was not put on permanent public display until nearly a century after its creation (see colour plate section). Perhaps part of the problem was that Courbet, ignoring what his peers and society taught him, went to the heart of the matter in naming his respectful portrayal of the vagina 'The Origin of the World'. Ingres' 'La Source' (1856) reveals a similar sentiment.

The western world's reluctance to look at positive images of female genitalia is perhaps summed up by one of the most famous journals in the world, Anne Frank's *The Diary of a Young Girl*. When it was originally published in 1947, many passages were omitted, amongst them several which focused on Anne's sexuality and her genitalia. At the time of publication, these entries were deemed to be too open about sex for a book which would be read by young adults. Anne Frank's diary was finally published in its entirety at the end of the twentieth century, following the death of her father. The following, written when Anne was fifteen, was one of the deleted passages. It is remarkable in its honesty, frankness and level of knowledge for a girl of her age in her society.

Friday, 24 March 1944

Dear Kitty,

. . . I'd like to ask Peter whether he knows what girls look like down there. I don't think boys are as complicated as girls. You can easily see what boys look like in photographs or pictures of male nudes, but with women it's different. In women, the genitals, or whatever they're called, are hidden between their legs. Peter has probably never seen a girl up close. To tell you the truth, neither have I. Boys are a lot easier. How on earth would I go about describing a girl's parts? I can tell from what he said that he doesn't know exactly how it all fits together. He was talking about the '*Muttermund*' [cervix], but that's on the inside, where you can't see it. Everything's pretty well arranged in us women. Until I was eleven or twelve, I didn't realise there was a second set of labia on the inside, since you couldn't see them. What's even funnier is that I thought urine came out of the clitoris. I asked Mother once what that little bump was, and she said she didn't know. She can really play dumb when she wants to!

But to get back to the subject. How on earth can you explain what it all looks like without any models? Shall I try anyway? Okay, here goes!

When you're standing up, all you see from the front is hair. Between your legs there are two soft, cushiony things, also covered with hair, which press together when you're standing, so you can't see what's inside. They separate when you sit down, and they're very red and quite fleshy on the inside. In the upper part, between the outer labia, there's a fold of skin that, on second thought, looks like a kind of blister. That's the clitoris. Then come the inner labia, which are also pressed together in a kind of crease. When they open up, you can see a fleshy little mound, no bigger than the top of my thumb. The upper part has a couple of holes in it, which is where the urine comes out. The lower part looks as if it were just skin, and yet that's where the vagina is. You can barely find it, because the folds of skin hide the opening. The hole's so small I can hardly imagine how a man could get in there, much less how a baby could come out. It's hard enough trying to get your index finger inside. That's all there is, and yet it plays such an important role!

Yours, Anne M. Frank

Anne Frank is to be applauded for her innocent teenage act of *anasuromai*. More are needed. In the twenty-first century, we live increasingly in a world where the most common image of female genitalia is the one pushed by the pornography industry – and is a negative, shaming one. This representation – styled by men for men – bears scant resemblance to the varying beauty of unadulterated vaginas. Typically shorn of pubic hair, labia snipped into regular lengths, sanitised, neutered and surgically enhanced, pornography creates effigies of female genitalia. And for many men and women, such cunt caricatures are coming to be seen as a normal view of the vagina.

This is a sad, narrow and small representation of this amazing female organ of sexual reproduction and pleasure. Yet it seems that this journey – from the sacred to the profane for the origin of the world – is the one that will be made, unless we stop being ashamed and scared of what is really between a woman's legs. The way to alter this shameful attitude is to look at all the varying views of the vagina in an attempt to understand and appreciate what female genitalia actually embody – past and present, in art, history and science, and across cultures and languages.

2

FEMALIA

'. . . so he started playing the water over my legs and then directly on my . . . femalia, and I held my lips open so that he could see my inner wishbone, and the drops of water exploding on it . . .' These are the words of the female protagonist of *Vox*, Nicolson Baker's erotic, arousing paean to phone sex. 'Femalia' is just one of the words invented in an attempt not to spoil the spoken sexual flow and throw an on-line orgasm off-course (there's 'strum' for masturbate and 'tock' for ass too). Femalia is also the word chosen by Joani Blank to title her fantastic book, which is full of colour photographs of female genitalia. Baker and Blank aren't alone in finding common terms for female genitalia too restrictive. For many, the conventional sexual lexicon is deeply unsatisfactory. Vulva, it's moaned, is too clinical, while vagina, others murmur, smacks too much of passivity. Pussy and other slang expressions, well, they suffer from being too laden with sexual stereotype, and cunt is just too hard to be heard. And then there's the fact that words for female genitalia often overlap and vary in meaning. Vulva generally describes the external female genitalia, but not always, while vagina can encompass all parts of the female sexual anatomy, minus the uterus, or refer specifically to the interior muscular organ.

So why, in the west, is the selection of suitable sexual terms to describe female genitalia so small and lacking in specificity? For starters, the naming of any object is a tricky business – be it a child or a body part. What to focus on? There's so much to consider. Names say a lot, and what they convey can be of vital importance. An appropriate name can have great influence, but choose the wrong title and you may offend. Names should also stand the test of time. Yet fashion is fickle: plump for popularity and the title could all too quickly fall from grace; decide on a mouthful of a monicker, and the term may never take off. Interestingly, though, the fact that there are so many influences on the choice of a title means that language is capable of being a unique barometer of a society's attitudes. If you look closely, it can even expose how a society views the vagina – whether it's vaunted or vilified lexically. And if you get really close up, the history of sexual language can also explain the nature of the English sexual lexicon.

Names often reflect the beliefs and ideas of the time, and the field of sexual anatomy is no exception in this. For example, the term 'renal' is used today to denote an association with the kidneys (*renes*). However, the kidneys got their Latin name because it was believed that *rivi ab his obsceni humoris nascuntur* – the stream (*rivus*) of semen (*obscenus humor*) flows from them. This reflects the ancient theory that seminal matter (both the female variety, *sperma muliebris*, and the male form) was perfected in the lumbar region of the spine and kidneys (after originating in the brain). From ancient Greece through to the seventeenth century, *nymphae*, meaning 'water goddesses', was a common name for a woman's inner labia. This accepted medical term stemmed from the idea that the labia's fluted design and position, surrounding a woman's vaginal and urethral openings, guided the gush and flow of both semen and urine away from female genitalia. It also reflected the practice in pre-Christian Greece of placing statues of nymphs near public fountains. As midwife Jane Sharp explained helpfully in *The Midwives Book* (1671): 'these wings are called Nymphs, because they joyn the passage of the Urine, and the neck of the Womb, out of which as out of Fountains . . . waters and humours do flow, and besides in them is all the joy and delight of Venus'.

Some names either attempt to explain what an organ does or paint a mental picture of the part, often badly and baldly. Take *cunnus interior* and 'the king's highway' – both ancient expressions for the vagina. A woman's perineum, as it is known today, was formerly dubbed the *interforamineum*, literally, 'the space between the two holes' – vagina and rectum. Genital labia were sometimes referred to as the *orae naturalium* – 'the edges of the natural parts' – while other anatomists preferred the more cumbersome monicker, the *genitalis muliebris ambitus*, the 'periphery of the female genital part'. In men, the *vas deferens* – the duct that transports spermatozoa from the epididymis to the urethra – is made up of two Latin words. *Vas* is a duct or tube that carries a fluid, and *deferens* is the past participle of the verb *deferre*, which means to bear away. Simple and to the point, and this term is still used today, despite losing something in translation over the centuries. An earlier Greek term for the *vas deferens* – 'the swollen vein-like bystanders' – was far vaguer about function, and did not stand the test of time. The man who bestowed this graphic title, the Alexandrian anatomist Herophilus, also called a man's seminal vesicles 'the gland-like bystanders'. Perhaps Herophilus was suffering from anatomist's block.

Names can also be used to make a political point or emphasise a particular idea. The words 'genitals' and 'genitalia' derive from the depiction of these organs as parts of generation. It could be said there is a hidden agenda here, as such vocabulary places a specific function on genitalia. In this case the role rammed home is sexual reproduction, which is arguably not the predominant function of a person's genitalia. Conceiving children is certainly not the most common use the vagina and penis are put to. Significantly, what this terminology omits to mention is that these organs are also organs of ecstasy and pleasure, capable of generating orgasm as well as offspring.

Titles are often used to educate, and in some examples this education extends to prescribing what emotions are appropriate regarding particular body parts. In his medieval summing-up of ancient scientific knowledge, *Etymologiarum*, Isidore of Seville uses the term *inhonesta* – the parts which cannot honourably (*honeste*) be named – to describe female genitalia (*turpia* and *obscena* were other sex-negative Latin expressions for the genitals). Isidore also explains how 'The ancients called the female genitalia the spurium', and goes on to amplify that this is why illegitimate children, those that do not 'take the name of the father' are called *spurius*, because they are seen to spring solely from the mother. Today spurious commonly means not genuine or real. A term used today to describe a person's genitals (in particular female genitalia) – *pudendum* (plural *pudenda*) – irrevocably associates shame with genitalia, as it is said to be derived from the Latin verb *pudere*, to be ashamed. Modern shaming connotations also linger on in other European languages, notably German. Terms for the female genitalia include *Schamscheide* (literally 'the sheath of shame'); *Scham* (genitalia); *Schamhaar* (pubic hair) and *Schamlippen* (the labia).

One of the most interesting aspects of language is that it is mutable, that is, over time words can change in meaning as they shift to reflect the predominant attitudes of the day. In this context, it is significant that a look at more archaic epithets for the genitals reveals that prior to the shift to Christianity, the western world did not view a woman's genitals in an inherently negative manner. Indeed, Greek words to describe genitalia can convey positive overtones. In classical Greek, people such as Hippocrates, Aristotle and Homer wrote about female genitalia using the term *aidoion*, which does not contain an anti-sexual judgement, and, as noted earlier, derives from a word meaning to stand in awe or to fear or regard with reverence. Likewise the Greek word *verenda*, which was used extensively by Pliny as an equivalent of *aidoion*. *Verenda* or, as we would say today, vagina, means literally the 'parts that inspire awe, or respect'.

Natura, another Latin term for female genitalia, was neither overtly vulgar nor technical, and was generally acceptable in educated language. *Natura*'s origin is understood to lie in the word *nascor*, which indicates 'place of birth', i.e. the female genitalia. *Natura* in turn gave rise to *naturale*, which Celsus (*c.* 30 CE) used to describe the passageway of the vagina specifically. Etymologists also point out that even the word *pudendum* wasn't always read as a signifier of shame. When first used by Roman philosopher Seneca, it did not carry such connotations. Rather it was used to express seemingly indifferently the genitalia of both men and women. The western world has early Christians, such as Augustine, to thank for conflating human sexual organs, in particular the vagina, with shame. It appears that 'shameless' which can mean 'perfectly modest', was spun into something to be ashamed of, in order to stress a particular religious belief.

The stress of the name game often prompts some peculiar appellations. Many of these, it seems, spring from the fact that sometimes it's simpler to attach a term that sets out to describe what the object resembles. The newborn baby reminds you of your Uncle Bob, so why not call her Bobbina, or even better, Roberta? This simile method for naming objects is common in anatomy. Hippocrates referred to a woman's plump, pillowy outer labia using the Greek for 'overhanging cliffs', while a later term was *monticuli* – hillocks. In contrast, the inner, thinner labia were likened to wings in both Greek and Latin. *Mentula*, an early name for the penis, has its roots in the term for spearmint stalk. Likewise the penile phrase *caulis*, which stems from another stalk, this time that of the cabbage.

The word 'penis', peculiarly, has its origin in the male member's similarity to a piece of animal anatomy. Put plainly, penis was an archaic word for an animal's tail. However, today it is the standard term for a man's phallus. How come? It's suggested that the title was conferred in part because, like many animals' tails, the phallus could stiffen and rise, as well as hang down. (An understanding of this etymology of penis adds some resonance to the phrase 'sending someone away with their tail between their legs'.) Moreover, when first coined, penis was an exclusively obscene term for the phallus, not a conventional one. *Cauda*, the classical Latin word for tail, was also used in a similar way. And for whatever inexplicable reasons, penis is the simile that has stuck, while *mentula*, *caulis* and *cauda* fell from grace.

Of sheaths and scabbards

The word 'vagina', too, has its origins in the anatomical habit of using resemblances to bestow titles. In Latin, the word originally implied a sheath or scabbard, the protective covering for a sword. During the sixteenth century, though, this meaning began to change, and the word started to be used in conjunction with a specific portion of female sexual anatomy. The first person to apply vagina in this way is believed to be the Italian anatomist Matteo Realdo Colombo. In 1559, Colombo, writing in his manuscript *De Re Anatomica*, described a woman's interior erectile muscular sexual organ as 'that part into which the mentula [spearmint stalk/penis] is inserted, as it were, into a vagina [sheath/scabbard]'. As this Renaissance man saw it, this particular part of female sexual anatomy enveloped the penis just as a sheath or scabbard covers a sword. Hence to him it was a vagina.

It took nearly a hundred years, though, before the word vagina started to be used as a standard anatomical term. Its first appearance in this sense is credited to Johann Vesling, who in 1641 used it in his text *Syntagma Anatomicum*. Its take-up as a medical term appears to be fairly rapid after this. In 1682 vagina was used in English for the first time, and by the turn of the century the term (or its equivalent, such as *vagin* and *Schiede*) had entered European vernacular. From

1700 onwards, it became the term of choice in childbearing guides, such as Pierre Dionis' 1719 *A General Treatise of Midwifery*. Dionis describes how the vagina 'receives the Sword of the Male, and becomes a case to it, and therefore is call'd the Vagina, that is to say, its sheath'. The vagina had arrived. From conception to public acceptance in approximately 150 years. So, thanks to similes and early anatomists, humans have sex with sheaths and tails. It could have been worse, though; it could have been a combination of the king's highway and cabbage stalks.

However, the roots of some genital terms remain hazy. One of these is 'vulva'. According to the medieval manuscript *De Secretis Mulierum* (*Women's Secrets*) by Pseudo-Albertus Magnus, 'the vulva is named from the word *valva* [folding door] because it is the door of the womb'. Seventeenth-century anatomist Reinier de Graaf agreed with this etymology, but added that others thought the derivation was 'from *velle*, "want", on the grounds that it has a great and insatiable want of coitus'. This recalls the infamous verse from Proverbs, Chapter 30: 'There are three things that cannot be sated ... Hell, the mouth of the vulva and the earth.'

Isidore of Seville (*c.* 560–636) used the term *valvae* (doors) to describe a woman's labia, while the Babylonian Talmud (fourth century CE) used an expression for hinges. Others state that vulva means wrapper or covering. This alternative meaning is thought to derive either from the occasional use of the word in Roman times to describe the membrane which surrounds a developing foetus, or from its use as a term for the uterus. It's certainly the case that the archaic meaning of vulva was the uterus of an animal. More specifically, in the old dialect of Sassari, Sardinia, vulva was a culinary term for a sow's uterus, which was considered a delicate dish in Roman times. The word uterus, meanwhile, is thought to have its origins in the Roman word for belly (*venter*), and could be applied to men as well as women. Shades of this uterus/belly conflation can be found in the still common habit of saying a woman has a baby in her tummy.

Defining the vagina

Sometimes it's impossible to pin down why some names endure and others don't. To my mind, Colombo's vaginal conception may well have been successful because it fulfilled a particular and timely need – namely providing a specific term for a particular area of female sexual anatomy. Prior to this, the female genital lexicon in the sixteenth century appeared designed to confuse rather than clarify. Some vaginal phrases, like *sinus pudoris*, 'the hollow of modesty', were vague, while elsewhere words for the vagina, uterus and vulva overlapped in meaning. In the Latin of late antiquity, for example, vulva had various meanings. In some cases it implied the chamber of the vagina and the vestibule. In other situations, it implied the external female genitalia. The word vulva could also signify the uterus, or describe the uterus, vagina and vestibule as one entity.

From Aristotle onwards, however, it was how the uterus was conceptualised that was one of the commonest sources of genital confusion. Uterus was typically applied to describe the entirety of female genitalia, both outside and in, yet in some cases its meaning was the one it has today – namely, the womb, the organ that is home to a developing embryo. Uterus, though, could also imply the vaginal passageway, hence the description by one anatomical tome of how, in virgins, the hymen 'prevents the penis from being inserted in the uterus'. As well as being both an all-encompassing genital term and a singular one, the uterus was also used as a reference point for the remainder of female genitalia. As a result, reading old anatomical texts is like swimming in an increasingly complex uterine sea. There's the mouth of the uterus, the neck of the uterus, the *fundus*, the horns of the uterus, the entrance of the uterus, the boundary stone, the *pudendum* of the uterus and the *latera*. Sometimes it seems that many anatomists were themselves unsure which bit of a woman's body they were discussing as they got lost in uterine terminology. To me, it sounds like the western world's antipathy towards women, sex and the vagina resulted in a severe lexical deficit surrounding female genitalia.

Not surprisingly, when vagina is used for the first time as a medical term (by Vesling), it is in a uterine context. For him the uterus comprised three portions – the fundus of the uterus, the neck of the uterus and the vagina of the uterus. However, not everyone agreed with his use of the word vagina. Many anatomists continued to refer to the vaginal chamber in a wholly uterine context – although it seems that no one could agree whether the vagina was the neck of the uterus, the mouth of the uterus, or the entrance of the uterus. In time, though, the introduction and acceptance of the word vagina did settle the uterine confusion, and talk of the vagina as the neck, mouth or entrance to the womb began to fall out of fashion. While thanks for this clarification must go in part to Colombo, another person deserves credit too.

That man is the seventeenth-century Dutch anatomist Reinier de Graaf (whose name now graces a female's Graafian follicles). De Graaf's 1672 *magnum opus* on female genitalia, *The Treatise Concerning the Generative Organs of Women*, set the Renaissance gold standard in understanding female sexual anatomy. In fifteen chapters, de Graaf set out to describe in detail a woman's genitals in terms of structure, language and function. In Chapter I, 'Setting Out the Topics', after commenting: 'It will be obvious to everyone . . . how various is the use of the term uterus', he provides a breakdown of the female genital parts in tabular form. Chapter VII, entitled 'Concerning the Vagina of the Uterus', contains a discussion of vaginal vocabulary, both past and present, and all the potential pitfalls that vague and overlapping terminology can lead to. Critically, before beginning a vivid description of the vagina's design, position and proportions, he states: 'For this reason, so as to leave no room for confusion, we shall call this channel, in the following discussion, the vagina of the uterus. This is an appropriate name, since the part encloses the male member within itself, receiving it as a scabbard does a sword or knife.'

How the uterus got its horns

The distinct sexual lexicon created and promoted by de Graaf, Colombo and their contemporaries filled a much-needed gap in the language of female genitalia. Moreover, on close inspection the way that these men described women's sexual organs reveals another key aspect of the mutable nature of language. Fashion, favoured and then defunct theories, and a society's morals, all influence whether a certain word remains in common use. But there is another major reason why terminology fluctuates over time – human error. Sometimes it's clear how such mistakes occurred. Some slips were made as texts were translated over the centuries from Greek to Latin, or, more typically, from Greek to Arabic and then to Latin. Other shifts in sense are harder to pin down. And while some permutations are minor, others have altered meanings radically.

'Cervix' is one modern female genital term that bears the scars of human error made at some stage in its history, mistakes that changed its meaning drastically. In modern medical terminology, it is a term that is understood as meaning the short, thick tube of smooth muscle which surrounds the narrow channel (the endocervical canal) which leads from the vagina through to the uterus. The lower end of the cervix dips into the vaginal chamber, and is called the external os (opening, or mouth), while the upper uterine end of the cervix is known as the internal os. The intimate connection between the cervix and the uterus is highlighted in the full title of the cervix, the cervix uteri, which means the neck of the womb or neck of the uterus – a phrase that many medics continue to use (although the uterus is distinct from the cervix in terms of tissue type). Indeed, in medical terms, the term cervical is understood in general as referring to the neck; for example, a person's cervical vertebrae are the top seven spinal bones – those in the vicinity of the neck.

Curiously, though, the word cervix did not originally mean neck. *Collum* is the Latin for neck. De Graaf uses the word *collum* when talking about the neck of the uterus (the cervix as we know it today). As de Graaf explains: 'The uterus is linked to the vagina, the rectum and the bladder by that part of it which is properly called the collum, neck.' Elsewhere he adds: 'The real collum of the uterus is the one where the narrow little hole is . . . The semen proceeds through it into the fundus of the uterus.' De Graaf wasn't the only anatomist to call the neck of the uterus the *collum*. So do earlier anatomists, such as the second-century scientist Soranus, in his immensely influential book *Gynaecology* – the major source of information regarding female genitalia for the following fifteen centuries.

So if the neck of the uterus was known as the *collum* what was, or is, the original cervix of the uterus? The source of the word cervix lies, surreally, in the curving, crescent-shaped horns of many mammals. And curiously, although this horn meaning was somehow lost in human anatomical vocabulary, it survives today in animal physiology. A cervid is any ruminant mammal of the class *Cervidae*, mammals that are characterised by the presence of horns or antlers (in Latin, *cervus* means deer). It is still common today for scientists to talk of uterine horns, in particular when discussing animal anatomy although this is true of human anatomy too. As yet, it is unclear how *collum* became transposed with cervix.

What is certain, though, is that the belief that a woman's uterus had horns, as did the wombs of many other mammals, including cows, ewes, goats and rabbits, is a long-held one. Aristotle talks of the two horns of a woman's womb. So too do medieval anatomical manuscripts such as the *Pantegni*, which relates: 'The womb (matrix) is like the bladder in shape, for both of them are very deep, but it is different in its two extensions which are similar to horns.' The notion of the horned womb was also used to explain how an embryo's sex was determined. The left horn of the uterus, it was said, was responsible for the creation of female offspring, while the right resulted in boys. Hence the advice to women to lie on their left side during and after sex if they wanted to produce a girl.

The yoking of horns to a woman's uterus was accepted for centuries, as seventeenth-century descriptions of what we now call ectopic pregnancies make clear. In his text *Anthropographia*, anatomist Jean Riolan states:

> As I write this, 10 years have passed since a surgeon in Paris, with physicians present, found, in a dead woman he had dissected, a very small foetus excellently formed in the right horn of the uterus ... We have, too, the recent example of the laundress of the Queen's bed linen. Some years ago there was found in her body a foetus of the length and thickness of a thumb and well formed, resting inside one horn of the uterus. For 4 months it caused such cruel pains that at last the woman exchanged life for death, in the seventh month of her pregnancy.

The modern term for these uterine horns is, of course, the Fallopian tubes. Even the man whose name would later be applied to them – Gabriel Fallopius – described them in his manuscript, *Observationes Anatomicae*, in terms of their horn-like design. He comments how 'that thin and rather narrow seminary passage originates, nervous and white, in the horn of the uterus itself and when it has got a little way away from the horn gradually widens and curls itself like a vine-tendril until near its end'.

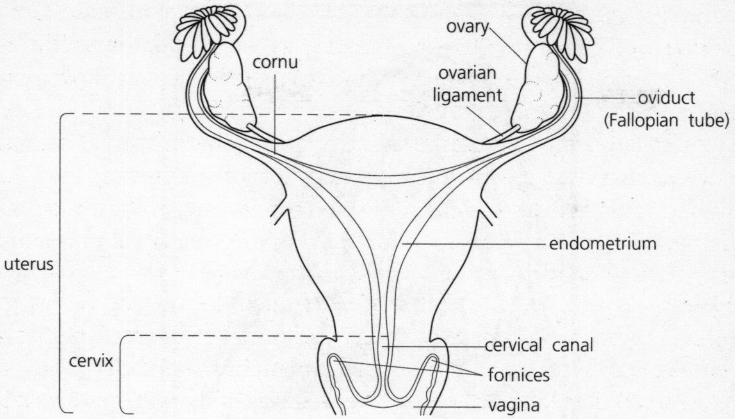

Figure 2.1 A woman's uterus and Fallopian tubes. It's striking how the exterior of the uterus does trace a bull's head shape with the Fallopian tubes in a position akin to where a bull's horns would be.

A bull's head with horns

The conception of the Fallopian tubes as horns of the uterus is easily understood. A look at any modern illustration of a woman's uterus, or the real thing, reveals the source of the idea. Fallopian tubes do trace a graceful horn-like curve, and are positioned in conjunction with the uterus in such a way that it's not too fanciful to see them as mirroring the horns and antlers of deer or bulls (see Figure 2.1). The shape of the exterior of the uterus is also suggestive of a bull's head, being wider at the top than the bottom, thus adding weight to the idea of uterine horns. This structural similarity in outline, coupled with the ancient notion that the uterus had horns, is presumably the driving force behind the decision of Renaissance anatomists to depict women's uteri as two-horned organs.

Images of slender, curving, antler-like Fallopian tubes appear on the pages of Belgian anatomist Andreas Vesalius' pioneering anatomical text *De Humani Corporis Fabrica* (1541), while shorter, thicker uterine horns adorn Jacopo Berengario da Carpi's illustrated anatomy book. Another of Berengario's drawings depicts an astonishingly

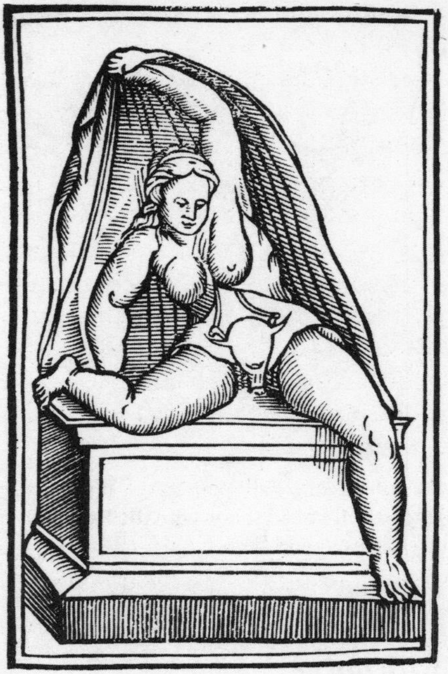

Figure 2.2 The uterus as bull's head with horns (from Jacopo Berengario, *Isagoge brevis*, 1522).

bull's-head-like uterus, complete with horns (see Figure 2.2). Indeed, during the sixteenth and seventeenth centuries, when anatomical texts began to be illustrated for the first time, it seems routine to depict a woman's uterus with horns. This artistic habit, of course, in turn gave further credence to the scientific notion that uteri did have horns. Berengario's text labels the uterine ligaments as *Ligamentum cornulae* (*cornu* is Latin for horn, while *korone* is the Greek for anything curved), while the Fallopian tubes themselves are entitled the *vas spermaticum* – the semen-delivering vessels – reflecting the contemporary belief in their female-semen-delivering function (of which more later).

The connection between female genitalia and horns is an ancient one. As we've seen, one of the earliest stone carvings of women, the prehistoric Venus of Laussel (*c.* 24,000 BCE) depicts a woman, one hand holding a horn with thirteen grooves, and the other hand pointing to her genitalia. Fast forward approximately eighteen thousand years, and the association between women, horns, fertility and female genitalia is still being spelt out, this time more strongly. The early Neolithic community of Çatal Hüyük, on Turkey's Konya Plain, flourished from *c.* 6500 BCE for around ten centuries. Archaeological evidence from this important Stone Age site has revealed that for this culture the two most common religious icons are images of goddesses and, in conjunction with them, illustrations of bull's heads and horns (the archaeological term is *bucranium*). The goddess and her *bucrania* are found embellishing temples, shrines and the walls of ordinary buildings too. One beautiful temple painting shows female torsos with bull's head and horns in place of their uterus and Fallopian tubes. The connection is unequivocal. On some images it even appears as if the artist has tried to represent the flower-like ends of the Fallopian tubes, as rosettes appear on the horns. The concept of reproduction was certainly known in the culture of Çatal Hüyük, and is pictorially explained on a grey stone plaque. One side depicts the bodies of two lovers, the other a woman holding an infant.

The later Greek Minoan civilisation (2900–1200 BCE) also has at its centre the same two iconic images – the figure of a goddess and her bull's horns – with both found adorning altars, shrines, sealstones and the walls of buildings. The presence of Minoan horns, which are known as horns of consecration, has come to be recognised as a clear indication of a shrine, and the double axe (the *labrys*) that the goddesses commonly hold aloft is seen as a symbol of power in Minoan religion. In some images, the Minoan goddess wears a crown made of bull's horns. Although gods do appear in Minoan images, when gods and goddesses appear together, the goddess is always larger than the male.

The archaic association between horns, fertility and the uterus is also reflected in ancient and modern language – both written and gestural. The Egyptian hieroglyph for womb is a two-horned bovine uterus, while the word cornucopia – 'the horn of plenty' – means both a great abundance, and a horn-shaped container. The horn of plenty is also read as a symbol of fertility, and in Tibet is associated with the white moon-cow goddess. In Italy, if a man is given the sign of the horn (index and small finger extended, the others folded in), it is one of the worst insults possible. The implication of this gesture is that his wife is unfaithful to him, he is being cuckolded (another man's sperm could be in the horns of her uterus). Moreover, the Italian verb *cornificare* means to be unfaithful to, while *cornuto* means cuckolded.

The association between a man being cuckolded and horns is prevalent across all of southern Europe. In Portuguese (*cornudo* or *cabrão*); Spanish (*cornudo*); Catalan (*cornut* or *cubron*); French (*cocu*) and Greek (*keratas*), the word for cuckolded means 'the horned one', someone 'who wears the horns'. In England, *cornute* was introduced as a word during the Norman Conquest and remained in use until the sixteenth century. It was then to be replaced by 'cuckolded', a word which derives from cuckoo – the bird that lays its eggs in others' nests. Tellingly, cuckolded is a term that is applied to men, not women. That is, of course, because women cannot be cuckolded; it is a unique male fear that they cannot be certain that a child is theirs. Other connections between horns, fertility and the uterus remain. For the English, to be horny is, of course, to be sexually excited. According to scientific studies, a woman's libido often reaches a peak when an ovum is released into her uterine horns. Cornification is the medical term for the change in structure of the outer layer of vaginal epithelial cells that occurs during oestrus and ovulation.

The vagina is a penis?

The notion that women had horned uteri was not the only one to be overplayed in anatomical illustrations and scientific theory. Renaissance medicine was also under the apprehension that the vagina was equivalent to an interior penis, and medical drawings depicted this vagina/penis conception with a peculiar precision. These illustrations, rather startlingly, outline the difference between female and male genitalia as a spatial, rather than a structural one. One of the most astonishing visual renderings of the vagina as a penis is by Vesalius, and features in his text *De Humani Corporis Fabrica*, the founding work of modern anatomy (see Figure 2.3). Indeed, the vagina is represented as a penis in all three of Vesalius' works. Moreover, as these manuscripts were all widely plagiarised by other anatomists, the habit of representing the vagina as an interior penis became routine in Renaissance anatomical texts. Vesalius' drawings comparing side

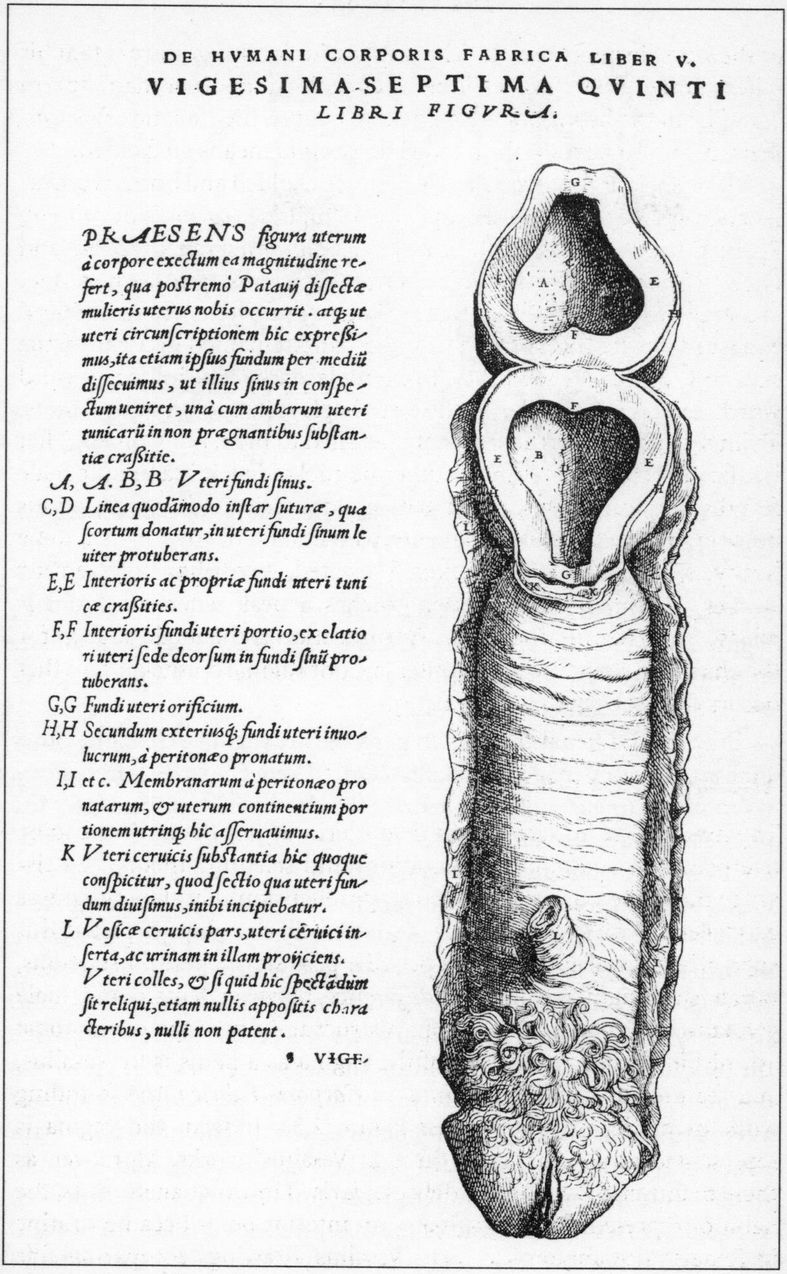

DE HVMANI CORPORIS FABRICA LIBER V.

VIGESIMA SEPTIMA QVINTI LIBRI FIGVRA.

PRAESENS figura uterum à corpore exectum ea magnitudine refert, qua poſtremò Patauij diſſectæ mulieris uterus nobis occurrit. atq; ut uteri circunſcriptionem hic expreſſimus, ita etiam ipſius fundum per mediū diſſecuimus, ut illius ſinus in conſpectum ueniret, unà cum ambarum uteri tunicarū in non prægnantibus ſubſtantiæ craſſitie.

A, A. B, B Vteri fundi ſinus.

C, D Linea quodāmodo inſtar ſuturæ, qua ſcortum donatur, in uteri fundi ſinum leuiter protuberans.

E, E Interioris ac propriæ fundi uteri tunicæ craſſities.

F, F Interioris fundi uteri portio, ex elatiori uteri ſede deorſum in fundi ſinū protuberans.

G, G Fundi uteri orificium.

H, H Secundum exteriusq; fundi uteri inuolucrum, à peritonæo pronatum.

I, I et c. Membranarum à peritonæo pronatarum, & uterum continentium portionem utrinq; hic aſſeruauimus.

K Vteri ceruicis ſubſtantia hic quoque conſpicitur, quod ſectio qua uteri fundum diuiſimus, inibi incipiebatur.

L Veſicæ ceruicis pars, uteri cēruici inſerta, ac urinam in illam proijciens.

Vteri colles, & ſi quid hic ſpectādum ſit reliqui, etiam nullis appoſitis characteribus, nulli non patent.

§ VIGE-

Figure 2.3 The vagina as penis: Vesalius' view of the vagina (1541).

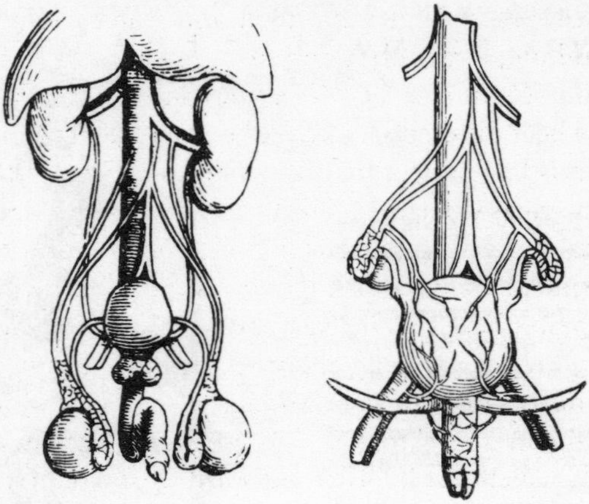

Figure 2.4 How female and male genitalia were seen to compare – male *left*, female *right* (from Vesalius, *Tabulae sex*, 1538).

by side a woman's female sexual anatomy with that of a man (see Figure 2.4) were also reproduced cheaply in a format that was available to non-academics, and so this idea of the vagina as an interior penis entered public consciousness too.

But why did Renaissance men perceive the vagina to be none other than an interior penis? This phallic-centred belief has a lengthy history. Its roots are in antiquity, in theories that both Aristotle and later the physician to the gladiators, Galen (*c.* 129–200), propounded. According to Aristotle and his followers, heat, or more precisely how much heat a person possessed, was the factor determining whether an individual ended up female or male. Males, these minds opined, had more of this precious heat than females, a fact which made them men. Objects, too, were given a gender according to their heat or fire factor. In this system, the fiery hot and dry sun was seen as masculine, while the moon, on account of its cold and moist properties, was viewed as feminine. Heat or fire was just one of the four elements that ancient scientists saw as making up the natural world. The others were air, which was understood as moist and hot; earth – cold and dry; and water – cold and moist. However, these four elements were not seen as equal. Fire was rated ahead of the other three as it was both hot and dry – things hot and dry were superior to those that were cold and moist. Hence, fire or heat came first, and water last – a completely arbitrary ranking, it must be stressed.

In *On the Usefulness of the Parts*, Galen enunciates how this female/male heat differential affects the sexes' genitalia, commenting: 'The woman is less perfect than the man in respect to the generative parts. For the parts were formed within her when she was still a foetus, but could not because of the defect in heat emerge and project on the outside.' Women, Galen is saying, do not possess the necessary heat to unfurl their phalluses. Instead, because of their cooler, moister nature, they are left with an interior, un-pushed-out penis. As the men of antiquity saw it, in essence, vagina and penis were alike. It was their position in space that separated them, not their underlying structure. As Galen put it: 'Turn outward the woman's, turn inward, so to speak, and fold double the man's [genitalia], and you will find the same in both in every respect.' This vagina/penis analogy explains why many genitalic terms, such as 'spermatic vessel', and the Latin *veretrum*, could be applied equally to the vagina or the penis.

Using a man's genitals as the yardstick with which to grade a woman's genitalia was not the only outcome of the heat differential theory. This entirely arbitrary hierarchy of elements also gave the authorities of the day (who were male) a system within which they could rate man above woman. Man became the measure of woman and all other things. Women were defined inferior because of this lesser 'heat' in relation to men. The whimsy of placing fire above water in an elemental scale meant that Aristotle could rationally say: 'For the female is, as it were, a mutilated male.' This subjective superiority scale has also led to, and underscored, a multitude of other misogynies.

Many male minds have used Aristotle's heat theory of sexual difference to put forward their own deranged and deeply distorted views of women. Galen explains his view of how heat grades human and animal life in the following way: 'Now just as mankind is the most perfect of all animals, so within mankind, the man is more perfect than the woman, and the reason for his perfection is his excess heat, for heat is Nature's primary instrument.' In the medieval text, *Women's Secrets*, the author states of female offspring: 'If a female results, this is because of certain factors hindering the disposition of the matter, and thus it has been said that woman is not human, but a monster in nature.' From a mutilated man to a monster, and all because of an arbitrary scaling system.

When girls become boys

The theory that it was a matter of heat that was at the root of the difference between men and women had consequences other than imagining the vagina was an interior and inferior penis, and that women were less evolved than men. One notion that followed on from the theory of fire was that it was possible for women to turn into men. Medical documentation from the first century through to the seventeenth contains many examples of cases where such a sex transformation was seen to occur. One of these is the story of Marie Garnier, a servant in the employ of France's King Charles IX. According to the king's chief surgeon, Ambroise Paré, at the age of fifteen Marie showed 'no mark of masculinity'. However, while in the 'heat' of puberty, Marie was chasing pigs through a wheatfield, and, while jumping a ditch, sprouted an external penis; or as Paré put it: 'at that very moment the genitalia and the male rod came to be developed in him, having ruptured the ligaments by which they had been held enclosed'. Marie returned home to his/her mother, who took her child to a bishop, who proclaimed Marie to be a man. And so Marie became Germain, or Marie-Germain.

Marie-Germain's crime, and the reason why she changed sex, was, authorities explained, to indulge in inappropriate behaviour, moving in such a swift and violent (read unladylike) way that she shook out her internal genitalia. According to the heat theory, this occurred because 'the heat, having been rendered more vigorous, thrusts the testes outward'. Another account of Marie's sex transformation added ominously that in that part of France there was now 'a song commonly in the girls' mouths, in which they warn one another not to stretch their legs too wide for fear of becoming males, like Marie-Germain'. Fortuitously for men, however, they did not have to watch their stride in the same way, as such sex transformations were perceived to be one-way only. As the anatomist Gaspard Bauhin (1560–1624), explained it, 'we therefore never find in any true story that any man ever became a woman, because Nature tends always toward what is most perfect and not, on the contrary, to perform in such a way that what is perfect should become imperfect'. Woman was put firmly in her place yet again – beneath man, and with her legs placed carefully together.

Science would today suggest that the cases of girls who became boys at puberty were in fact feeling the effects of a genetic hormonal imbalance. This imbalance is known as 5–alpha-reductase syndrome, and results from a failure to produce the enzyme 5–alpha-reductase (which converts testosterone into 5–alpha-dihydrotestosterone). Although defined as genetically male – i.e. they have an X and a Y sex chromosome – such children are born with external genitalia that resemble female genitalia. This 'female' appearance occurs because their testes remain undescended, inside their body, leaving their scrotal sac looking like outer labia, and their penises are typically so short and stubby that they seem to be akin to a large clitoris. The only clue that this is not a typical clitoris is that they urinate through it.

These children 'become' boys at puberty, when steep hormonal changes cause the male genitalia to continue developing – their 'labia' swell and sag, testes descend, and the phallus lengthens. After puberty, their genitalia do not appear too different from other males, and many individuals go on to father children. In fact, in some areas of the Dominican Republic, this condition is so common that there is even a colloquial name for the affected children – *guavedoces*, 'eggs at twelve'. Interestingly, the idea of a third sex is accepted here without social stigma. One reason for this is probably the prevalence of *guavedoces*. Doctors in the region are also adept at recognising which girls will become boys, so the affected children do not have to suffer the shock of swapping sex unexpectedly.

Women have testicles too

Another consequence of the ancient habit of viewing the vagina as the penis was that other genital congruences could be called into play in the anatomy game. In this strange one-sex scenario, where the vagina was seen as an interior penis, it was also argued that the uterus was a scrotum, a woman's inner labia were equivalent to a man's foreskin, and the ovaries were testicles. As Galen commented: 'All the male genital parts are also found in women . . . you could not find a single male part left over that had not simply changed its position.' To illustrate his point of view, Galen gives a step-by-step account of how the two sexes' genitalia measure up:

> Think first, please, of the man's [external genitalia] turned in and extending inward between the rectum and the bladder. If this should happen, the scrotum would necessarily take the place of the uterus with the testes lying outside, next to it on either side; the penis of the male becomes the passageway that the hollow creates, and the part situated at the tip, now called 'prepuce', becomes the external genital parts of the woman.

He then continues with a mental manipulation of a woman's genitalia.

> Think too, please, of . . . the uterus turned outward and projecting. Would not the testes [ovaries] then necessarily be inside it? Would it not contain them like a scrotum? Would not the neck [the cervix and vagina], hitherto concealed inside the perineum but now pendant, be made into the male member?

This anatomy of female/male genital correspondences, using man as the measure of woman, was, in fact, the prevailing one in scientific lore for at least two thousand years – from the third century BCE through to the seventeenth and eighteenth centuries CE. (Some argue that it is still the case today.) It's important to realise, though, that Galen's confidence about the structure of female genitalia was not based on actual dissection experience. He had examined dead male gladiators, yes, but his experience of dissecting the female of the species was confined to pigs, goats and monkeys. Instead of direct evidence, Galen based his theories on the work of the anatomist Herophilus, who lived and worked in Alexandria in the third century BCE. Herophilus had viewed a woman's internal sexual anatomy; indeed, it was he who discovered a woman's ovaries. However, steeped as he was in Aristotelian ideas of man as the measure of all things, with women simply a lesser version of this perfect male human blueprint, Herophilus chose to see the ovaries as a version of a man's testicles. Galen, with no physical evidence to the contrary, in fact, no physical evidence at all, appears to have simply gone along with Herophilus' hypotheses, fitting as they did with his own world view – that women were an imperfect version of men because of their lesser 'heat'.

While Galen's persistence in seeing woman as an inverted man is perhaps understandable in light of the lack of physical evidence to the contrary, the confidence with which Renaissance anatomists continued to repeat this dogma is disturbing. From the fourteenth century onwards, female bodies were made available for dissection. Pioneering sixteenth-century anatomist Vesalius is known to have based his drawings of female genitalia in *De Humani Corporis Fabrica* on at least nine female bodies. 'The books contain pictures of all parts inserted into the context of the narrative, so that the dissected body is placed, so to speak, before the eyes of those studying the works of nature' is his boast of his illustrated anatomical texts. Yet what the reader actually saw was the product of Vesalius' prior ideologies, not the product of accurate observation, as we've seen.

For Vesalius and his peers, seeing was most definitely not believing. These anatomists may have been Renaissance men in that they lived through this period of time; however, the majority of them were still in large part simply sheep, following old doctrine blindly, and held in sway by the scientific and religious conventions of the day. The science of anatomy suffered for this. No image, verbal or visual, existed independently of an 'authority' decreeing why it should be so. For Aristotelians it was the lack of 'heat' that made women inferior to men; later, the Christian church promoted the view that sexual differentiation was a result of Eve's actions in the Garden of Eden, i.e., women had fallen from grace and it showed in their stunted genital shape. Renaissance anatomists promulgated and gave credence to both these absurdities. And so women continued to be viewed as just a lesser version of men.

Is it a bursa or a scrotal bag, ovaries or testes?

The idea of women as inverted men had a staggering – and extremely confusing – effect on the western world's sexual lexicon. Not only were female genitalia seen as a stunted version of the male's, they were referred to by the same names too. The name Herophilus bestowed on a woman's ovaries was *didymi* – the Greek word for 'twins' – because they always came in pairs. *Didymi* was also the standard term at the time for what we call today a man's testicles. Echoes of these twins remain in modern male anatomical terminology. The epididymis – the twisted sperm-carrying tube that runs along the posterior edge of each testicle – derives from *epi*, near or close to, and *didymi*, the twins.

Remnants of another bisexual Greek testicular term, *orcheis*, which Hippocrates and later Galen used, are also found in modern medical terminology. Inflammation of the testicles is known as orchitis, while orchidectomy is the surgical removal of the testes. Orchids, members of the plant species *Orchis*, are reputed to have received their name because they excite the 'Venereal appetite', and assist in conception because of 'their similitude of the Testicles' and because 'they also have the odour of the Seed'. Orchids were also believed to increase the production of semen.

In Roman times, *didymi* slipped from currency as the term for the ovaries. One replacement was *testis* (the Latin for 'witness'), or its diminutive *testiculus*. The modern term, testicle, derives from this diminutive, with testis (plural testes) remaining the same. *Testis* was the word bestowed on a woman's pair of ovaries and a man's twin testicles because in Roman times, for testimony to take place, it was ruled that there must be at least two people. This idea that there must be at least two people (witnesses) in order to bear testimony legally is still found today in modern legal settings, such as marriage ceremonies or will-making. 'Stones' was another term straddling both sexes. Even today, ovaries and testicles share a medical term – gonads, which derives from the Greek word for seed, *gonos*.

The conception of women as imperfect men, albeit with all the requisite parts, also had knock-on effects on theories of genital function. While both Galen and Herophilus regarded a woman's ovaries as analogous to men's testicles, Galen went a step further with his comparisons. Not content with a structural analogy, he postulated that men's and women's testicles shared the same function, namely to produce semen. However, women's semen was, of course, not as thick and hot as a man's because of her inherent cooler nature. 'Forthwith of course the female must have smaller, less perfect testes, and the semen generated in them must be scantier, colder and wetter (for these things too follow of necessity from the deficient heat),' Galen explains.

The uterus also bore the brunt of the male-centric way of looking at female sexual anatomy. Despite its thick, muscular structure in contrast to the thin skin of the scrotal sac, and despite its unique role in gestating a child, it was consistently perceived of as a simple scrotum (a word which is thought to have its roots in the Greek term for a leather bag). As one sixteenth-century Frenchman put it: '*La matrice de la femme n'est que la bourse et verge reversée de l'homme*' – 'The matrix [uterus] of the woman is nothing but the scrotum and penis of the man inverted.' And as with the vagina/penis theory, this uterus/scrotum analogy was promulgated pictorially as well as lexically.

During the Middle Ages, the word bursa, which implies a bag, purse or sack, was used to describe the womb as well as the scrotum. One of the most popular medieval sex manuals, *De Secretis Mulierum*, explains how, after a man ejaculates, the woman's uterus 'shuts like a bursa [purse]'. In Renaissance England, 'purse' was commonplace as a term for both uterus and scrotum. 'The uterus is a tightly sealed vessel, similar to a coin purse,' states an anonymous German text. However, in the French word, *bourse*, which implies a place where moneymakers gather as well as a purse or bag, there is some sense of the uterus being a place where something of value is produced. This sense is also present in *matrice*, or the English version matrix, a word for uterus which derives from *mater*, meaning mother. A matrix is a place where something has its origin, where something of value is produced. Matrix (and fundament), unlike other uterine and scrotal epithets, applied only to the female.

A vaginal renaissance?

The seventeenth century was a good one for female genitalia. Not only was it the period in which the word vagina came into its own as a specific anatomical term, this was also the century that first heard opposition to the 'woman is an inverted man' theory of genitalia. Some brave scientists dared to state what they saw, rather than repeat the accepted and ancient viewpoints. One non-conformist was the English anatomist Helkiah Crooke, who argued in 1615 against 'any similitude betweene the bottome of the womb inverted, and the scrotum or cod of a man'. According to Crooke, the skin of the 'bottom of the wombe is a very thicke and tight membrane, all fleshy within', while 'the cod is a rugous and thin skin', hence the two should not be seen as analogous. The seventeenth-century Danish anatomist Kaspar

Bartholin was another dissenter, arguing astutely: 'We must not think with Galen . . . and others, that these female genital parts differ from those of men only in situation.' To do that, Bartholin suggested, would be to fall in line with an ideological plot 'hatched by those who accounted a woman to be only an imperfect man'. Meanwhile, the Dutch anatomist Reinier de Graaf wrote: 'The notion of some people that the vagina corresponds with the penis of males, differing only in being inside rather than out, we say is ridiculous. The vagina bears no similarity at all to the penis.'

De Graaf also observed that women's 'testicles' did not look like men's testicles, and, more importantly, he said so. 'The testicles of the female differ greatly from those of the male . . . in their position, shape, size, substance, integuments and function. Their position is not outside the abdomen, as in men, but right inside the abdominal cavity, each one about two finger-breadths from the fundus of the uterus.' Partly backed up by research from his peer, Jan Swammerdam, de Graaf went on to refute the conventional function of a female's 'testicles', as well as their structure. This was not semen production, he suggested, but egg (or ova) formation. 'The common function of the female testicles is to generate the eggs, foster them and bring them to maturity. Thus, in women, they perform the same task as do the ovaries of birds. Hence they should be called women's ovaries rather than testicles, especially as they bear no similarity either in shape or content to the male testicles properly so-called.'

So a woman's gonads had a name of their own for the first time in their history, as well as a unique function ascribed to them – one that it was recognised men did not possess. By the eighteenth century, de Graaf's new ovarian terminology had taken hold, and women's testicles were no more. The word vagina had appeared, and along with the word came the conception of this muscular organ as a separate entity, and one that was not just an imperfect interpretation of the penis. Added to this was the fact that the uterus stopped being referred to using scrotal language. Although it may have looked and sounded as if a vaginal Renaissance was finally taking place, the tradition of seeing woman as a stunted version of man had not been lost completely. One genital congruence did not fall by the wayside, and as the habit of viewing the vagina as an interior penis lost resonance, another raised its head – namely, the clitoris was a penis. An undersized, unevolved penis. This, sadly, is still a theory that is given credit today.

Quite how this clitoral/penile idea came about is unclear. Some researchers point to language, to errors in the translations of anatomical texts, others to the erectile capacity of both organs, how sexual arousal stiffens them both. The most famous British sex advice manual, *Aristotle's Masterpiece* (published in different forms from the seventeenth century through to the nineteenth), wrote of how the 'use and action of the clitoris in women is like that of the penis or yard in men, that is, erection'. In Latin, *virga*, meaning rod, could be the clitoris or the penis. For some anatomists, the clitoris was simply the *membrum muliebrum*, the female member. It's also hard to break habits, so for some it must have been simpler to see the clitoris as a penile equivalent than a genital entity in its own right. Perhaps laziness played a part, allowing man to continue to be the measure of woman.

When women had two penises

The habit of using a man's penis to grade a woman's genitalia led to some strange genital scenarios. Some manuscripts seemed to declare that women had two penises – a vaginal penis and a clitoral one too. Thomas Bartholin's 1668 *Anatomy* was one of these – despite his defence of women's genitalia differing from men's. For Bartholin, the vagina 'becomes longer or shorter, broader or narrower, and swells sundry ways according to the lust of the woman'. It 'is of a hard and nervous flesh, and somewhat spongy, like the Yard'. However, the clitoris is also for Bartholin akin to 'the female yard or prick', as it 'resembles a man's yard in situation, substance, composition, repletion with spirits and erection', and it also 'hath somewhat like the nut and foreskin of a Man's Yard' (see Figure 2.5). Elsewhere, the seventeenth-century English midwifery manual, *The Midwives Book*, by Jane Sharp, talks on one page of how the vagina, 'which is the passage for the yard, resembleth it turn inward'. Yet in another paragraph, it states that it is the clitoris that resembles a penis, as 'it will stand and fall as the yard doth and makes women lustful and take delight in copulation'. The truth about the clitoris, as we'll see later, is something else altogether.

But first, why the word clitoris? It's such a particular term, so precise, and yet today it appears to convey very little of the nature of the subject. What does the word mean? Various sources are cited.

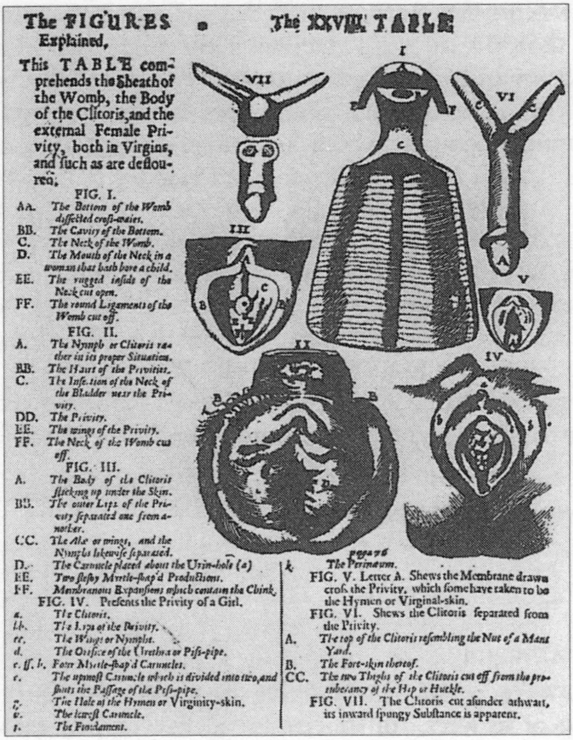

The FIGURES Explained,

The XXVIII TABLE

This TABLE comprehends the Sheath of the Womb, the Body of the Clitoris, and the external Female Privity, both in Virgins, and such as are deflour'd.

FIG. I.
AA. The Bottom of the Womb dissected cross-waies.
BB. The Cavity of the Bottom.
C. The Neck of the Womb.
D. The Mouth of the Neck in a woman that hath bore a child.
EE. The rugged inside of the Neck cut open.
FF. The round Ligaments of the Womb cut off.

FIG. II.
A. The Nymph or Clitoris rather in its proper Situation.
BB. The Hairs of the Privities.
C. The Insertion of the Neck of the Bladder near the Privity.
DD. The Privity.
EE. The wings of the Privity.
FF. The Neck of the Womb cut off.

FIG. III.
A. The Body of the Clitoris sticking up under the Skin.
BB. The outer Lips of the Privity separated one from another.
CC. The Alæ or wings, and the Nymphs likewise separated.
D. The Caruncle placed about the Urin-hole (a)
EE. Two fleshy Myrtle-shap'd Productions.
FF. Membranous Expansions which contain the Chink.

FIG. IV. Presents the Privity of a Girl.
a. The Clitoris.
bb. The Lips of the Privity.
cc. The Wings or Nymphs.
d. The Orifice of the Urethra or Piss-pipe.
e. ff. h. Four Myrtle-shap'd Caruncles.
e. The upmost Caruncle which is divided into two, and shuts the Passage of the Piss-pipe.
g. The Hole of the Hymen or Virginity-skin.
h. The least Caruncle.
i. The Fundament.
k. The Perinæum.

FIG. V. Letter A. Shews the Membrane drawn cross the Privity, which some have taken to be the Hymen or Virginal-skin.

FIG. VI. Shews the Clitoris separated from the Privity.
A. The top of the Clitoris resembling the Nut of a Mans Yard.
B. The Fore-skin thereof.
CC. The two Thighs of the Clitoris cut off from the protuberancy of the Hip or Huckle.

FIG. VII. The Clitoris cut asunder athwart, its inward spungy Substance is apparent.

Figure 2.5 The clitoris as penis (from Bartholin's 1668 *Anatomy*).

Many etymologists claim that it is connected to *kleitys*, the Greek word for hill or slope, recalling the *mons Veneris*, the mount or mountain of Venus that it is said lovers of women must scale. Some wordsmiths point to clitoris being related to the Greek *kleitos*, meaning 'renowned, splendid or excellent'. Others suggest the Greek verb, *kleiein*, 'to close', or the Greek word for key, *kleis*, making the clitoris the key, catch or hook with which one can open a door to pleasure (and bestowing an additional meaning on the phrase 'the key to the door'). Another possible association is the Dutch *keest*, meaning 'kernel or core'.

What is certain is that the word first appeared as an anatomical term in the writings of Rufus of Ephesus in the first century CE. Rufus also explained how clitoris, the word for the sexual organ, gave rise to the verb clitorising, meaning 'to make voluptuous strokings of the clitoris'. The German verb *kitzlen*, to tickle, and a colloquial term for clitoris, *der Kitzler*, 'tickler', are suggested to stem from this etymology. In this sense, clitoris stands out in the western world's lexicon of female genitalia. Unlike many other vaginal terms, it, and many of its nicknames, has associations with female sexual pleasure. For example, past clitoral descriptors include the *amoris dulcedo*, 'the sweetness of love'; the *sedes libidinis*, 'the seat of love'; the *oestrus Veneris*, 'the gadfly of Venus'; the *Wollustorgan*, 'the ecstasy organ'; and the *gaude mihi*, 'great joy'. Then there's the fury and rage of love; the ear-between-the-legs; and the myrtle-berry, so named because the myrtle was sacred to Aphrodite and Venus, the goddesses of love in Greek and Roman mythology respectively. In modern times, it is French clitoral terminology that conveys the sweetness and pleasure of the part with sobriquets such as *bonbon*, *praline* (sugared almond), *framboise* (raspberry), *grain de café* (coffee bean) and *berlingot* (humbug). My favourite French clitoral confection is *la praline en délire*, a phrase which translates as 'a delirious sugared almond', and implies a deeply aroused clitoris, one that is about to burst into orgasm.

Terms of endearment

While the history of vaginal language in the west is – in the main – characterised by a lack of words, both in terms of number and specificity, the same cannot be said of eastern cultures. As the ancient sex manuals of China, India and Japan show, when a culture's imagination soars, unfettered by repressive notions of sexuality, a wealth of vaginal language emerges. For instance, words describing female genitalia are commonly appellations of beauty and pleasure, reflecting a sense of delight in the visual, physical and olfactory aspects of the *yoni* or vagina. Chinese and Taoist vaginal terms include the 'doorway of life'; 'lotus of her wisdom'; 'love grotto'; 'open peony blossom'; 'treasure house'; 'inner heart'; and 'heavenly gate'. *Yoni*, the eastern word for vagina, itself encompasses the meanings of womb, origin and source (as previously discussed). Moreover, the Sanskrit term *bhaga*, which means womb or *yoni*, also means wealth, luck and happiness. Significantly, its root, *bhag*, forms the core of words for both female genitalia and bliss and power. These include clitoris (*bhagshishnaka*);

mons pubis (*bhagpith*); ecstasy (*bhagananda*); Divine One (*bhagwan*); mother or divine consciousness (*bhagavat-cetana*); divine power (*bhagavatisakti*) and devotee (*bhagat*). *Bhaga* is also said to signify that aspect of humans that is the 'divine enjoyer' of things both erotic and non-erotic, the *bhagavat.*

In the west, if one didn't know better, a look at centuries of paintings of naked woman would suggest that female pubic hair did not exist. For some reasons, pubic hair was problematic in the west – probably because it implied an animal sexual nature, which wouldn't fit with preconceived and moralistic notions of female sexuality. In stark contrast, in China, abundant luxurious pubic hair is a sign of passion and sensuality in a woman, and pubic hair that forms an equilateral triangle with an upward-directed growth is read as a sign of beauty. *Yinmao* is the common name for female pubic hair; if a woman has no pubic hair she is known as a 'white tiger'. Perhaps expressing the positive feelings about pubic hair, Chinese terms for it are particularly poetic. Phrases such as 'fragrant grass', 'black rose', 'sacred hair' and 'moss' elicit a sense of somewhere soft, sprung and scented, and reflect the fact that the area that is covered by pubic hair contains scent glands. The glands that are scattered throughout a woman's vulval skin, and are suggested to play a role in perfuming the pubis, are in Chinese called by the terms 'sun terrace', 'mixed rock' and 'infant girl'. In India the Sanskrit term *purnacandra*, meaning full moon, is the phrase for the vaginal glands, which are said to be filled with the 'juice of love'. Other Chinese terms for the vagina that carry aromatic overtones include 'pillow of musk', 'pure lily' and 'anemone of love'. However, how the vaginal phrase 'purple mushroom peak' came about is unclear.

'Hill of sedge' – a Chinese term for the mount of Venus, the cushion of fatty tissue that covers a woman's pubic bones – shares some similarity with the west, in that it too recalls the *mons*' appearance as a hill or mountain. However, 'hill of sedge' has other resonances. Sedge is any grasslike plant which typically grows on moist or wet ground. Moreover, another feature of sedge is that it has triangular stems, making the phrase hill of sedge particularly appropriate for a woman's pubic triangle. Botanical phrases also flourish in terminology for the small hood-like fold of skin just above the clitoris. In Chinese, this clitoral hood, which moves freely under a finger, and can cover the clitoral tip either partially or completely, is called the 'dark garden', 'god field' and 'grain seed'. There is no particular word to describe it in English. The highly sensitive area just below the tip of the clitoris, where the labia minora appear to meet, is known in China as the 'lute or lyre strings' (in English it is the frenulum, a word which originally meant 'the corner of the mouth where the lips join'). The lower meeting point of the inner labia is referred to as *yü-li* – the 'jade veins'. The labia minora themselves are known as 'red pearls' (*ch'ih-chu*) or 'wheat buds'.

Just as in the west, many oriental genital terms owe their name to ideas of sexual function. These ideas, though, are not necessarily the ones espoused elsewhere. In Chinese thought, for example, it is the ovaries that are considered to contain a woman's yin energy, and are understood to contribute most of their energy during sexual arousal. They are the 'ovarian palace', the *Kuan-Yuan*. For men, the seat of male or yang energy is the testicles. However, the Chinese view another part of a female's sexual anatomy as being a seat of female, or yin, sexual energy. This other site is the perineum, or the *Hui-Yin*, the collection point of all yin energy. It is also known as the 'gate of death and life' (recalling the ancient ideas of female genitalia as the sacred gateway between worlds). Yet the perineum is an area which for the western world is not usually regarded as an important part of female genitalia, although it is exquisitely sensitive and is all too often cut unnecessarily during childbirth. In India too, the perineum is viewed as a centre of female sexual energy, and its Sanskrit name is *yonisthana*, the *yoni* place.

Gold, cinnabar and jade

As we've seen, names say a lot. So how about the following Taoist term for the uterus – the 'precious crucible'. What kind of message does that convey? The place where a unique, magical, life-giving transformation takes place, perhaps? This uterine phrase is, to my mind, light years away from the west's desire to see the womb as nothing more than an inverted scrotum and penis. Along with other eastern genital terminology, it reveals very clearly the different attitude to sex and female genitalia. As has already been noted, Taoism sees sex as sacred, whereas Christianity viewed it as sinful and still perhaps does. Significantly, other Chinese and Taoist words for the womb also convey the sense of a special or valuable site. These uterine terms include the 'children's palace' (*tzu-tung*), the 'palace of yin', 'the red chamber' (*chu-shih*), 'the jewel enclosure,' 'the heart of the peony', the 'inner heart' and the 'cinnabar cave'. 'Flower heart' and 'innermost knot' are two Chinese names for the cervix or, more specifically, the cervical orifice.

Some common ideas emerge in the orient's general lexicon. One of these is the prominent role given to jewels and precious metals, minerals and stones as descriptors of female genitalia. For example, in Japan, the vagina is the 'gate of jewels', and according to Japanese folk belief there were three precious stones inside the vagina which moved during sex. It's also said that up until the nineteenth century, Japanese women carried a pearl inside their vaginas, and folklore warned that if it was taken out it would cause their death. Turning to minerals, cinnabar is the commonest denominator by far. We've already seen the 'cinnabar cave' as a term for the uterus; the vagina is also referred to as the 'cinnabar cleft', the 'cinnabar hole', the 'cinnabar gate' and the 'cinnabar crevice'. For the Chinese, cinnabar was significant as a descriptor of female genitalia for two main reasons. First, its colour – a lustrous red or reddish-brownish hue, which recalled that of female genitalia and blood. Most important, though, was cinnabar's alchemical role. For in Taoist alchemy, cinnabar was one of the key symbols of transformation, which makes it a perfect word for describing female genitalia, which transform base matter into new life.

In terms of precious metals and stones, the Chinese favoured gold and jade as genital terms. Gold, of course, has been seen as an object of beauty, something to treasure, in the majority of world cultures. To use gold in conjunction with the vagina is therefore to acknowledge the precious nature of female sexual anatomy. Consider the following ways of describing the vagina: 'golden gully', 'golden doorway', 'golden gate', 'golden lotus' and 'golden furrow'. However, there is another reason for the frequent use of gold, and as we'll see, it ties in with the third typical genital descriptor – jade. This semi-precious green stone, a silicate of calcium and magnesium, is also found in many vaginal terms, including 'jade door', 'jade gate', 'jade cavern', 'jade gateway', 'jade veins', 'jade pavilion', 'pearl on the jade step' (clitoris) and 'jade chamber'. The 'jade chamber' is an ancient phrase for the vagina, and appears in the title of two of China's oldest extant sex manuals, *Important Matters of the Jade Chamber*, from the Pre-Sui Dynasty (*c.* fourth century, but before 581 CE), and *Secret Instructions Concerning the Jade Chamber*, which also dates from the Pre-Sui Dynasty. Moreover, as well as having jade genitalia, women are said to produce 'jade juice' too, a fluid which promotes longevity in the man who can gather it with his 'jade stalk' (once again men have stalks for penises).

It is longevity that is the key to understanding the use of gold and jade as genital terms. For according to ancient Chinese thought, both gold and jade protected the body from decay – even after death. That is, they promoted longevity. Significantly, this idea ties in with ancient Taoist thought, which teaches that the vagina is the source of the elixir of life, and hence sex is a way of cheating death. This belief in the power of jade can be seen in many aspects of Chinese culture. The *I Ching*, the Taoist *Book of Changes*, states that 'Heaven is Jade.' And as the Chinese viewed jade as the key to everlasting life, the stone was ground into a powder and drunk or eaten as a literal elixir of life. Concubines also used jade as part of the tricks of their trade, because ground jade potions were said to have the power to improve sexual potency.

The associations between jade and genitalia go further than you might imagine. It's intriguing to see that the roots of the word jade are associated with sexual anatomy; that is, sexual anatomy as defined by Chinese medicine, which views the kidneys as sexual organs. One of the two varieties of jade, nephrite, is known as the kidney stone, because of the long-held belief that it was beneficial in treating kidney and sexual disorders. In fact, the word jade was coined by a sixteenth-century Spanish doctor and derives from the phrase *piedras hijades*, 'the colic stone' or literally, 'the stone of the flank' (the hips), because it was believed to cure renal colic and all known kidney ailments. In Chinese medicine the kidneys (including the adrenals) are considered part of a person's sexual geography, because they are understood as one of the principal storage sites of sexual energy (or *jing*), and hence have a key role to play in sexual arousal.

This linking of jade with the kidneys and sexual energy may also help to explain why 'to be jaded' means to be exhausted. It also recalls ancient western medical thought, which connected a person's kidneys with their sexual energy and semen. (Intriguingly, western medicine now recognises that there are a number of connections between the kidneys and sexuality, both hormonal and structural. For example, in embryonic life, an individual's gonads, be they ovaries or testicles, grow in intimate association with the kidneys, even incorporating unused renal pieces into them.)

Finally, and touchingly, in this look at the east's vaginal lexicon, there are some similarities in the different approaches to christening parts of female sexual anatomy. In both hemispheres, east and west, names for the clitoris focus on sexual pleasure and the importance of this sexual organ. Chinese clitoral phrases include 'seat of pleasure', 'pleasure place', 'golden tongue', 'golden terrace', 'jewel terrace' and 'jade terrace', while the Chinese ideogram for clitoris combines the words *yin* and *tee*, as the stem (*tee*) of an aubergine is said to resemble the clitoris. In Japan, the clitoris is *hoju*, a term that in Buddhism also signifies the 'magic jewel of the dharma [the essential principle of the cosmos]'. In western sexual anatomy, a woman's vestibule is the oval-shaped entrance to her vagina and urethra which is visible when her inner vaginal lips are parted, while in architecture, a vestibule is a small hall or lobby at the entrance to a building or passageway. The Chinese language plays with similar associations, with phrases for this vaginal entrance including 'heavenly court' (*t'ien-t'ing*), 'secluded valley' (*yu-ku*) and 'examination hall'.

First impressions

A view of the vagina by taking a tour of its lexical history would not be complete without considering 'cunt'. Although a remarkably direct expression, cunt has multiple meanings, depending on the country you find yourself in. In Spain, if you wish to express your delight in a delicious experience, a suitable comment might be that it is *como comerle el coño a bocaos* ('like eating cunt by the mouthful'). If you're in Britain, though, this phrase would not go down so well. Cunt, one of the oldest words for female genitalia, is also the most taboo. Yet in Spain it's not. In fact, *coño* is so common a word in Spain (albeit an expletive) that just as the English have been dubbed *les fuckoffs* by the French, in Chile and Mexico, Spaniards are known as *los coños*. The Spanish seem to have had fun playing with their *coño* phrases. *Otra pena pa mi coño* – 'another pain in my cunt' – is said when one is faced with something extra to contend with. If you're fed up with something or someone, you can be *estoy hasta el coño*, 'up to your cunt with it'. And if you want to get across the fact that a place is completely out of the way, i.e. it is the back of beyond, you can use the common Spanish expression *en el quinto coño* – 'the fifth cunt'. It remains a mystery as to why a particularly remote area should be described as 'the fifth cunt'.

The dichotomy of the significance of cunt is visible elsewhere across Europe. In Italy, *figa* (cunt) is not an insult or an ugly word. Rather, it is a common expletive (after *cazzo*, 'prick', it is probably the most used). *Figa* is the spoken form, *fica* the more common written term. *Che figa!* is actually a light-hearted expression. It can be applied to people – 'Che figa', 'What a looker!'; to objects – *Che festa figa!* – 'What a great party!'; and to situations – for example, 'Che figa' can mean 'What good luck!' And although at times men can use it in a sexist way, akin to English men saying 'chick' or 'pussy', Italian women have reclaimed the word, making it applicable to men as the masculine noun, *figo*. So if you fancy an Italian man go ahead and say, admiringly, '*Che figo!*' If something is excellent it is *figata*. However, in Germany, like Britain, cunt, or *Fotze*, reigns supreme as an extreme taboo word. Yet *Fotze* is also an old word for mouth, and in expressions such as *Halt dei' Fotze!* 'Shut your trap!' and *hinterfotzig* 'two-faced', it loses some of its impact.

Like Italian and Spanish, the French equivalent of cunt, *le con*, is not taboo. Rather, it is used as an affectionate insult, as in *vieux con* ('old fool') or *fais pas le con* ('Don't play the fool'). *Con* to the French isn't necessarily any stronger than calling someone a fool or an idiot. *Le roi des cons* ('king of cunts') implies a total idiot, while '*Quelle connerie!*' means 'What rubbish!' In Danish the word for cunt, *kusse*, has acquired no additional emotional baggage. The word conveys merely what it describes – female genitalia. In Finland, while *vittu* is still considered as a strong expletive, it's flexible and various in the ways it is applied. You can tell someone to go get lost in Finnish by saying *Vedä vittu päähäs!* ('Go pull a cunt over your head!), It can be used as an adjective, as 'bloody' is in English, in the form *vittumainen* ('cunt-like'). And there is a past participle, *vituttaa*, meaning 'to be annoyed'.

In England, cunt has been considered taboo in print and speech since the fifteenth century. Prior to this, though, it was an accepted enough part of English vernacular that it featured in the names for public thoroughfares. In about 1230, Gropecuntelane was a London street; other cities too, including Oxford, York and Northampton, possessed Gropecuntelanes in the thirteenth and fourteenth centuries. In Paris, there was rue Grattecon (Scratchcunt Street). Today, all that remains of the too-lewd lane names are truncated versions – Grove Street (Oxford) or Grape Lane (York).

Yet from 1700 to 1959, cunt was considered so obscene that it was a legal offence to publish the word in its entirety. This meant that lexicographers had a problem. The first edition of Francis Grose's *Dictionary of the Vulgar Tongue* (1785) bleeped it out with four stars, ****, three years later, the second edition, incredibly and offensively, defined cunt, or c**t, as 'a nasty name for a nasty thing'. Amazingly, the *Oxford English Dictionary* did not permit cunt's entry into its hallowed pages until 1976. The entry then read: '1. The female genitals, the vulva. 2. A very unpleasant or stupid person.' In the twenty-first century, cunt is still not a word that 'authorities', be they media-based or political, allow an individual to say freely. It remains the most taboo and insulting word in the English language.

When considering the etymology of cunt, it's hard to ignore the tone of the word. Whether it begins with a hard c, k or q, the sound of cunt is particularly distinctive. A quick trip around old and modern Europe gives a veritable concerto in C, as well as an impressive history. As well as the cunts listed above, there are: *cunte* or *counte* (Middle English); *kut* (the Netherlands); *kunta* (Old Norse); *queynthe* (Middle English); *qwim* (sixteenth-century England); *cunnus* (Latin); *cona* (Portuguese); *cont* (Wales); *cunnicle* or *cunnikin* (nineteenth-century England); *kunte* (Middle Low German); *cut* (eighteenth-century England) and *chuint* (Ireland). Outside Europe, this refrain continues. There's the Sanskrit term *kunthi*; the Indian words for cunt, *cunti* or *kunda*; and also Arabic and Hebrew, where cunt is *kus*. In these latter two languages, the word for cunt is said to be related to those for cup and pockets, making it some kind of receptacle. This idea of a vessel or container ties in with the suggestion that cunt is linked to the Old English word for womb, *cwithe*.

Other etymologists cite the root *cwe* (*cu*) as the connection between the words cunt and *cwithe* and a host of other words, such as queen, kin, country and cunning (which derives from the Old English *cunnende*). This *cu* root, it is said, signifies 'quintessential physical femininity'. It's certainly the case that the basic term, *kuna*, meaning woman, is found in a startlingly large and geographically widespread number of languages, and language families. Some of the language families *kuna* is represented in are: the Afro-Asiatic (for example, in the Cushitic language Oromo, *qena* means lady); the Indo-European (in the English word queen); the Amerind (Guarani *kuña* means female); and the Indo-Pacific (the Tasmanian for wife/woman is *quani*).

Does cunt derive from a global word for woman – *kuna*? Some scholars suggest it does. They point to ancient Egyptian writings, such as the maxims of Ptah-Hotep, where the word for cunt is synonymous with that for woman. However, it should be made clear that for this culture, cunt was in no way an insult; rather it was a word of respect. The Egyptian for mother, *k-at*, literally 'the body of her', also means the female genitalia or vulva. An ancient Indian goddess provides another link between words for woman and words for cunt. *Kunthi* is both a Sanskrit term for the vagina, and the name of an ancient Indian mother goddess. Kunti, a goddess of nature, was said to be able to take innumerable men into herself without altering her essence, just like the earth. She features in the epic Sanskrit poem of India, the *Mahabharata*. The ancient Anatolian goddess Kubaba, the 'Creatrix of All', also shares the *cu* root.

Although the etymology of cunt is disputed, the most accepted and cited explanation again ties it to words for woman. This explanation is also the one that seventeenth-century Dutch anatomist Reinier de Graaf gives in his treatise on female genitalia. However, in order to understand how de Graaf viewed the word (*cunnus* in Latin), a question needs to be asked: what is cunt? In the twenty-first century, according to the dictionary, cunt refers to the female genitals (collectively), or a very unpleasant or obnoxious person. However, when de Graaf was writing, cunt had another meaning, that is, it was perceived in another way. And it is in de Graaf's view of cunt, I feel, that the true etymology of the word can be found. This meaning also explains why cunt wasn't always heard as a swear word, as it was merely a way of describing a specific part of female anatomy. For de Graaf, *cunnus* was the word used to describe 'the great cleft'. But what is 'the great cleft'?

This great cleft is simply the area of a woman's genitalia that is visible to an onlooker when she has parted neither her outer nor inner labia. Looking face on, what is visible is a pubic triangle, with a line running down the middle. *Cunnus* just describes what you can see when you first look at female genitalia. This is what de Graaf meant by the great cleft, and he explains this clearly in Chapter II 'Concerning the Female Pudendum', when he says: 'The great cleft is called . . . the cunnus, because it looks like the impress of a wedge (cuneus).' Cuneus, the term for the impress of a wedge, is, I feel, the true origin of the word cunt. Moreover, this etymology is underlined by ancient Sumerian pictorial writing, cuneiform (*c.* 3500 BCE). In cuneiform, the impressed word symbol for woman or female is the image of cunt – a downwards-facing triangle with a line cleft down its middle. It seems it's hard to separate cunt from woman. Woman with her cleft cunt and horned uterus. Devil-woman. Is it any wonder then that cunt went on to be considered such a wicked word?

Outside in or inside out?

The following lines are from an eighteenth-century edition of that most famous British sex advice manual, *Aristotle's Masterpiece.* The author of the poem, who remains unknown, wrote:

> Thus the Women's Secrets I have surveyed
> And let them see how curiously they're made:
> And that, tho they of different sexes be,
> Yet in the Whole they are the same as we:
> For those that have the strictest Searchers been,
> Find Women are but Men turned Outside in:
> And Men, if they but cast their Eyes about,
> May find they're Women with their Inside out.

Casting your eyes about is the key to understanding. It's all too easy to get stuck in one safe, socially acceptable point of view, be it man as the measure of woman, heat as the most important element, women with unevolved male genitalia inside them, or the uterus with horns. It's significant that the theory that ovaries are testicles, the uterus is a scrotum and the vagina is a penis took approaching two millennia to be overturned. Despite physical evidence to the contrary, anatomists continued to 'see' what the religious and scientific authorities of the day wanted them to see. They did not cast their eyes about, but kept them firmly on their preconceived, conventional notions. It was safer and simpler to do so. The Polish-German physician and philosopher Ludwig Fleck (1896–1961), who used images of female genital anatomy to illustrate the cultural conditioning of scientific knowledge, summed this attitude up when he said: 'In science, just as in art and in life, only what is true to culture is true of nature.' One result of this is that the history of female sexual anatomy and language is, to date, characterised by outdated, erroneous ideas and absent or misleading information, be it in terms of words or pictures.

It would be pleasing to think that in the twenty-first century, humankind is not so hung up on ancient dogma and doctrine. Unfortunately, this is not the case. Cunt continues to be an extremely offensive word for many people, but again this is just getting stuck in centuries-old emotions and ideologies. Sadly, science does not fare much better at the art of casting its eyes about. Most researchers remain focused on their one narrow discipline. Science is also, to a large extent, still fixed on seeing man as the measure of woman. This is underlined by the vast number of people who take it for granted that the clitoris is analogous to the penis. Yet casting one's eyes about reveals a very different picture, as we will discover.

3

A VELVET REVOLUTION

Sexing spotted hyaenas is not straightforward. The usual suspects – genitalia, size and social status – do not supply any easy answers. Highly aggressive predators, both sexes of spotted hyaena are recognisable by their dappled dirty saffron-yellow fur. Both female and male rely on fresh kills to survive. With their formidable teeth and bone-crushing jaws, they are the only carnivores that can ingest a carcass in its entirety. But in the fierce, competitive and bloody environment that is the world of the spotted, or laughing, hyaena, it is, intriguingly, the female of the species that is the leader of the pack. In comparison to males, females are considerably bigger, heavier and more brutal. Males defer to their dominance. Even the lowest-ranking female can displace the highest-ranking male and for the female spotted hyaena, role reversal doesn't end there, because these feisty females have phalluses too.

Courtesy of its genitalic aspects, the spotted hyaena is one of the most misunderstood and maligned species on earth. Ancient naturalists were so puzzled by the social set-up and apparent sexual ambiguity of these prairie-dwelling carnivores that they wove stories to explain their strange genital apparatus. The spotted hyaena, it was said, was a hermaphrodite – capable of sporting both female and male genitalia. Seen as neither wholly female or male, the hyaena was deemed an unclean beast – and held responsible for desecrating graves in its search for the flesh of buried bodies. Hyaena mythology also talks of the carnivore's magical properties – hyaenas can render other animals immobile by walking around them three times, while merely touching a hyaena's shadow can cause a hunting dog to lose its bark. Hyaenas, it was also said, had the ability to imitate the human voice, and used this mimicry to lure unsuspecting shepherds to their death. The spotted hyaena's laugh – its infamous mocking cackle – was seen as an expression of the creature's mischievous glee at shifting sex. This bizarre genitalic arrangement, which no one could explain satisfactorily, meant that beliefs in the biological bisexuality and monstrous magical nature of spotted hyaenas survived for centuries.

It's now known that spotted hyaenas are not hermaphrodites, yet what is between the female's hind legs is still a source of bemusement for biologists and zoologists alike. This is not surprising. The clitoris of the female spotted hyaena is a truly stunning attribute. Enormously elongated, it extends away from her body in a sleek and slender arc measuring, on average, over 17 cm from root to tip (see Figure 3.1). Just like a penis, this colossus of a clitoris is fully erectile, raising its head in hyaena greeting ceremonies, social displays, games of rough and tumble or when sniffing out peers. Just like the male, the female has small spines on the glans, or head, of her erectile organ, making the clitoris tip feel like soft sandpaper. And in the centre of the clitoris, traversing its entire length, is the urethra, so the female, like the male, urinates through her phallus.

What lies beneath the female spotted hyaena's penis-like projection is just as bewildering. Where other female mammals have a vulva – a vaginal opening framed by labia – the female spotted hyaena does not. Her labia are completely fused together, from perineum to clitoris. Padded with fat and connective tissue, these wrinkled labial pouches look for all the world like the male's scrotal sac. Greater size, social status and conventionally male genitalia too – it's hardly surprising that the female spotted hyaena is the source of so much historical sexual confusion.

Up close, very close, subtle differences between the two sexes' members emerge. Females typically have a thicker, but slightly shorter organ. In general, female genitalia have more flappiness, folds and excess skin – a flaccid clitoris is less clearly defined than a flaccid penis. When erect, variations in the contour of the glans, the head of the clitoris or penis, are also visible. The *glans clitoridis* is flatter and rounder, the glans penis is more angular, or pointed. But these differences, while definitive, are not clear-cut enough to distinguish one sex from another at a distance. Hence the strength of hermaphrodite rumours through history.

Possession of this queenly clitoris is not without its drawbacks, though. With her vulval opening fused to form a labial pouch, the

a)

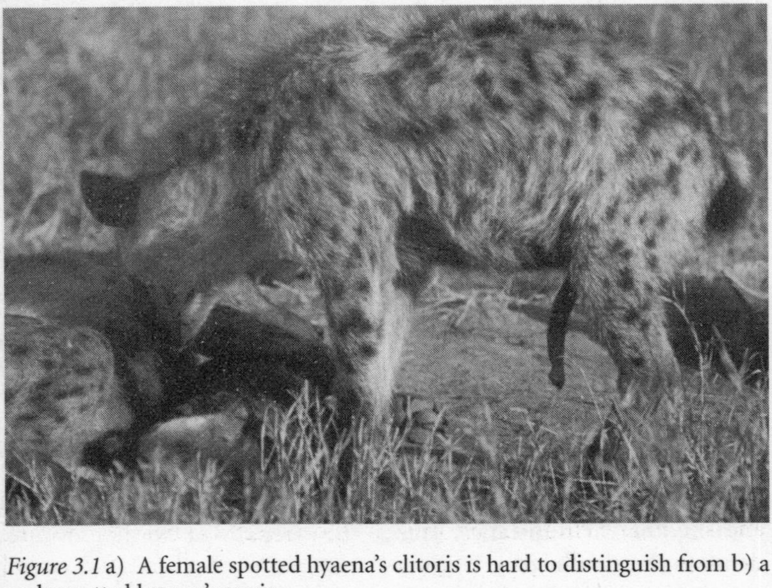

b)

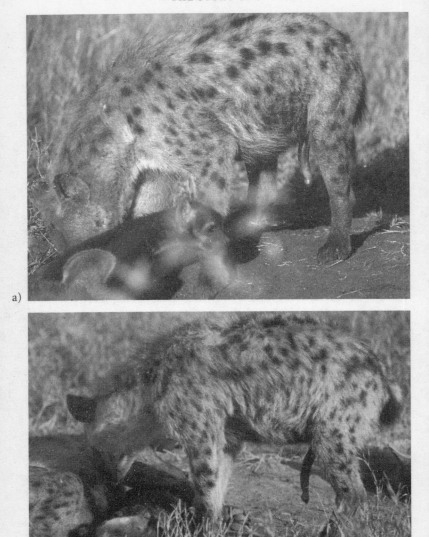

Figure 3.1 a) A female spotted hyaena's clitoris is hard to distinguish from b) a male spotted hyaena's penis.

spotted hyaena is forced to conceive and give birth through her clitoris. As a result, she endures one of the most painful and puzzling parturition experiences witnessed in the animal kingdom. For first-time mothers, and first-born pups, birth is far too often a fatal affair; almost one in five first-time mothers dies as a result of the searing, tearing trauma of giving birth. The outcome for first-born pups is even worse. The majority – over 60 per cent – will die while being born. Both mother and offspring are killed as a result of the strange and deadly design of the female spotted hyaena's genitalia.

Although not easily viewed, the internal genitalia of the female spotted hyaena are just as complex and perplexing as her extraordinary external apparatus. To the descending ball of flesh and fur that is a hyaena pup, the hyaena's unusual and convoluted birth canal presents a formidable obstacle course. Typically in a mammal of the hyaena's size, the distance from womb to outside world is around 30 cm. Yet the hyaena's birth canal measures twice this. In a cruel and unique evolutionary twist, the long and narrow canal contains a 180–degree hairpin bend halfway along. If cubs manage to negotiate the kinks and curves of the birth canal, they still face death by suffocation, for a hyaena's umbilical cord is only 12–18 cm in length – less than a third of the length of the the birth canal, and definitely not long enough to stretch from womb to outside world. Long before the hyaena is born, the cord either breaks or pulls the placenta with it. Either way the pup is left marooned and oxygenless to negotiate the final hurdle of birth. Many suffocate in their mother's genitalia and are stillborn.

Expelling a 1.5 kg hyaena pup headfirst through her slender clitoris is not easy for the mother. Its length may look impressive, but widthwise the clitoris is not the best structure for giving birth through (the opening is 2 cm wide). Cubs commonly get lodged, and die, in its tight embrace. The eye of a needle is the phrase that springs to mind. But the clitoris, with its central urogenital canal, is the only route out. Throughout and after delivery – a process that can take up to forty-eight hours – the female steadily licks her clitoris, and howls. The normally rugose clitoral skin stretches until it is greatly swollen, taut and shiny. The clitoral shaft must balloon until it is twice its normal diameter, while the glans engorges to a sphere three times its normal size. But even this distension is not enough. Two minutes before birth, the clitoris abruptly tears. Only then can the cub emerge. If the mother survives this searing tearing process, she will be scarred for life. While the edges of the birth wound will heal, they do not seal, leaving any living hyaena mother with a vivid pink streak of scar tissue coursing the underside of her clitoris. Sexing hyaenas is then a simple matter.

The genitalic conundrum

The bizarre genitalic arrangement of the female spotted hyaena is an extreme example of what it takes to reproduce successfully by internal fertilisation in the animal kingdom. It's a reproductive design that is both life-giving and deadly. Yet despite the appallingly high reproductive cost associated with first-time cub birth through a clitoris, spotted hyaenas survive and thrive as a species. Reproductive and evolutionary biologists are at a loss to explain satisfactorily why the spotted hyaena's internal and external genitalia should be shaped just so. The female spotted hyaena presents an unsolved painful genitalic puzzle.

This lack of understanding of vaginal design is not confined to the spotted hyaena. Science's appreciation of why species that reproduce by internal fertilisation have genitalia shaped just so is minimal, brief to say the least. Despite the importance of female sexual anatomy in sexual reproduction and pleasure, knowledge of its true structure and function remains in its infancy. Vaginas may be much penetrated physically, but from a design perspective they remain remarkably impenetrable. It seems that in design, as well as many cultures, a female's genitals remain shrouded in mystery, elusive and enigmatic, hidden from view.

The allure of the phallus is partly to blame for the lack of appreciation of the vagina. One element of this fascination is the obvious nature of the male structure – being exterior rather than interior makes it easier to approach. Yet the net result is that since the design rationale of genitalia was first considered, it is the penis, its engineering and prowess, the feats it can perform, that has been the focus of reproductive and evolutionary biologists. Look in any textbook, scan the internet. While the majority of books and articles describing animal genitalia typically devote pages to the variation in penis shape and size across the animal kingdom, the genitalic contribution of the female is generally summed up in a couple of sentences about flaps and flanges. A terse (and erroneous) statement about female reproductive organs not being as complex as those of the male is commonly added. Penises are indexed, vaginas hardly ever. The electronic database the Zoological Record lists (for 1978–97) 539 articles dealing with the penis, while just seven discuss the clitoris. A casual reader could all too easily draw the conclusion that either female genitalia have never evolved and that all vaginas are the same, or that the scientific world knows nothing about the evolution of the vagina and its variation among species. The former statements, of course, are not true, but the latter, until very recently, was.

Just a quick look reveals that vaginal variety across species is stunning. Some vaginas are expansive, some dead-ended. Many are ribbed. A sow, if you could see it, has a spiral-shaped cervix akin to a hollow screw thread. The vaginas of large aquatic mammals, like toothed whales, seals and dugongs, are long and winding, with well-developed hymens. Female pipefish and a sister piscine species, the Japanese sea raven, have extendable genitalia that they use to pinch sperm from male partners. Some species have more than one vagina. Some have none. Platypuses, like spotted hyaenas, are essentially devoid of a vagina, and, intriguingly, only their left ovary is functional. Some reptile species have a split, or bifurcated, vagina. When it comes to vaginal quantity, wallabies win hands down. Wallabies have a complex of vaginas – three in total. The first is in essence a vaginal cul-de-sac which, amazingly, opens at birth. The other vaginas have twin cervices and paired, but separate, wombs. This twin womb feature of wallabies and other marsupials (pouched mammals) means they are known as didelphic (two-wombed). Some primates, such as ring-tailed lemurs, also have two wombs, although the majority, including monkeys, apes and humans, are monodelphic, meaning we make do with a unified uterus.

Points of entry are flexible. Cow elephants have extremely low-slung vulvas, shifted from under their anus to beneath their baggy bellies. Some species, including guinea-pigs and bushbabies, have vaginas that only open for business during oestrus – at other times they remain sealed by a thin tissue membrane. Chickens have a composite organ – the cloaca, an orifice which is vagina, urethra and anus rolled into one. In an amazing party trick, chickens are capable of using their cloaca to selectively void unwanted sperm. Although many vaginal attributes are tucked away neatly inside the body, some females flaunt their sexual apparel. The external genitalia of some of our sister primates are truly awe-inspiring. Bonobos sport huge, glistening, cherry-pink clitorises and labia, baboons prominent peony-red perineal protrusions. Even some birds, such as the Japanese accentor, brandish bright vermilion external protuberances. Beautiful, bizarre, baffling, bloody: the vagaries of the vagina are all of these things. But a one-size-fits-all vanilla vagina simply does not exist. Females have evolved elaborate and diverse genitalia.

The vagaries of vaginal design

The big question is: why? What drives the female of the species to evolve such a striking degree of complexity in vaginal design? The conventional view of the function of female genitalia of internally fertilising species is no help. First formulated centuries ago, it has changed little since. The genitals of females, it supposes, are designed to act as a conduit for sperm and any subsequent offspring. Females simply provide the external and internal structures which sperm must pass through in one direction, and offspring in the other. Until the eighteenth century, with the realisation of the role of the egg in fertilisation, females were presumed to contribute nothing to the makeup of any offspring. They were merely the suppliers of the inert incubation apparatus.

At the start of the twenty-first century, however, it is increasingly apparent that this perception of the vagina as a passive vessel uninvolved in the reproductive process cannot begin to explain the complexity of female genitalia, or why such variety in vaginal design exists across so many species. The vagina, it seems, is far more than its simple title of sheath implies. Understanding the rationale behind the design and engineering of the vagina, however, requires nothing less than a complete reassessment of the role of internally fertilising genitalia. It is only by setting aside age-old assumptions about the vagina, and considering once again what female genitalia are actually designed to do, that the role that the vagina plays in sexual reproduction and pleasure can be revealed.

One approach to unveiling the significance of possessing internally fertilising genitalia is to look at species that use alternative reproduction strategies, such as those species that use the waters of the oceans as their womb. External fertilisation – the act of releasing gametes (egg and sperm) into surrounding water and hoping for the best – is practised by many, but not all, water-bound creatures. Fish, starfish, sea urchins and anemones are among those that broadcast their spawn to all and sundry. But as a reproductive strategy, this ancient procreation process has many pitfalls. In the vast sexual arena that is the sea, finding someone to spawn at, or with, is a hit-and-miss affair. Release your eggs at the wrong time, and they will soon be washed away. In the depths of the ocean it is very unusual for all of an individual's eggs to be fertilised.

In a bid to improve their reproductive odds, many broadcast spawners choose to take their reproductive cue from the moon, metronome of the ocean's high and low tides. The Palolo worm, a South Pacific marine worm, gets just one shot a year at reproductive success. One week after November's full moon, and for the space of little more than one hour, the worm's discharged gametes transform the Samoan Islands' sea into a milky, glutinous vermicelli soup. This breeding broth produced by synchronised mass spawnings is the Palolo worm's best bet to ensure any offspring. Sex here has nothing to do with meeting the right mate. For external fertilisers, any gamete will do.

There are, however, design limits to external fertilisation. Successful spawners are those that can produce the most eggs, or sperm. A female oyster, for instance, will shed a staggering 115 million eggs in just one spawning session. To ensure at most a couple of offspring, she must repeat this virtuoso performance five or six times a year. But producing 700 million eggs a year requires a gargantuan investment in gametes. Not surprisingly, in the battle to survive as a species, many ocean-dwellers become little more than gonads with fins. The gonads of both female and male starfish make up more than one third of their total body weight.

In contrast, keeping all your eggs in one basket – a womb inside you – neatly sidesteps the location and production problems of the broadcast spawner. The internally fertilising female, courtesy of her genitalia, does not need to invest so heavily in egg production. Her eggs are not fated to be tossed away by the tide, and she does not need to fling them at all comers in the vicinity. A vagina, or its equivalent, makes sure that not all males have access to a female's eggs. In doing so, internal fertilisation hands a female the capacity to control which sperm get to fertilise her eggs. This is a very important ability. Courtesy of internally fertilising genitalia, the female of many species can exercise reproductive choice. She can be selective.

There's more to the vagina than meets the eye

Features common to the genitalia of internally fertilising species also provide clues as to the true function of a female's genitals. In internally fertilising females, it is an almost universal fact that sperm are never deposited directly on top of the female's eggs. Instead, internally fertilising females typically separate the sperm deposition site (the vagina in humans, the uterus in pigs, and the *bursa copulatrix* in insects) from that of fertilisation. In this basic way, the design of female genitalia simply and effectively uncouples copulation from fertilisation. The act of depositing sperm does not ensure sperm will reach the correct destination for reproductive success. Another result of this separation of the two sites is that reproductive ducting – the lengths of internal tubing or canal connecting vagina with uterus, or oviduct (egg tube) with ovary – is an elementary feature of female genitalia. Hidden from view, these internal tunnels, or genitalic plumbing, map out the subterranean route sperm must progress along if they are to reach a female's eggs.

The style and shape of the reproductive tracts of internally fertilising females tells another important story. If the idea of female genitalia as passive vessel – structured merely to assist and smooth the passage of sperm to egg – is correct, then the design of female reproductive canals appears perverse in the extreme. In no sense can their architecture be described as tracing the easiest, or straightest, route from A to B. Figure 3.2 shows the spectacularly tortuous, highly coiled ducts of two hydraenid beetles. Snaking round in slender sinuous spirals, looping and entwining, the reproductive ducts of these stream-dwelling beetles seem designed to impede, not progress, the passage of sperm. Similar intricate internal curls and coils – to my mind organic curving works of art – can be seen in many species of spiders and insects.

Not only are these ducts extremely narrow and extraordinarily convoluted in design; they also place a female's eggs far beyond the

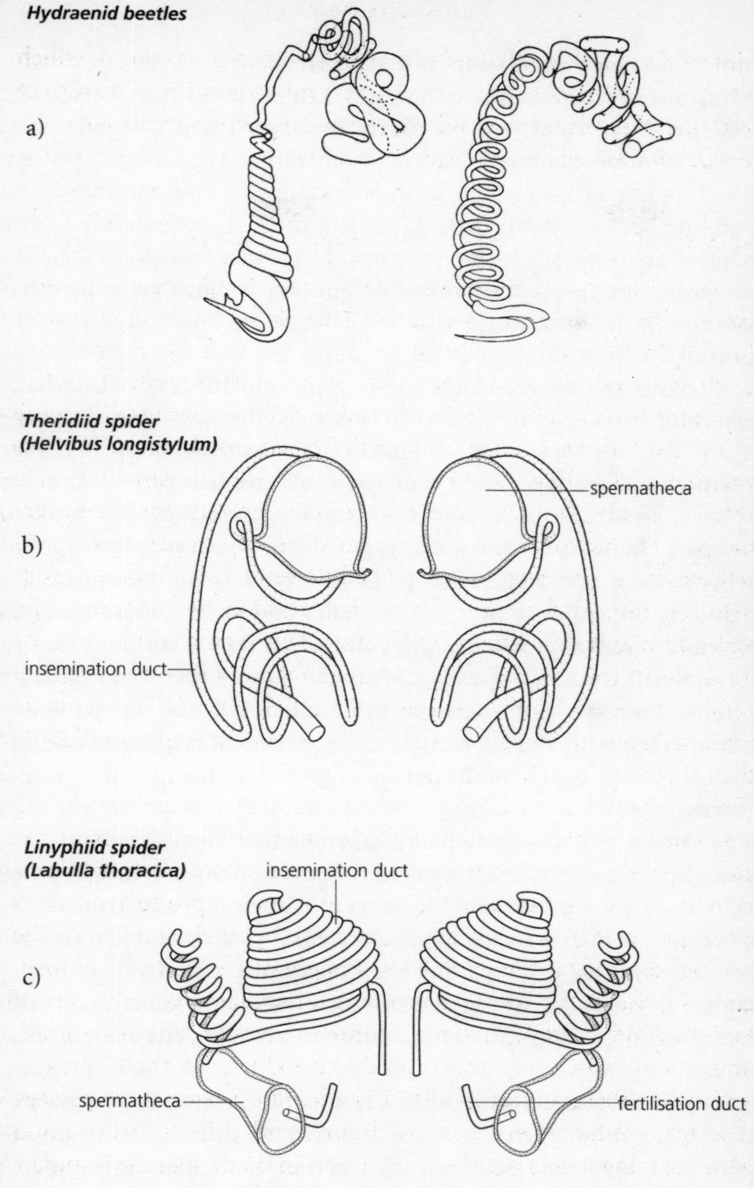

Figure 3.2 a) the fantastically twisted reproductive ducting of two hydraenid beetles; b) and c) spiders too have tortuous and complex internal genitalia. Note in c) how the insemination portion (entrance) of the reproductive duct is far longer than the fertilisation section (exit), suggesting that females' genitalia have evolved to exercise extra control over sperm here.

immediate reach of sperm. In female elephants, the distance from vulva to ovary can measure more than three and a half metres. Yet beetles manage to take the biscuit for distance. The tiny female plant beetle (*Charidotella propinqua*) has such a long, twisted duct system, spiralling one way and then another, looping around and frequently doubling back on itself, that, if it is stretched out, it measures more than twenty times the length of her body. From a transport efficiency viewpoint, it appears the general design of a female's genitalic ducts does not fit the theory of female genitalia acting as a straightforward conduit for sperm and offspring.

A further puzzling, and again common, genitalic trait of internally fertilising females is the presence of spermathecae – sperm storage organs or reservoirs (see Figure 3.2). Spermathecae (singular spermatheca) are specialised genitalic structures that provide females with the capacity to store sperm for varying periods of time prior to the sperm being used to fertilise eggs. Although it's now known that spermathecae are a standard genitalic attribute in many species, including the majority of insects, reptiles and birds, these structures incredibly went unnoticed until 1946, when they were described in the domestic chicken. Typically spermathecae are situated in a separate location from the spot where sperm are deposited, and the site where they are fertilised, and are connected to the rest of the female's reproductive tract by means of the female's typically thin and winding duct system.

Spermathecae, like a female's reproductive ducts, seem to have very little to do with enabling direct access to her eggs. Instead, they seem to offer another way for females to manage and control the movement of sperm inside themselves. Like a siding where trains are shunted until it's time for them to be put into service, or a money bag for depositing cash, sperm storage organs provide females with the option of storing sperm for a later date, rather than using it all at once.

Amazingly, females who possess spermathecae have the capacity to store sperm from hours, to days, to weeks, to months, to years (see Table 3.1). While all birds can store sperm, the turkey is the medal winner. Female turkeys typically store sperm for forty-five days, but have been known to manage 117 days; in contrast, pigeons can only notch up six days, on average. Months is the norm for spiders, while

Table 3.1 Sperm Storage in the Genitalia of Female Animals

Taxa	**Duration stored**
Insects	
Fruit fly	14 days
Water strider	30 days
Stick insect	77 days
Grasshopper	26–113 days
Reptiles	
Crocodiles	7 days
Lizards	30–365 days (1 year)
Turtles/tortoises	90–1460 days (4 years)
Snakes	90–2555 days (7 years)
Birds	
Finch	8–16 days
Chicken	21–30 days
Canary	68 days
Turkey	56–117 days
Mammals	
Mouse	6 hours
Marsupials	0.5–16 days
Human	5–8 days
Bats	16 days–6 months
Fish	
Shark	Up to several years

Adapted from Neubaum, Deborah M., and Wolfner, Mariana F., 'Wise, winsome or weird? Mechanisms of sperm storage in female animals', *Current Topics in Developmental Biology*, 41 (1999), 67–97; and Birkhead, T. R., and Møller, A. P. (eds.), *Sperm Competition and Sexual Selection*, London: Academic Press, 1998.

some insects can make a single insemination last years. Females of the seed beetle (*Callososbruchus maculatus*) are extremely parsimonious, and can store enough sperm from a single mating to last a lifetime. Prolonged sperm storage reaches its peak in reptiles. These cold-blooded creatures have prodigious sperm-storage abilities. Virtually all female reptiles can store sperm for at least some weeks. Storing sperm from one year to the next is standard for terrapins and swivel-eyed chameleons.

However, the reptilian record for sperm storage must go to the snake. Some species typically store sperm for two to three years, and one, the Javan wart snake, is credited with hoarding sperm for seven years before using it to produce fertile eggs. Although most mammals do not possess specialised sperm storage structures, insectivorous bats are one exception, and are capable of storing sperm over the winter, ready for fertilisation when they ovulate in spring. However, despite the lack of spermathecae, female mammals do have the capacity to keep sperm viable for short periods of time. In women, the maximum recorded is eight days.

Design-wise, sperm storage sites range from relatively simple sacs or pouches, to highly convoluted organs. In mammals, the cervix and uterus are used. And although it's still not clear precisely how some females manage to achieve the miraculous feat of keeping sperm viable for months on end, some aspects of spermathecal engineering suggest possible nourishment, protection and anchoring mechanisms. The spermathecae of many insects and spiders have fine striae, ridges or grooves, and scale- or hook-like projections, lining their interior surfaces. In the sperm storage organs of the female fruit-feeding fly, *Drosophila wassermani*, sperm are typically to be found wrapped around curved hooks near the spermathecal entrance. In some species, like the bat, it's suggested that sperm obtain sustenance from the female by attaching to the epithelial lining of her spermatheca. In birds, it's thought fluid produced deep in the sperm storage tubules, which is then washed over the stored sperm, may provide some sort of nutrition. Cervical mucus or other genital fluids may also play a role.

The way in which different species store sperm varies dramatically. Like a miser hoarding discrete amounts of cash all over the house, birds plump for storing small amounts in a vast array of sperm storage tubules. The number of tubules employed is staggering, varying between 300 and 20,000 in differently-sized species, with larger birds having more tubules. Most bird sperm storage tubules are long, thin and blind-ending, resembling a single sausage-shaped tube, but some are branched. The female dunnock, a small drab brown bird that routinely mates up to twenty times a day, has a phenomenal total sperm capacity, and can pack up to 500 sperm in each of her 1,400 sperm storage tubules, giving her a total sperm capacity of over 700,000. The common chicken, or domestic fowl, has so many sperm tubules clustered tightly around the neck of her oviduct, at the junction of the vagina and uterus, that it appears as if her oviduct is wearing an Elizabethan ruff.

Lizards, the nearest relatives to birds, use a similar safety-in-numbers storage strategy, and it's thought dinosaurs did too. Spiders also have multiple spermathecae, with some spider species squeezing over a hundred spermathecae into their compact bodies. Insects choose an alterative approach, storing a massive sperm pile in one place – an insectean bank vault strategy. In some insects, wall flexibility is key; for example, the spermatheca of the female walking cricket (*Gryllus bimaculatus*) is so elastic it can expand to accommodate over thirty ejaculates. Flies and mosquitoes usually have two or three sac-like spermathecal structures, while dragonflies and their close relatives, damselflies, store sperm in their *bursa copulatrix* and a T-shaped spermatheca. Crustaceans, millipedes, mites and beetles possess at least two sperm storage pouches, and sometimes more.

The bedbugs' new genitals

The curious case of the bedbugs' new genitals adds further weight to the idea that there is more to female genitalia than providing sperm with easy access to eggs. Bedbugs, and other cimicid bugs, are an oddity – both female and male. Instead of inseminating females via the usual route, males use hypodermic insemination to get their sperm to a female's eggs. A male bedbug, as many articles are at pains to point out, has developed genitalia capable of injecting sperm directly through the female's body wall into her body cavity. The male bedbug's sperm are also able to negotiate their way through the female's body cavity to her ovaries. This male's sperm can move not only within the spaces between cells but also through cells.

But hypodermic insemination is not the end of the bedbug story, although most chronicles of bedbug genitalia leave the tale there. In an astonishing retort to the spermatic shenanigans of the males, female bedbugs have evolved a new set of genitalia (para, or secondary genitalia) at the point where males penetrate. The new set of genitalic structures, called the spongy spermalege, is a complex and sophisticated structure. The external part, the ectospermalege, is designed to receive the stabbing insertions of the males' genitalia, while the internal portion, the mesospermalege, receives and routes the injected semen.

The mesospermalege has another role too – that of sperm destroyer. The sperm receptacles and ducts that form the female bedbugs' second reproductive system are derived from cells and tissues that are normally used to combat invasions of pathogens and foreign materials. Their common effect is to kill sperm. Sperm that are not destroyed are stored and conducted slowly, via a 'conductor cord', where still another portion of the sperm is resorbed before it can reach the female's oviduct. Only a few sperm ever leave the female bedbugs' conductor cord intact, and even these must pass through a sperm-destroying synctial body before arriving at fertilisation sites near the bedbugs' ovaries. Most sperm are left dead along the way.

The reinvention of reproductive tracts in bedbugs and their relatives suggests that female bedbugs prefer the male's sperm to be routed in a manner dictated by female biology, not the male's whim. Far from ensuring sperm reach fertilisation sites, the bedbugs' new genitalia turn a stream of sperm into a trickle. The evidence strongly suggests that bedbug paragenitalia evolved as sperm-killing and deactivating organs. This is in complete contrast to the conventional view of female genitalia as a simple conduit for the safe passage of sperm and offspring. What is going on?

In fact, the idea of the female and her vagina as a passive vessel for sperm is one of science's greatest misconceptions. As more investigations into the structure and function of female genitalia are undertaken, it is becoming increasingly clear that there is far more to female genitalia than meets the eye. Indeed, what is exciting evolutionary biologists today is the realisation of the active participation of the female and her genitalia in controlling a species' successful copulation, conception and birth of offspring. Science is undergoing nothing less than a revolution in the way females, their genitals and their sexual habits are viewed. It is a twenty-first-century sexual revolution. A vaginal revolution. A velvet revolution.

Freed from the confines of convention, the true function of female genitalia is finally being unveiled. The vagina, it seems, is designed to enable females to exert an extraordinary influence over which sperm will successfully fertilise their eggs. A female's genitals are not a simple thoroughfare for sperm, but comprise an exquisitely structured organ with the complexity and sensitivity to determine the paternity of a female's offspring. Indeed, it is now realised that it is the drive to determine paternity that has led to the evolution of a female's amazing, beautiful, awe-inspiring internally fertilising genitals. Astonishingly, female control of paternity can be wielded either before, during or after copulation.

In stark contrast to her previous incarnation as a passive creature, the picture that is emerging of the internally fertilising female is of a supremely successful sexual and reproductive strategist. Across different species, female traits influence who gains access to their gametes in a myriad subtle, yet striking ways. Copulation, insemination and fertilisation all take place within the female's body, on her turf. Consequently, it is her sexual biology and sexual behaviour that set the ground rules for successful sexual reproduction. In this game of life, it is the female's big brooding body against a mass of minuscule sperm. It's her long ovarian obstacle course that the male's spermatozoa must traverse on their odyssey to the egg. Hence it is female genital structure that lies at the heart of reproductive control. Courtesy of their sensitive, muscular, complex genitalia, females control the paternity of their offspring.

Female control

Female birds do it. Female bees do it. And close examination reveals that both do it on their own terms. Contrary to popular belief and previous assumptions of sexual behaviour, it is now known that it is the female of the species that controls whether copulation occurs or not, and who it occurs with. Females have the choice of initiating, granting or refusing copulation, and for the majority of species, declining to copulate is a simple matter. Indeed, apart from within human societies, rape is extremely rare. For the majority of insects, with their many genitalic parts, coupling is so complex that it is impossible without the female's full co-operation. Butterflies signal no by bending their abdomens upwards, out of reach. The female honey bee and the flower-eating rose chafer beetle have various internal vaginal valves which the female must open for sex to be possible. Other insects simply shut the genital aperture at the apex of their abdomen. Walking away is often a clear enough message.

Species-specific manoeuvres vary. For the small Scottish Soay ewe, holding her tail firmly downwards is sufficient to thwart unwanted attentions. Female warthogs and collared peccaries refuse to copulate in a similar manner – covering their vulva with their tail and tightening their leg muscles upwards. For birds, copulation is all about 'cloacal kisses' – achieving contact of the cloaca, the female and male sex organ. Any female bird that is uninterested in sex, or that particular suitor, can turn down the opportunity by refusing to evert, turn inside out, her cloaca. Without her input, sex is an impossibility. Even those male birds that possess the beginnings of a phallus, such as the vasa parrot, need the female's full assistance. For a sexual encounter to occur and sperm transfer to be successful, the female vasa parrot must extend and envelop the male's genital protuberance with her everted cloaca.

The need for the female's full co-operation is illustrated beautifully by our friend the spotted hyaena. As the dominant sex, female spotted hyaenas are in complete control of all copulations, and if they're not interested in a male's attempts to mount them, they simply walk away. Added to this, their extraordinary external genitalia effectively bar access to all males other than the ones they want. For not only does the female have to urinate and give birth through her elongated clitoris, she also has to have sex through this slender stalk. The way she does this is unique. In order to receive the male, the female has to form a makeshift vagina. She achieves this by flexing the robust retractor muscles of her genitalia, which retract her clitoris up into her abdomen, just like a shirt sleeve being rolled up. However, because of the angle of the dangle of her clitoris, the opening of her urogenital canal faces forwards, away from the mounting male, making mating an even more precarious process. One wrong move by the male, and the female is away. In spotted hyaena society, it is the nature of the female's relationship with a male that determines whether mating occurs, and if it is successful.

Across the kingdom of internal fertilisers, the design of female genitalia effectively dictates what a male must do if he is to have a chance of gaining entry to a female's body, and access to her eggs. For male insects this can mean tapping, rubbing, vibrating or stridulating the female repeatedly near or around her genital opening. In other species, gaining entry can be even more involved. The vaginal complexity of many females leads to breathtaking performances from ardent males. In order for rabbits to copulate, the female (like many mammals) must be in what is known as the lordosis position, with her back arched in a concave curve. Only then can the male enter her. This is because lordosis effectively elevates and rotates the rabbit's pelvis, shifting the vagina from a position inaccessible to the male (pointing towards the floor) to one tilted towards him.

Female rabbits, though, will not assume the lordosis position unless the male can persuade them to do so. This is no easy matter for the male rabbit, because what a female rabbit requires is rhythm, and lots of it. If the doe is to adopt the lordosis position, the male rabbit must first perform up to seventy rhythmic constant-amplitude, high-frequency extra-vaginal thrusts (that is, against the vulva). Low-frequency and non-rhythmic thrusting will not do, and rarely or never elicits lordosis, even in highly oestrous does. Female rabbits know what they like.

Female mites and ticks do, too, and what these tiny parasites require if they are to open up to sex is lengthy oral genital manipulation. Like many insects, the mating strategy of ticks and mites does not involve the transfer of free-flowing sperm to the female via a phallus. Instead, the male produces a sperm packet, known as a spermatophore, which he must persuade the female to take up into her vaginal opening. Both of these steps – the production of his pre-packed ejaculate, and the relaxing of the opening to the female's vulva – rely on the male inserting some or all of his mouthparts into the female's vagina.

In some mite species, the male inserts and withdraws his mouthparts repeatedly. In others he moves them back and forth in her vagina, sometimes rubbing there for hours at a time, as if feeding. Gradually, under the weight of this oral onslaught, the female's genitals start to swell. Only then does the male produce a spermatophore from his own genital opening, and only then, after much stimulation, will the female's vagina be ready to have his sperm package inserted into her. For mites and ticks, oral sex is not a hoped-for part of foreplay, but an essential ingredient in ensuring a successful sexual encounter.

Gaining entry is not enough

It is significant that gaining entry to a female's body is generally not enough to ensure sperm will be deposited inside the female –

copulation does not as a matter of course lead to sperm transfer. Indeed, it is common for females of many species to terminate sexual sessions before ejaculation has occurred. For some females, such as the spotted hyaena, the slant of their genitalia means they simply walk away from unsatisfactory sex. However, many females – including bees, beetles, birds and women – have another trick up their sleeves: their vaginal muscles.

This musculature can be used in different ways – to prevent copulations occurring, to terminate copulations that have already begun, and because typically sperm transfer does not take place until minutes or sometimes hours after copulation commences, a female's vaginal muscles can also be used to prevent insemination. It's even thought that in the case of the honey bee, the female's vaginal muscles may also be responsible for triggering the male honey bee's ejaculation, while in birds, it appears to be the female's genital musculature that is responsible for successful sperm transfer. Studies of Adelie penguins and pigeons show that it is the rhythmic muscular pumping movements of the female's cloaca that draw sperm deposited on the outside of her everted cloaca into her reproductive tract.

The leaf-eating beetle (*Macrohaltica jamaicencis*) is one female that uses her muscular wherewithal to prevent unwanted males from inseminating her, and she can do this even after a male has already inserted his genitalia into her vagina, or bursa. This tiny beetle avoids insemination by contracting her powerful bursal muscles so tightly that the bursa appears to have an internal plug. Squeezing the bursa tight shut stops insemination occurring in two ways. First, it blocks entry to the passageway leading to the female's sperm storage site, which is situated at the inner end of the bursa. Secondly, the female's vaginal contractions prevent the male from inflating his genitalic sac, a move which is necessary if he is to form a sperm-containing spermatophore in her bursa. Males typically thrust for about a minute under these female-induced conditions but, faced with a vaginal wall of steel, they are forced to give up, and pull out prior to insemination. As well as beetles and bees, internal vaginal contractions strong enough to force males out of the female have been seen in the tsetse fly. This can also happen with humans.

Even if a female allows the male to deposit his sperm inside her, it is quite often the case that insemination will still be unsuccessful because the male has not left his sperm at the right site within her. Unfortunately for males, it can sometimes be difficult to reach the correct sperm deposition site, which is often deep within the female. Typically, females will only permit such deep penetration if the male can provide a particular type of stimulation. Deep penetration is a necessary requirement for guava-devouring Caribbean fruit flies to reproduce successfully. However, the female Caribbean fruit fly possesses a particularly convoluted reproductive structure. The entrance to her vagina lies at the tip of her abdomen, which is long and extensible. When not extended, this genital opening remains hidden, and inside her, her long vagina remains folded into a tight 'S'. Deep at the end of this S-shaped vagina is the fruit fly's bursa – the site where a male fruit fly needs to deposit his sperm. And if he cannot penetrate her deeply enough, successful sperm transfer will not occur. In this way, the external and internal genitalic complexity of these females allows them to control whether or not sexual activity occurs, and with whom.

Bizarrely, song is the key to negotiating the female fruit fly's deep, sinuous passages. So, Orpheus-like, the male Caribbean fruit fly charms the female with music and song. Mounting her, he must sing, sing, sing, to persuade her to let down her abdomen and expose her genital opening. If he is successful, he threads his long, flexible phallus, called an aedeagus, through this tiny tip. And he continues to sing. It's then believed he coaxes her with song to extend her long curved vagina, so that his aedeagus can reach through to the deep recesses of her bursa.

Female fruit flies are very choosy about the songs they like. If a female doesn't appreciate what she hears, she uses vigorous movements to knock the disappointing male off her back. The songs of males who are rejected during mounting are typically tunes that are less powerful, comprising both lower sound pressure levels and less total energy, than the songs of successful males. The suitors that are successful in negotiating the female's internal complexity are the males who sing the most intense songs. This mounting ballad, which the male Caribbean fruit fly produces by fanning his wings, usually continues until his aedeagus is deep in its final position. If a female grows restless, he must sing again, or he will be rudely removed.

Female philanderers

Even after insemination has taken place, and in the right place, a female, if she wishes, has many options with which to scupper a sperm's chance of fertilising her eggs. As previously noted, a female's reproductive geography dictates that males do not deposit their sperm directly on top of a female's eggs. Just as copulation does not necessarily lead to the male transferring his sperm to the female, neither does insemination lead directly and inevitably to fertilisation of a female's eggs. In fact, examination of the genital structures of female animals with internal fertilisation strongly suggests that copulation seldom leads directly and inevitably to fertilisation. Many couples trying to get pregnant can testify to this. Copulation is an act that is uncoupled from fertilisation, and females can, and do, make the most of this fact.

Post-copulation, one of the simplest ways in which females can influence whether or not that male's sperm will sire their offspring is by choosing to mate with another male. Polyandry, the practice of mating with multiple males, is not just one of the most straightforward methods of confounding paternity, it is also an extremely widespread sexual strategy of the female. Incredibly, though, it wasn't until the 1970s that scientists began to realise that polyandry, and not monogamy (the practice of having only one mate), was the norm for female animals. It has taken approaching three decades, and an overwhelming mountain of evidence pointing to both the sexual flexibility of females and the common occurrence of offspring with different fathers (mixed paternity broods), but the verdict is now in. Polyandry is the norm for the female of the species; the idea of the monogamous female is erroneous.

In fact, the myth of the monogamous female was a product of its time, of misplaced Victorian moralities. It also serves as a warning, an example of how scientists can see only what they want to see, and nothing else; it is yet another scientific notion driven by ideology not evidence. In this case, for a period of over a hundred years, mainly male scientists said that they saw females of all species studied practising monogamy. Sadly, it wasn't until female scientists entered this field of research that the polyandrous nature of female sexuality emerged. It's now believed that a mere 3 per cent, if that, of all females are monogamous. Science, it seems, is still capable of being as subjective, and as sexist, as any other discipline.

One of the basic lessons from the discovery of widespread female polyandry is that females must benefit more from insemination by multiple mates than previously thought. There must be a clear evolutionary advantage underpinning the routine multiple mating that the majority of females go to great lengths to practise. It's not just the number of males a female is sexually active with that is puzzling, though, it's also the frequency with which many females copulate. Female sheep, the subject of many a sexual joke, are phenomenally sexually active. One account of their sexual appetite records the Scottish Soay ewe mating an amazing 163 times, with seven different rams, in the space of five hours. Many males cannot keep up with the females' sexual appetites and run out of sperm before the end of the mating season.

Replenishing sperm supplies is one of the suggestions put forward to explain why females have sex so frequently. Yet in many species of birds, where females control the frequency and success of copulations, and require only a few inseminations to fertilise their entire clutch of eggs, the copulation frequency rate is even more staggering. The migratory songbird, Smith's long spur, the nondescript dunnock and its small, dark grey relative, the alpine accentor, all copulate up to several hundred times per clutch, when just a couple of times would suffice. In the primate world, female rhesus macaques enjoy so many copulations back to back that they commonly experience a phenomenon known as vaginal overflow – their vaginas literally overflow with sperm as a result of their multiple matings.

Insemination does not always lead to fertilisation

One answer to why females routinely copulate multiple times with multiple males is thought to lie in the fact that insemination does not always lead to fertilisation. It's known that in some cases multiple mating by females results in high levels of multiple paternity in their broods, while in other situations it doesn't. The female Columbian ground squirrel is sexually active for just four hours a year, and typically uses her short oestrous period to copulate with several males. While, on average, these female squirrels will copulate with 4.4 males over four hours, not all litters will be multiply sired. In comparison, with female side-blotched lizards, multiple mating results in high rates of multiple paternity (81 per cent).

The female tree swallow, however, reveals a curious aspect of multiple mating and how copulation does not always lead to conception. Like most birds, female tree swallows have a complex social and sexual life. The females pair up with a male within their nesting area, co-operating with this partner in rearing offspring, but also mate with many other males, typically leaving their territory to do so, and initiating these away-from-home sex sessions. Intriguingly, the copulations with males from outside their nesting area are far more likely to produce offspring than copulations with their nesting partner. One study of the sexual habits of these small greenish-blue birds showed that although one female mated an average of 1.6 times an hour with her nesting partner, all her offspring were the result of sexual activity outside the nest. Another female tree swallow in this study mated 1.2 times every hour with her rearing partner, but produced a brood which was in the main sired by other males (over 60 per cent). Other research shows that in some tree sparrow populations, 50–90 per cent of all nests contain offspring that are not those of the female's regular mate.

Chimpanzees provide another very striking example of how the frequency of a male's copulatory activity does not tally with the likelihood that a female will be fertilised by his sperm. Researchers estimate that female chimpanzees copulate 135 times for every conception – a fact that clearly demonstrates that gaining sexual access to a female does not guarantee male reproductive success. Studies of the sexual lifestyles of chimpanzees suggest that mating style may influence reproductive outcome. The mating habits of chimpanzees are extremely flexible, with adults of both sexes choosing to engage in any of three different patterns. These sexual systems are dubbed opportunistic mating, possessive mating and consortship mating.

Opportunistic mating typically involves a female mating repeatedly, up to fifty times a day, with all of the males that accompany her in the troop. With possessive mating, a female pairs off with one male for a period ranging from one hour to five days. This type of sexual activity does not necessarily preclude the female from mating with other males; however, males typically try to prevent copulations with lower-ranking males. The third type of chimpanzee mating arrangement, consortship mating, occurs when a female and a male choose to leave the group together for a period of between three hours and four months. During this time they maintain exclusive sexual access with each other.

One study of the eastern common chimpanzee (*Pan troglodytes schweinfurthii*) counted the number of times that chimpanzees copulated. Counts were conducted when all females were at the peak of their oestrous cycle, which coincides with maximum genital tumescence. This count of chimpanzee copulations showed that of 1,137 copulations, the majority were opportunistic (73 per cent), 25 per cent were possessive matings, and only 2 per cent of all recorded matings occurred within consortships. However, despite the far lower frequency of consortship matings, it was this pattern of sexual activity that led to the greatest number of pregnancies. In this particular study, 2 per cent of the copulations led to 50 per cent of the pregnancies, and longer consortships were also more likely to result in pregnancies than shorter ones.

These results suggest that a female chimpanzee is far more likely to become pregnant when she is copulating with a male she has chosen to pair off with above all others. The big question is how consortships, which typically involve five or six matings a day, lead to conceptions more often than group mating situations, where females copulate much more frequently (up to thirty times a day). In both the chimpanzee and the tree swallow examples there is an apparent correlation between paternity bias and overt female preferences for males. Can females, courtesy of their sexual behaviour and genitalia, directly influence which inseminations turn into fertilisations, and which don't? Do females have the controlling hand in determining successful sexual reproduction internally as well as externally?

The oviductal obstacle course

The answer to whether, during and post-copulation, females can and do influence which male will father their offspring lies within the female's internal genitalia. Consider the female/sperm asymmetry. The contest is between one large complex, dynamic female and masses of minuscule delicate sperm. Internal fertilisation means the female is always playing at home. This doesn't mean that males and their sperm are completely powerless, but it certainly gives the female the upper hand about what happens next. By dint of her morphology – the structure of her genitalia – and her physiology – the functions her reproductive tract is designed to perform – the female of the species represents a formidable opponent. Ejaculates can contain hundreds of millions of sperm, yet the vast majority will fail to reach the female's ova. Typically only between two and twenty sperm get anywhere near the vicinity of a female's eggs. A female's reproductive tract functions very efficiently as a chemical and physical deathtrap for sperm.

The fairy tales of the Brothers Grimm offer a reproductive analogy. In one fable, a beautiful princess has too many suitors to choose from. To help her in her decision, she sets each prospective prince a series of tasks. Only the man who successfully completes each assignment is deemed worthy to gain her hand in marriage. Likewise with a female and a male's sperm. In order to weed out the unsuitable fertilisation candidates, the female's vagina presents a series of genitalic hurdles in the shape of her oviductal obstacle course. Only the sperm that can overcome all of these will have a chance of fusing with her egg. It's not an easy task.

Post-ejaculation, females set to work immediately to bring sperm numbers down. In many insects, birds and mammals, the vagina, the immediate environment sperm find themselves within, is no safe haven. On the contrary, the vagina is an extremely hostile acidic arena, which easily destroys newcomers. It has to be if it wants to be selective. If low pH doesn't pulverise the sperm, then killer cells appear to digest the intruders. Digestion of sperm by spermicidal phagocytic cells occurs in insects, worms, fish and mammals. As well as possessing sperm storage pouches, many snails and slugs have specialised sperm-digesting pouches, while other molluscs have gametolytic (gamete-eating) glands in their *bursa copulatrix*, which mop up excess sperm. In some species the spermicidal properties of the female's reproductive tract fluctuate during her reproductive cycle.

The sperm that survive the chemical warfare within the vagina now face a veritable odyssey – the biological equivalent of many a mythological journey through the underworld. Their goal is to meet an egg coming down the female's curving uterine horns. To get there, however, they must negotiate the female's internal labyrinth. Some sperm have further to go than others. The sperm of pythons is eight metres from its goal; that of geckos just 20 mm. In humans, the distance from entrance to eggs is between 15 and 20 cm. Most sperm, though, never get further than the spot where they fell. Summary expulsion is their fate.

A cunning stunt

Sperm ejection is one of the most vivid and dramatic ways a female can rid herself of unwanted sperm. This cunning stunt, like many other vaginal attributes, is a facet of female behaviour that has only recently begun to be explored in depth. It is possible that sperm ejection by females was noticed years ago, but was dismissed as not important. An 1886 study of the female alpine or mountain grasshopper (*Podisma pedestris*) detailed 'faeces of a special character' being voided by the female just before copulating, but no further observations were made. It is now becoming increasingly clear, however, that sperm ejection or dumping by females is a common occurrence.

Spiders, snakes, insects, parrots, poultry, pigs, mice, sheep, cattle, rabbits, humans: all these and more have been observed ejecting surplus sperm. Indeed, sperm ejection seems to be the rule in mammals. A slick, quick and effective method, up to 80 per cent of the ejaculate is known to be expelled in this way by female rabbits, pigs, cattle and sheep. In some cases, this represents a voluminous voided volume. The female Grevy's zebra, the largest and most narrowly striped of zebra species, sheds up to a third of a litre of superfluous sperm (see Figure 3.3). Sperm expulsion times vary across species. Sperm dumping can occur during copulation (previously stored sperm is rejected), immediately after, or, in the case of one leaf-eating beetle, up to a day after sexual activity.

Strong genital musculature, leading to pressure changes in the vagina, is the mechanism believed to underpin many females' sperm removal technique. A study of the small soil nematode worm (*Coenorhabditis elegans*) provides a dramatic and almost violent example of the contractile forces involved in voiding sperm. Under the microscope, sexual activity involving virgin female soil worms revealed that in 42 per cent of 102 copulations, the female apparently rejected some or all of the recently deposited semen from her uterus.

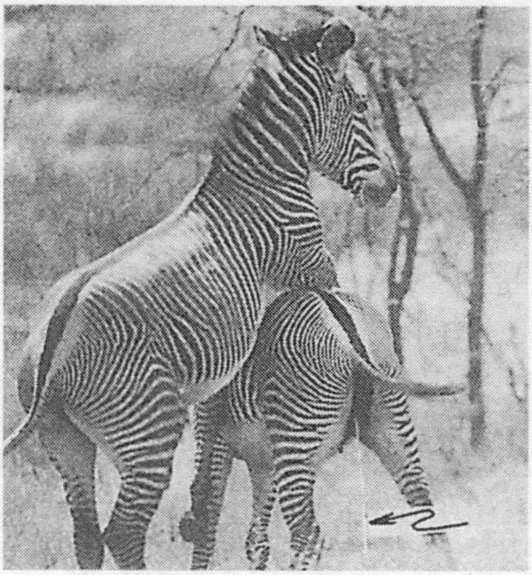

Figure 3.3 The female Grevy's zebra ejects up to a third of a litre of superfluous sperm.

'The vulva would open and the entire mass of seminal fluid would appear to be blown out of the uterus under pressure. This usually resulted in the spicules [phalluses] of the male also being blown out of the vulva,' commented the researchers.

Sperm removal manoeuvres also differ depending on the consistency of the sperm deposited. In those animals that receive sperm in the form of packages, or spermatophores, or those who receive sperm that coalesces into a solid plug, the trick is to reach down to the vagina and gnaw or tug the plug out. Squirrels pull sperm plugs out with their teeth, while rats gnaw away at an inserted plug, and ease its removal by shedding their vaginal lining. Many insect females simply devour pre-packed ejaculates. Immediately after copulation, female Anolis lizards wipe their cloaca by dragging it along the ground.

The precise role of female expulsion of sperm is still unclear. This is not surprising given that recognition of the phenomenon is very much in its infancy. One suggestion is that female ejection of sperm could provide females with a way of rejecting a male as a potential father, even after accepting him as a copulation partner and taking his sperm. Evidence is now accruing that some females do seem to eject sperm selectively, thus using the manoeuvre as a way of biasing paternity. For female chickens, social status appears to be the deciding factor. After a cockerel has deposited about 100 million sperm in her cloaca, the female feral fowl is more likely to walk away squirting 80 million sperm back out of her cloaca if she was inseminated by a subordinate, rather than a dominant, male.

Selective sperm expulsion is also known to be practised by the female fresh-water damselfly (*Paraphlebia quinta*). As usual, females control both the initiation of copulation (the female has to bend her abdomen forward to a 'wheel position') and the termination point. However, for this species, sperm dumping occurs during copulation and is the product of previous sexual activity. Curiously, it appears that it is the male's sexual style that influences whether a female will dump previously stored sperm. That is, if his copulation performance is up to scratch, then he has a better chance of fathering offspring. Studies show that emission of stored sperm during copulation is more likely to occur when females copulated with clear-winged damselfly males – who tend to copulate for twice as long (on average forty-one minutes) as their darker-winged brothers. For female damselflies, the mechanism of sperm ejection seems to allow them to change their minds when someone 'better' comes along.

Sisters are doing it for themselves

If a male's sperm have not been summarily digested, destroyed or ejected, they are ready to have a shot at determining the paternity of a female's eggs. However, while accounts of this stage of the sperm's odyssey typically evoke images of valiant sperm battling to be the first to reach the treasure trove of the female's eggs, or describe the heroic endeavour of a spermatozoa as it struggles to swim vigorously onwards and upwards, such imagery is fallacious. Sperm do not get to the egg under their own steam; rather, females must actively transport sperm. It is the female's body which is the prime mover at this stage of sexual reproduction too. Although sperm do have a bit part to play in getting to the egg, sperm motility, the little independent motion sperm possess, is not thought to kick in until later in their vaginal voyage, and is triggered by female fluids present further up her reproductive tract. Instead, an array of animals, including insects, mammals, birds, spiders, molluscs, lizards and nematode worms, are known to rely on the female's morphology and physiology to transport sperm.

Female-mediated sperm transport is a sophisticated affair, consisting of a series of interactions, controlled predominantly by the female's nervous system, which together tug and pull sperm to the target of the female's choosing. Depending on the female, the sperm's destination could be her sperm-storage sac, her sperm-digesting pouch, her fertilisation site or the exit to the outside world. For example, female snails store the sperm of some males, while the sperm of others will be sent to the sperm-digesting pouch. The female's reproductive ducts, her long and convoluted subterranean system connecting the various sites (insemination, fertilisation, storage and digestion) within her body, are of particular importance in selectively transporting sperm. When viewed as a device simply for connecting sperm with eggs, their design does not make sense, but when viewed as a structure to selectively transport some sperm, and not others, the engineering of this internal duct system begins to make sense. As well as weaving and winding tortuously towards a female's eggs, in some insects and spiders the female's duct system is often slender to the point of being nothing more than a straitjacket for sperm. The ducts of the tiny mite *Caloglyphus berlesi* are so narrow that only a single sperm can pass through at a time. Such tight environments effectively silence the one-tailed swimming efforts of sperm, leaving them at the mercy of the machinations of the female's body.

Muscles placed strategically along the female's duct system, and her spermatheca, underpin the female's ability to move sperm. Waves of muscular contractions (predominantly moving in the direction of the uterus) typically force sperm along the female's coiling reproductive tract. However, a female's duct musculature can be an obstacle too. Contractions of the duct muscles of one parasitic wasp (*Dahlbominus fusipennis*) constrict sperm movement into or out of a sharp bend in her reproductive canal. Once again, this female's reproductive canal is so slender that only a single sperm can pass at a time. Muscular valves preventing or allowing upstream flow along the female's reproductive tract are also in place. Dogs provide an awesome illustration of the contractile forces that a female's reproductive tract can muster. About one minute after copulation is over, a bitch's uterus begins to contract in a powerful pulsing movement. Like an internal ejaculation, the contractions of uterine muscle shoot sperm towards her oviduct. These muscular compressions are so strong that they produce sufficient pressure to shoot streams of semen a distance of between 20 and 25 cm.

Also manipulating the movement of sperm is the suck and push of the absorption and secretion of vaginal, cervical or spermathecal gland fluids. These female fluids sometimes smooth the sperm's passage, but can also coagulate and accumulate, effectively smothering sperm. Working in conjunction with the female's muscular contractions and fluid secretions and absorptions is the rhythmic beating and beckoning of the fine ciliary hairs that line the internal labyrinth duct system. Bands of these waving cilia create currents flowing either upstream towards the egg, or downstream, flushing sperm out. The net result, from the female's perspective, is a finely tuned transport system. From the male's perspective it is more of a headache. One flex of muscle, or beat of cilia, and some sperm will be shunted into storage, while others will be headed for a digestion pouch, or ejection. It's up to the female. A more appropriate spermatic image that has been suggested is that of a school of tiny fish swirled by the ebb and flow of the waves, and often dashed against the rocks.

The ovum, the female's egg, represents the final obstacle that the sperm must negotiate on its vaginal voyage. This is the pivotal point of the process – the moment when the large egg meets the small sperm (eggs are approximately eighty thousand times bigger than the sperm). Like many other aspects of internal fertilisation this event is typically misrepresented. Usually described as the moment when the sperm penetrates the egg, a more correct description of the processes involved (which are still not fully understood) is one of the egg 'swallowing and then gently coddling' the sperm. Even at the level of fusion, the egg is much more active than the sperm. Indeed, without the initiation of active processes by the egg, sperm are essentially helpless. It is the egg's responses to nearby sperm that are critical in pulling sperm towards and inside the egg, and once embraced, enveloped and then engulfed by the enormous egg, sperm are reliant on the egg's interior resources to first decondense or unravel their nucleus, and then reactivate the sperm's DNA.

Hints are also emerging that, during the final stages of fertilisation, the female is still sizing up which combination of gametes (egg and sperm) she prefers. Just prior to fusion occurring there is a major difference between the egg and sperm pronuclei sitting within the ovum. Sperm cells are haploid – containing only a single set of chromosomes – whereas egg cells are diploid – containing a double set of chromosomes. So, for fusion to take place, the female has to make a choice: one set of her chromosomes must be rejected, and the other retained and used to fuse with the sperm's set. This final step, choosing which set of her chromosomes to pair up with the male's single chromosome set, is, some scientists suggest, one last way in which females control the genetic make-up of their offspring. If this is the case, female choice and control over sexual reproduction is truly far-ranging – operating far further than ever imagined.

A muscular marvel of engineering

One of the most important realisations of the vaginal revolution in reproductive biology is that female genitalia can never be looked at again as simple passive vessels for sperm and offspring. As more and more aspects of vaginal architecture are uncovered, the remarkable feat of engineering that internally fertilising genitalia represents is finally being revealed and appreciated. It's a story of an astonishingly complex and sensitive subterranean system, of sperm-storage sites, coiled and curving canals, of strategically placed muscles and valves, all delicately tuned to support optimal sexual reproduction. Take the female marsh-dwelling bug (*Hebrus pusillus*). This insect illustrates and encapsulates beautifully the importance of female genital architecture and musculature in achieving exquisite control over the movement of sperm. Not only are this tiny bug's steely genital muscles brought into service for transporting sperm; she also uses them to suck sperm from the male's phallus, and to route sperm into storage sites.

The result is impressive: the female's genitalia controls not just sperm transport, but also sperm transfer and storage. How the semi-aquatic bug achieves this level of control is astounding. The first step is harvesting the male's sperm, which takes place in the bug's gynantrial complex or sac. Harvesting is completely under the female's control, because the male does not possess a sperm pump. Instead, the walls of the female's gynantrial sac are lined with numerous dilator muscles, arranged in such a way that their contractions suck sperm out of the male's genitalia with a vigorous pumping action as he withdraws at the end of a copulation bout.

The second step is to transport sperm from the gynantrial sac to

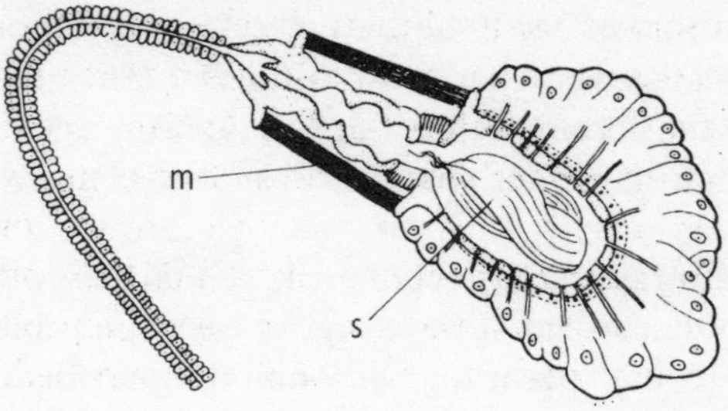

Figure 3.4 A muscular marvel of engineering: when this *Gramphosoma* insect's spermatheca compressor muscles (m) contract, they shoot sperm (s) down the spermathecal duct.

her spermatheca. Muscles strung along the coils of the spermathecae (which loop round and round an average thirty-nine times) contract and relax, causing the spermathecal coils to compress and extend, pulling in sperm. A muscular pump at the entrance to the spermatheca also helps to transport the sperm into the spermatheca, as perhaps does sperm movement itself. Once stored, sperm stay here until an egg is close by. Finally another set of muscles in the bug's fecundation canal come into play. These muscles stretch and release the fecundation canal, positioning its opening opposite the opening (the micropyle) in the bug's egg. Finally, her spermathecal muscles contract and relax again, pumping sperm out of storage and on to her egg. It's an impressive, muscular yet mind-boggling female-dominated sperm transport system. Who would have thought that female insects had such intricate reproductive machinery and were so in control?

Muscular mechanisms for moving sperm into and out of storage exist in many animal groups. Many insect females alter the shape and volume of their spermathecae by contracting or relaxing muscles arranged around the spermatheca and the bursa (vagina). In this way storage pouches can expand to accommodate greater amounts of sperm, and contract to release sperm. The need for female genitalia to be able to transport and store sperm has resulted in one heteropteran insect (*Gramphosoma*) having a remarkable syringelike spermatheca (see Figure 3.4). In this insect, the strong compressor muscles surrounding the spermathecal opening contract, shooting sperm out of storage and down the spermathecal duct. In other species, including spiders, the entrance (insemination duct) to a female's spermatheca is separate from the exit (fertilisation duct). In such species, the insemination duct is typically more tortuous in design, making entry to the sperm storage site far more difficult than leaving.

The increasing appreciation of female genital design has also led to the realisation that sperm-storage organs are responsible for far more than simply storing sperm and decoupling insemination from fertilisation in time and space. Indeed, it's becoming apparent that spermathecae have been designed with another function in mind too – namely, the selective (as opposed to random) transport and use of sperm. In fact, possessing a spermatheca appears to offer one of the best opportunities for females to use sperm selectively, and thus manipulate paternity by biasing which sperm will sire her offspring. If a female has more than one spermatheca, and many do, the pattern in which her sperm sacs are filled can make a reproductive difference.

The female fruit fly, *Drosophila melanogaster*, like many flies, has three spermathecae. Two are slightly smaller, and the female fly typically fills these two pouches up first, before using the larger central sac. However, the sperm in this last-to-be-filled-up organ are the first to be used when the female fertilises her eggs. Female dunnocks, the birds that mate at least twenty times a day, leave some sperm storage tubules empty, while others nearby are packed full. Other species, including the green anole lizard and the Japanese quail, have also been shown to exhibit marked variations in the degree of filling of different storage tubules.

Studies also show that females may copulate with one male to ensure a supply of sperm, but if what she perceives as a 'better' male comes along, she will copulate with him, and preferentially use his sperm to fertilise her egg. One recognised mechanism for selectively using sperm is to pack a particular male's sperm in one sac, and that of a different partner in another, something that the humble yellow dung fly, *Scathophaga stercoraria*, has been spotted doing. The female yellow dung fly has three muscle-lined spermathecae, each with its own duct. Two of the spermathecae form a pair, surrounded by a common envelope and partly connected by muscles. The third spermatheca is a singlet. However, this small fly does not store and use sperm equally. She prefers to fertilise her eggs with sperm that she earlier stored in her paired spermatheca. Intriguingly, studies show that after mating with more than one male, the female chooses to store the sperm of her larger mating partner in her paired spermatheca, thus biasing paternity towards larger males. Whether factors other than the size of the male are important in determining which spermatheca sperm are stored in is as yet unclear.

Female side-blotched lizards provide a stunning example of how stored sperm can be used selectively – and how larger is not always better. These lizards, which are the most common in the American west, typically mate with five or six males during a particular reproductive cycle, storing this sperm in their spermathecae for up to two months before using it to fertilise their eggs. Incredibly, though, female side-blotched lizards are able to use sperm selectively from large male lizards to sire sons, and sperm from small male lizards to father daughters. That is, their genitalia are capable of both recognising and sorting X-chromosome (female) sperm from Y-chromosome (male) sperm, as well as choosing the genes of large lizards to make sons and small lizards to make daughters.

As yet, however, neither the physical mechanism for sorting different-sized males' sperm, nor the method of differentiating between 'male' and 'female' sperm is clear. What is known is that females selectively fertilise their eggs with sperm from different-sized males because there is an evolutionary advantage associated with this practice. Putting the genes of large males into male offspring, and the genes of small males into female offspring, results in sons and daughters with high levels of fitness (genes for large male body size are in sexual conflict when put into daughters and vice versa). Hence it makes evolutionary sense for the females to have the ability to selectively use sperm, and to have multiple mating partners.

The intelligent vagina

Although not often viewed or described as such, female genitalia are incredibly efficient and precise hot-blooded sperm-sorting machines. In fact, courtesy of their reproductive geography, with its carefully placed muscles, valves, tortuous bends, narrow ducts and storage and digestion sites, many females are capable of almost unbelievably fine control over the movement of sperm. This is despite the fact that males display a great deal of seminal exuberance, typically depositing millions of sperm at a time, many more than are necessary, and forcing females to downsize sperm numbers drastically. Yet females are so internally flexible that they are able to perform such a selective and destructive deed, routinely, without compromising their fertility. For example, the female golden or Syrian hamster achieves fertilisation rates of nearly 100 per cent, despite only ever transporting a tiny fraction of the hundreds of millions of sperm deposited to her ampulla, her fertilisation site. It is still not clear how her reproductive tract is flexible and fine-tuned enough to hold back hundreds of millions of sperm, while at the same time always letting a few through. Similarly, in insects like the fruit fly, a 40 per cent reduction in ejaculate size does not reduce female fertility.

The vagina also seems to be able to sense how much sperm it has retained. Indeed, studies of moths and butterflies (*Lepidoptera*) show that females have evolved several mechanisms to detect and gauge the volume of sperm received, including the presence of sensitive stretch receptors in the walls of their *bursa copulatrix* (vagina). Incredibly, the vagina is intelligent enough to recognise if a male deposits too few sperm. Faced with a famine, rather than feast, of sperm, the female reproductive tract makes precise adjustments to increase the number of sperm retained. Rabbits are among the mammals that demonstrate precise regulation of sperm numbers. Post-copulation, which in the rabbit induces ovulation ten hours later, sperm numbers are reduced by a factor of about 10,000 as sperm are moved from the vagina into the oviduct. This 10,000–fold reduction typically brings the number of sperm in the rabbit's oviduct to between 1,000 and 2,000 sperm. These numbers then stay remarkably constant while ovulation occurs. Even when indulging in multiple, as compared to single, matings, female rabbits keep the number of sperm retained in their oviduct in the same narrow range.

Female genitalia need to be able to exercise such exquisite precision over the movement of sperm for a number of reasons. As well as avoiding too many sperm reaching the vicinity of the egg, barriers in place along the female's reproductive tract must be able to filter out damaged, old, malformed or merely less competent, or unfit sperm and prevent them from reaching the egg. The successful sexual reproduction of a species relies on the vagina being able to perform this sorting and screening process effectively. Studies of the domestic chicken showed that when sperm from low-fertility cockerels is introduced into the uterus of females (bypassing the vagina), large numbers of sperm reached the chicken's fertilisation site (the infundibulum), and consequently large numbers of eggs were fertilised. However, a high percentage of these embryos died before any eggs were laid.

In contrast, when the same low-quality sperm was introduced into the bird's vagina, and the chicken herself transported the sperm (or not) to her infundibulum, only a few eggs were fertilised. Critically, though, those embryos that were formed were more likely to be normal, indicating the vagina's ability to screen and sort sperm. Studies involving 'normal' cockerel sperm also demonstrated this female screening ability. Typically 20 per cent of sperm shows some kind of structural defect, yet the sperm that females ferry to their sperm storage tubules are those without such flaws.

Mammals, including humans, also demonstrate vaginal screening properties. In all well-studied mammals, when fertilisation is carried out *in vitro* (outside the body and independent of female genitalia) it routinely results in large numbers of abnormal embryos. It is also now being realised that when such recently developed fertility techniques as intracytoplasmic sperm injection (ICSI) are carried out, they are far more likely to result in embryos with chromosomal abnormalities or embryo death. It is known that fertilisation is a complex and easily disrupted affair, and, as more and more studies show, without the assistance of female genitalia in selecting sperm, fertilisation all too easily goes awry. There is a warning here – science may well have taken the idea of the vagina as a passive vessel too far. In neglecting to consider the specialised role of female genitalia in selecting and transporting 'suitable' sperm, biological problems may be being bred. Human health may be compromised.

Finding Mr Right

The vagina's ability to select sperm goes far deeper than merely sorting the wheat from the chaff. Until recently it was assumed that because the DNA of sperm is so tightly wound and packed inside the sperm's head, the true genetic nature of the male was invisible, or unreadable to the female and her reproductive tract. An increasing number of studies suggest that this is not true, and that females have the ability to judge a male's potential as a father, not only by his external appearance and behaviour, but also at the level of his sperm, by assessing his internal genetic make-up.

Studies of the fruit fly, the world's most studied insect, highlight how female fruit flies can detect differences in the genetic make-up of sperm, and subsequently bias their treatment of sperm accordingly – some sperm is stored more rapidly and in greater numbers than others, some is used preferentially to fertilise eggs, while other sperm, on the basis of its genetic script, is rejected. The female fruit fly's genitals can distinguish both between sperm within a single ejaculate, and between sperm from different males. Incredibly, research suggests that once sperm with a particular genotype is discriminated against, female genitalia appear to be able to 'remember' the sperm type they have previously rejected, and will do so again.

Mice provide an even more remarkable example of how female genitalia appear to be able to read or size up sperm. Studies of female mice show that they possess an astounding and remarkable internal ability to choose the right father for their offspring. Female mice, it seems, are capable of choosing Mr Right Sperm from Mr Wrong. Research shows that they bias paternity by selecting the sperm of the male that is most compatible or complementary to them in terms of their individual genetic make-up. For mice, birds and other mammals, including humans, the major histocompatability complex (MHC), which is associated with resistance to disease, plays a vital role in choosing the right mate. Individuals with MHCs that are complementary to each other produce viable offspring, whereas the embryos of individuals with incompatible MHCs are aborted.

In mice, the ability of the female's reproductive tract to recognise which sperm are more compatible than others results in those complementary sperm being transported more quickly and in greater numbers to her Fallopian tubes. Sperm that the female reads as a bad match are left behind. In effect, a female's genitalia allow her to strip a male bare and see behind any artifice. By reading his DNA she can see what he's really made of. The vagina, more than any other arena, is where males are forced to reveal their true colours, and prove their fitness to be fathers.

Variety is the spice of life

For a female, possessing the genitalic power to select which sperm are more compatible to her is of utmost importance. The advent of DNA fingerprinting techniques is revealing that it is the genetic complementarity or compatibility of two individuals, rather than their size or status, that is of prime importance in determining the viability of any offspring they may have. In birds, research investigating the DNA fingerprints of female and male partners reveals that if a couple's DNA fingerprints are more similar (less complementary) it is far more likely that any eggs resulting from their sexual union will fail to develop or hatch. Likewise a study of sand lizards showed that females were less likely to produce offspring with males that were genetically more similar to them. The adage that there is strength in diversity is true.

The realisation that a female's genitalia are capable of selecting sperm, and thus biasing paternity, on the basis of whether or not the male's sperm is compatible with the female's own genetic make-up, has also supplied scientists with an answer to why females prefer to have multiple mating partners. Practising polyandry provides females with the opportunity to sample a variety of types of sperm, and select the ones that suit them the best. The more partners a female tries the more likely she is to find Mr Right, or, more correctly, Mr Most Genetically Compatible (and that should not be Mr in the singular). That is, the more mates a female has, the greater her reproductive success is likely to be.

Studies investigating the population of a group of adders in southern Sweden showed precisely this – multiple mating by females improved their reproductive success. The female adders that copulated with multiple males produced fewer stillborn or physically deformed offspring than the female snakes that had only a single partner. A recent study of pseudoscorpions, tiny tailless scorpions, illustrated remarkably clearly that increased female fertility is a direct consequence of practising polyandry. Virgin female pseudoscorpions that were mated with two males gave birth to 33 per cent more offspring than those females that were allowed only one partner (each female received the same amount of sperm).

Because female pseudoscorpions have transparent wombs, this research was able to reveal a more complete picture of what happens to developing embryos. Females that had enjoyed a selection of partners aborted 32 per cent fewer embryos than their single-partner sisters. For female pseudoscorpions, sampling the sperm of multiple males makes sound reproductive sense, as it drastically reduces the costly time and energy involved in producing, and then having to abort, an embryo. Indeed, many other studies involving other species have reached the same conclusion. Multiple mating – polyandry – is the best sexual strategy for a female in terms of ensuring her optimal reproductive success, because it enables her to choose her most complementary males.

The idea of the compatibility of two individuals being the key component in ensuring optimal reproductive success signifies an about-turn in understanding sexual reproduction. Scientists, and others, have been hung up for some time on the idea of the supermale, the male that can be everything to every female. Like the western world's favourite comic book hero, Superman, biology's supermale was seen as the male that every female wants, and that every male aspires to be. However, what studies of the multiple-mating practices of females and their resulting offspring show is that there is no such thing as this single supermale. What each and every female really, really wants if she is to enjoy optimal reproductive success is to find the males that she best measures up with. If, via her sexual behaviour and her intelligent vagina, she can find these best-matched fathers-to-be then she gives her offspring the best possible start in life. It seems that variety really is the spice of life – for both females and males.

This, then, is the true function of female genitalia – to enable females to sample and select the sperm of males in order to find the sperm that is most compatible with them. Far from being a passive vessel, female genitalia in fact enshrine one of the most important jobs of life – that of ensuring the optimum health of offspring, and thus the survival of a species.

4

EVE'S SECRETS

When last we looked at a woman's vagina the view was of the cunnus. But that is not the full view of a woman's external genitalia. Part a woman's external labia, her labia majora, and a vastly different sight emerges – take a look. Arranged in delicate curves, contours and folds, a woman's clitoris and inner labia glisten and shimmer. Some labia create beautiful heart-shaped forms, others more oval outlines. Tiny scalloped curves trace the point where labia and clitoris come closest together, as the inner labia become part of the clitoral crown. Rosy pink, russet brown, vermilion red, all these lustrous, vivid vaginal hues and more form a visual feast.

A delicious asymmetry is also here, with some labia longer or more curved than others. With some vulvas, clitorises nudge out from underneath their clitoral hood, others push forwards more prominently, some with a distinctive, delicious nasal aspect. All are unique. And right at the heart of each vulva, a woman's vestibule shines, whether aroused or not. The full vaginal picture is, I feel, an awe-inspiring rich work of art (see colour plate section), a glorious jewel. There is a delightful story to tell here too, a history full of twists and secrets. Eve's secrets. Importantly, it's a history that reveals the multiple facets of this vaginal vision. We'll start with the clitoris.

Imagine a wishbone, the two-winged seed of a maple tree or sycamore, an inverted Y, a tuning fork or the eleventh letter of the Greek alphabet, λ, lambda. Trace the shape, from the curved, delicate protuberant tip, across the crown, and down the shaft, to the point where the bifurcation begins, as the body separates into two legs or wings. This design – incorporating crown, corpus (body) and crura (legs) – is the blueprint of the clitoris. An elegant tripartite structure, with, surprisingly to many, far more to it than meets the eye. Indeed, only the clitoris' uppermost tip, the exquisitely sensitive crown, projects out and beyond the vulva, making it visible to any observer. To sense the rest of a woman's wishbone-shaped clitoris, touch is needed.

The body or shaft – a column of clitoral tissue – ranges upwards and backwards into the pelvic area, in intimate connection with the urethra. Its dimensions (between 2 and 4 cm long and between 1 and 2 cm wide) can't be seen, but a portion can be felt by applying rolling finger pressure around the area behind and around the clitoral crown. And tapering further back still, the long legs of the clitoris anchor this shockingly responsive sensual structure deep inside a woman's sexual heart. These legs or crura, which measure between 5 and 9 cm long, effectively embrace or straddle the barrel of the vagina, shooting out the erotic and sensual sensations that can make a woman quiver with delight.

The news that the clitoris was composed of crown, corpus and crura, and was a much much larger organ than previously imagined, made world news headlines at the start of August 1998. For the very first time in history, this much misunderstood, yet much loved mouthful of female sexual anatomy made the front page. The clitoris, an Australian urology and surgery team reported, is at least twice as large as anatomy textbooks depict, and tens of times larger than most people realise. The world's media (at least in the west) lapped up the words of discovery, and a myriad articles on clitoral size and structure were spawned.

For me, the steady stream of articles on the amazing size and structure of the clitoris was an occasion for celebration. This information about the clitoris in all its glory was news to me too. Yes, I'd known since I was a young girl that something particular about the outside of my vagina made it feel good to be touched. That was my first discovery of the clitoris – a physical one. However, the fact that there was a particular name attached to that section of my sexual flesh eluded me for years. I still can't remember for sure when I found out that the word clitoris existed, and I know I'm not alone in that uncertainty. I'm told that by eighteen I was conscious of this fact, and was passing on my knowledge. I wish I could remember when I made this, my second, and this time cerebral, discovery of the clitoris, but I just can't seem to recall where my information came from. Possibly a book.

But words can deceive, smear, confuse and con. As a child, with only my body to guide me, I'd conceived vaguely of the whole area as being ultra-sensitive and feelgood. For me at that stage it was a nebulous region. Then came the words and pictures, in my teens and twenties. But the words of this era, the time when I was sowing the seeds of my sex life, were sharp and pointed, reductive in their impact. Button, cherry, bell, spot, small, pearl. They reduced my idea of what the clitoris was to a confined and finite spot. A blob of tissue. All nerve endings crammed into this one small space. I, and others, consequently played with it as such – a knob to be twiddled, a button to be flicked, a third nipple to be tweaked. This source of pleasure became bounded. It took the words and pictures of an Australian research team to make me view my clitoris (and then the rest of my vagina) in a completely different light. Not as a button, bell or pearl perched atop the vaginal opening, or an isolated mass of nerve endings. No, this research stated, and showed me diagrammatically, that my clitoris was an incredible expanding, highly sensitive structure sunk deep, and tethered well, inside me. It was only then that my clitoris became a vibrant three-dimensional part of me.

Did Colombo discover the clitoris?

I am not alone in my multiple clitoral revelations. Indeed, multiple discoveries are one of the clitoris' key characteristics. History is littered with them. Take the Renaissance, a period when all and sundry seemed to be sticking their flagpole into a piece of flesh and naming or renaming it for their own. The clitoris was not exempt from this fashion. Science gave its greatest honours – the bestowing of your own special name on a piece of flesh (an organ to call your own) – to those who discovered previously unmanned, unmapped virgin territory. And so, approaching 450 years ago, the Italian anatomists Matteo Realdo Colombo of Cremona and Gabriel Fallopius, the man who gave his name to the Fallopian tubes, locked horns in a dispute over who was the first man to discover that special piece of female sexual anatomy.

Writing about the clitoris in his work *De Re Anatomica*, published in Venice in 1559, Colombo says: 'if you touch it, you will find it rendered a little harder and oblong to such a degree that it shows itself as a sort of male member. Since no one has discerned these projections and their workings, if it is permissible to give names to things discovered by me, it should be called "the love or sweetness of Venus" [*dulcedo amoris*].' He goes on to describe the clitoris as 'pre-eminently the seat of woman's delight', noting: 'You who happen to read these laboriously produced anatomical studies of mine know that, without these protuberances [the clitoris] which I have faithfully described to you earlier, women would neither experience delight in venereal embraces nor conceive any foetuses.'

Meanwhile, Gabriel Fallopius, one of Colombo's peers at Padua University, staked his claim to be the first to uncover the clitoris. In his *Observationes Anatomicae* published in Venice in 1561, one year before his death at the age of thirty-nine, Fallopius wrote:

> Avicenna ... mentions a part positioned in the female pudendum and calls it a penis or rather *al bathara* [the Arabic word translated as meaning the clitoris]. Albucasim ... calls it the tension. It sometimes can reach a growth so remarkable in some women that they can have coitus with each other, like men fornicating. This part is still called by the Greeks the clitoris, and from this term is still found the verb clitorising used in an obscene sense ... Truly our anatomists completely neglected it and do not even speak of it ... This small part corresponds to the male penis ... This very private part, small in size and hidden in the very fatty part of the pubis, has remained unknown to the anatomists, so that up to now from the preceding years I am the first to describe it, and if there have been others who have spoken of it or written about it, be it known that they have not heard it spoken of by me or by those who have heard me and, therefore, only for this reason, there is not a good knowledge about it. You will easily find the end of this kind of penis in the upper part of the external pudendum, exactly where the 'hanging wings' [the inner labia] ... come together or where they begin.

The third man to enter this clitoral fray in Italy was Thomas Bartholin, the son of the Danish anatomist Kaspar Bartholin (it is Thomas' son, Kasper II, whose name adorns a female's Bartholin glands). Fifty years after Fallopius' comments on the clitoris, Thomas Bartholin produced *Anatomy*, a revision of his father's anatomical manuscript, *Institutiones Anatomicae*. Figure 2.5 shows Bartholin's dissections and drawings of the clitoris and vagina. On the nature of the clitoris, he wrote that it was 'the female yard or prick' because it 'resembles a man's yard in situation, substance, composition, repletion with spirits, and erection', and because it 'hath somewhat like the nut and foreskin of a Man's Yard'. Tellingly, though, Bartholin's text also criticises both Colombo and Fallopius for their attitude in claiming the 'invention or first Observation of this part'. The man from Copenhagen noted that the clitoris had been known to everyone since the second century.

Bartholin was right to censure the two Italians. What they were squabbling over was not a new discovery, as Gabriel Fallopius so obviously understood with his comments on earlier references. Yet neither man was prepared to cede ground to the other. The period in which their dogfight took place was aptly named the Renaissance, for it was a period of rebirth, of rediscovering the highlights of the heyday of the Greeks and Romans, after being stuck in the mud of the Middle Ages. Yes, new discoveries and inventions occurred, but they were all rooted in understanding and appreciating what had gone before. Likewise with the clitoris. Although it may have appeared under different names through the preceding centuries, knowledge of the clitoris, its physical appearance and function was evident in both ancient literature and anatomical texts.

Enter the clitoris

Greek-born physician Galen, in his work *On the Usefulness of the Parts*, writes about a mysterious part which offers 'no small usefulness in inciting the female to the sexual act and in opening wide the neck of the womb [the vagina] during coitus'. Galen goes on to say that the part in question extends out to the pudenda, is sinewy and becomes straight during intercourse. He also describes a man's penis as being a sinewy body that becomes erect. Interestingly, Galen saw the clitoris as an organ which gave protection to the vagina, and compared this with the protection that the uvula – the small, fleshy, finger-like flap of tissue which hangs down the back of the soft palate – gives to the throat.

As above, so below analogies between the mouth, neck and throat and the uterus, cervix and vagina were common during Galen's time and survived for many centuries, with some still having resonance today (as we'll see later). Indeed, nineteenth-century medical illustrations emphasised how the view into the aperture of the larynx looks remarkably like a woman's vulva. Medical knowledge of the clitoris was not just confined to the western world. In his work *Of the Vagina*, which relies heavily on Galen's original ideas, the Arabic physician Avicenna (Ali ibn Sina), who lived from 980–1037, refers to the clitoris (*al bathara*) too.

One of the most detailed early descriptions of a woman's external genitalia and the various names of the parts, complete with the correct verb to use when talking about the clitoris, is found in the first-century writings of the Greek physician Rufus.

As far as the external genital parts of the woman are concerned, some refer to these as the pudendi, others as the pubis, the triangular extremity of the hypogastrium [abdomen]. The cleft is the opening of their external genital parts. The little piece of muscular flesh in its middle, called the nymphae, also the fruit of the myrtle, is the skin that is also named the clitoris, and one says clitorising to express the lascivious touching of this part. The lips of the myrtle [the outer folds] are the fleshy parts that detach themselves to each side; Euryphon names these also the steep slopes – today, on the one hand, one substitutes the expression hanging wings (pterigomata) for the outer folds, and, on the other, nymphae for the fruit of the myrtle [the inner folds].

The fact that the second-century doctor Soranus of Ephesus described the clitoris in his work *Gynaecology*, which was the major gynaecology reference text for the next 1,500 years, should have been enough for Colombo to realise that he couldn't take credit for discovery of the clitoris. Soranus used the archaic word *landica* (possibly derived from the Greek letter lambda) to describe the clitoris, commenting:

What is the woman's sinus [uterus]? A nervous membrane similar to that of the large intestine: very spacious on the inside, it is, on the outside – where coitus and the acts of love take place – rather narrow; it is vulgarly called cunnus; outside are the labia, called pterigomata in Greek and pinnacula in Latin; from the upper part there comes down into the middle what is called the landica [clitoris].

The fact that information about the clitoris must have been available to the Renaissance men is also highlighted by the words of Pietro d'Abano (1250–*c.* 1320), a physician at Padua University, some three hundred years before Colombo and Fallopius. In his major medical work, the *Conciliator Differentiarum*, d'Abano wrote: 'Women are driven to desire by having the upper orifice near their pubis rubbed; in this way the indiscreet bring them to orgasm.'

It seems that neither Colombo nor Fallopius had done their homework very thoroughly. The clitoris was known of and named long before either man set eyes on it. They were not the discoverers of the clitoris in the true sense of the word, although Fallopius did gain a clitoral first, in that he was the first person to perform and describe the dissection of the deep internal structure of the clitoris. Today it is his peer, Colombo, perhaps by dint of his discovery-oriented name, who is commonly credited with finding the clitoris. *The Anatomist*, a novel by Federico Andahazi, based in part on Colombo's publication *De Re Anatomica*, even expands on this discovery theme. However, Matteo Realdo Colombo as the discoverer of the clitoris is nothing more than a modern myth.

Lost and found

The tale of Colombo and the clitoris appears to have been re-enacted in very recent history. The announcement in 1998 that the clitoris was far larger than previously supposed, and composed of crown, corpus and crura, was not strictly a discovery. More accurately, it was another rebirth of knowledge, and one that was much needed. The shape and structure of the clitoris, as the twentieth-century anatomical team described it, had been depicted before, but, as with other aspects of clitoral knowledge, it had not been widely disseminated, taught or built on. As a result, this information was, apparently, forgotten.

Just eleven years before news of the clitoris' true size and structure made worldwide headlines, a book, *Eve's Secrets: A New Theory of Female Sexuality*, by Harvard graduate and medical researcher Josephine Lowndes Sevely (now out of print), was published. This book made very similar observations on clitoral structure to those of the Australian anatomists. However, Lowndes Sevely, in turn, also revealed how her observations about the design of the clitoris were not strictly a discovery. Instead, she illustrated how they were a reappraisal of an earlier work, by the seventeenth-century Dutch anatomist, Reinier de Graaf.

In 1672, de Graaf had a surprisingly clear understanding of the wishbone structure of the clitoris. His illustrations of the clitoris, dissected in different ways, are shown in Figure 4.1. Crown, corpus and crura are clearly delineated. De Graaf also appears to have appreciated the type of tissue the clitoris is composed of, as well as how deeply the organ is anchored internally. In Chapter III of his *Treatise on the Generative Organs of Women*, which is entitled 'Concerning the Clitoris', de Graaf writes:

> We are extremely surprised that some anatomists make no more mention of this part than if it did not exist at all in the universe of nature. In every female cadaver we have dissected so far we have found it quite perceptible to sight and touch. It is small in some women and larger in others ... The external part of the clitoris is covered by the same membrane as the labia of the pudendum ... The other parts of the clitoris lie hidden in the fatty region of the pubes and for this reason, says Falloppia, they have escaped even the notice of anatomists. We do not want them to escape our notice and shall examine them individually ... The most important in our opinion are two corpora nervosa (nervous bodies) ... they take their origin from the lower part of the pubic bones, each in a distinct place, proceed obliquely downwards on both sides beneath these bones, unite and form a third body ... the bifurcated parts of the clitoris are twice as long as the conjoined parts.

De Graaf considered clitoral function, as well as structure, ending his clitoral chapter by suggesting, significantly, that 'the function of the clitoris is ... to rouse torpid sexual feeling'. He enthuses about the 'sharp and perceptive sensitivity' of the clitoral crown, commenting that 'it is not without justice called the sweetness of love, the gad-fly of Venus'. He also ascribes a reproductive function to the erectile organ, concluding that 'If the clitoris had not been endowed with such an exquisite sensitivity to pleasure and passion, no woman would be willing to take upon herself the irksome 9-months-long business of gestation, the painful and often fatal process of expelling the foetus and the worrisome and care-ridden task of raising children.'

It seems that in the seventeenth century, knowledge of the clitoris was profound. Its existence had been written about and discussed for centuries, its role in sexual pleasure was rejoiced in, and the dimensions of its deep internal and tripartite structure were realised. Yet,

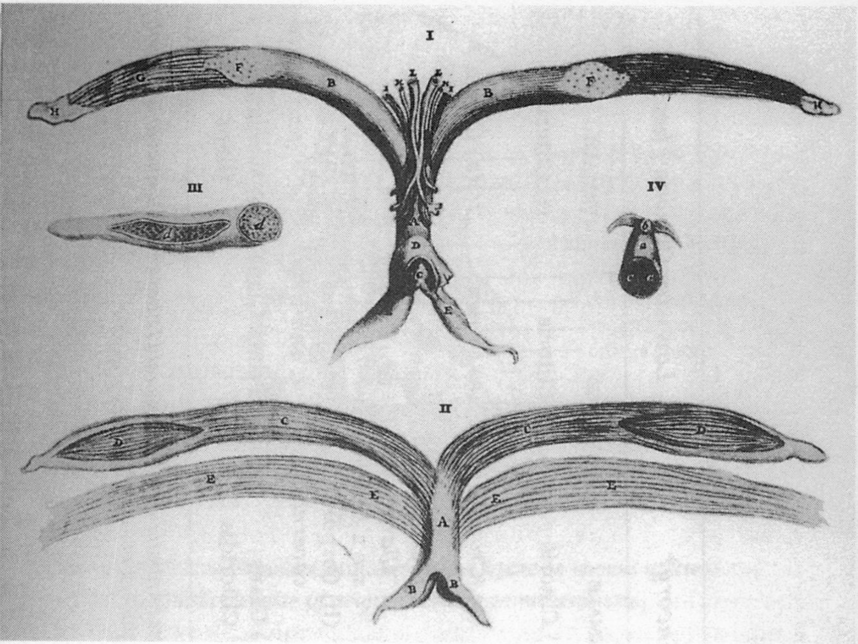

I shows the front of the clitoris

A *clitoris*
B *crura of the clitoris*
C *crown of the clitoris*
D *prepuce of the clitoris*
E *nymphae*
F *part of the periosteum by means of which the crura of the clitoris are connected to the lower part of the pubic bones*
G *muscles of the clitoris*
H *parts of the muscles which implant themselves in the bones of the ischium (or hip)*
I *nerves*
K *arteries*
L *veins*

II shows the back of the clitoris

A *clitoris*
B *nymphae inverted*
C *muscles running through the crura of the clitoris*
D *fleshy fibres of the same muscles forming cavities of a kind*
E *fleshy fibres of the sphincter, linked to the nervous substance of the clitoris*

III and IV show the clitoris dissected in different ways

a *clitoris*
b *crown of the clitoris with its nymphae*
c *spongy substance of the clitoris divided through the middle by the septum*
d *spongy substance of a crus divided through the middle by no septum*

Figure 4.1 The female clitoris: over three hundred years ago, the tripartite nature of the clitoris was appreciated – crown, corpus (body) and crura (legs) (de Graaf, 1672).

over the following three hundred years, each of these three areas of clitoral knowledge would be dismissed, overlooked or forgotten, instead of becoming common knowledge. When I was born, in 1968, anatomy books either overlooked the clitoris altogether, or rendered it as a minute blob of tissue, minus body and legs – a far cry from the generous detail provided by de Graaf. Why the misinformation in a scientifically driven century of information? Why not give the full and frank view available?

Although it is impossible to know for certain, and absolutely, why a large body of clitoral information disappeared sometime between 1672 and 1998, there are some clues. In de Graaf's day, it was felt that female sexual pleasure within marriage was morally acceptable, as female orgasm was understood to be essential for conception to occur (as we'll later see). In the same vein, male sexual pleasure and orgasm was deemed permissible by the religious authorities, as long as it was within the confines of sex for procreation's sake. And because it was viewed as a key to triggering female orgasm (and offspring), studying and disseminating information about the clitoris was sanctioned. However, this perspective on the clitoris (and other aspects of female genitalia) began to change in the late eighteenth century as the realisation that female orgasm was not necessary for conception to occur started to sink in. It took a while, but by the end of the nineteenth century, western medicine had done an about-turn, and the general consensus was that female sexual pleasure and orgasm did not play a role in sexual reproduction.

For the clitoris, this shift in scientific thinking regarding female orgasm meant that it was stripped of its role in reproduction. And without a reproductive function, the clitoris (and female sexual pleasure) could both be frowned upon freely by the Christian church. After all, sex was solely for procreation, not for pleasure. Other knock-on effects of this paradigm shift occurred. Some were broad, and are still with us today. Backed up by supposed scientific reasoning and religious ideology, many male medics went so far as to suggest that women were essentially passionless creatures, incapable of feeling sexual desire, pleasure or orgasm, or deviant if they did.

Other effects were more particular. In textbooks, clitoral anatomy was severely reduced or disappeared altogether. It is suggested that this happened because of societies' misplaced moral sensibilities. Scientific research could only be countenanced if it focused on a subject deemed decent by the authorities of the day (something that is still the case today). In the eighteenth and nineteenth centuries, genital anatomy that was involved in sexual reproduction just about passed the 'decency' test. However, genital anatomy that did not have a role to play in procreation was not a suitable subject. If the clitoris did not contribute to producing offspring, what was the point of representing it in a textbook talking about obstetrics, say, or reproduction? One major obstetrics textbook (published in 1794) chose to state that it would not spend time commenting on the clitoris or other aspects of external female genitalia as these were not pertinent to midwifery. In this way, defining the clitoris as a non-reproductive organ justified its deletion from medical diagrams and discussion. And slowly but surely, the organ itself began to disappear from common, as well as medical knowledge. Hence the lack of accurate clitoral information available to me as a child and young adult. Even in today's supposedly broad-minded western world, it is still difficult to find accurate representations, be it in words or pictures.

Prizing or purging

It is shocking to realise the clitoral downsizing of the nineteenth century was not confined to anatomy textbooks in the west. Redefined as a non-reproductive, i.e. non-essential sexual organ, this portion of the vagina became open to vilification – a scapegoat for supposed female sexual sins. It may seem ironic, but as science made mammoth strides in many fields of research, female genital tissue went from being seen as the seat of a woman's sexual pleasure to a scourge which should be excised in the name of science. Instead of being prized, the clitoris became something to be purged. In the second half of the nineteenth century, and over a period of ten years, the British surgeon Isaac Baker Brown performed clitoridectomies – removal of the clitoris – at his clinic, the London Surgical Home for the Reception of Gentlewomen and Females of Respectability suffering from Curable Surgical Disorders. Science sanctioned these excisions using the convenient 'theory' that removing the clitoris could cure conditions as varied as incontinence, uterine haemorrhaging, hysteria, and mania brought on by masturbation. Indeed, Brown was so renowned for his skills as a surgeon that in 1865 he was elected president of the Medical Society of London. The following year he produced a book promoting clitoral excision – *On the Curability of Certain Forms of Insanity, Epilepsy and Hysteria in Females.* A review of Brown's book in the Christian publication, *The Church Times*, contained the suggestion that the surgical procedure should be recommended to 'suitable' parishioners.

Records from 1879 for the Chelsea Hospital in London reveal that excision of the clitoris and labia became so prevalent that it was the cure of choice for a twenty-one-year-old single woman who was suffering from no more than irregular menstruation. Meanwhile, records also show that a nineteen-year-old girl underwent clitoridectomy for no apparent reason other than the fact that she was unmarried. While cutting out the clitoris was seen as one way of preventing women from masturbating, in the US, cornflakes king J.H. Kellogg had another remedy. He advocated applying 'pure carbolic acid to the clitoris', if girls would not stop pleasuring themselves. It is hard to imagine how anyone could have envisaged that such a cruel and damaging act could be in any way good or healthy for a person. These attitudes towards the clitoris and female sexual pleasure were found elsewhere in the west. Swiss anti-masturbation doctor Tissot pushed propaganda claiming that female masturbation was responsible for clitoral scabbing, and other female 'problems'. According to him, these included vapours, hysteria, incurable jaundice and a uterine fury that, 'depriving them of their modesty and reason, reduced them to the level of the most lascivious of brutes'.

Not surprisingly perhaps, the nineteenth-century fashion for surgically removing female genital tissue in order to correct what were seen as female diseases (but were in fact evidence of female sexuality) went further than excising the clitoris or labia. Ovaries came under the scalpel too. In just one year, 1855, over two hundred ovariotomy operations were carried out in the UK, with a death rate of approaching 50 per cent. Conditions indicating healthy ovary removal included 'masturbation, erotic tendencies, a troublesomeness, simple cussedness and eating like a ploughman'. The US, France and Germany also practised '*die castration der Frauen*'. Significantly, such was the craze for female genital mutilation under the banner of necessary medical surgery that in 1886, one doctor in a British journal wrote:

'... it will soon be somewhat rare to meet with a woman whose sexual organs are entire'. Unnecessary female genital surgery is still performed in the west today, as we shall see later.

Female genital mutilation

To prize or to purge? That it seems is often the question – at least, when it comes to the clitoris. Many cultures, spanning many millennia, have chosen the latter option – purgation, and, worryingly, this brutal and cruel act is still practised. In the world today, it's estimated that between 100 and 132 million girls and women have been forced to undergo female genital mutilation (FGM) as a part of their cultural heritage, and a further two million girls become at risk each year. FGM, which may comprise cutting off part of the clitoris, or part of the inner labia, and/or sewing the outer vaginal lips together, is a shocking world-wide problem. It is prevalent in twenty-seven African countries, in some Middle East and Asian regions, and increasingly in Europe, North America, Australia and New Zealand.

Although the women and men of many cultures which practise FGM are opposed to it, there are also many women and men who, for their own reasons, do not want this act removed. The argument most vociferously cited is that this mutilating act is part of many societies' cultural heritage. Therefore, the flawed reckoning goes, it should not be stopped. Others point out that stopping the practice will not help women because those females that are not cut will not be able to find a place in their society. To be ostracised or circumcised is the choice they are faced with, which is not much of a choice at all. The long history of FGM (some references to it date back to prehistory; for example, a Greek papyrus dated 163 BCE talks of girls from Memphis, Egypt being circumcised), coupled with the opposing views of all the peoples concerned, mean that excising FGM itself from the world's cultures is not a straightforward exercise.

While dubious and unfounded medical reasons were used to support the routine practice of FGM in the nineteenth century in the UK and the US, other societies have justified FGM using alternative arguments. One African belief is that sex with an uncut woman can result in the man suffering a puncture from the 'dart' (clitoris), a notion that contains echoes of tales of *vagina dentata* – the vagina with teeth (which we'll consider in Chapter 5). One Indian myth tells the story of a young man trying to seduce a faithful wife. However, to his dismay, the man discovers that the woman has a saw above her vagina, with which she cuts off his penis.

This idea of the clitoris that can prick, pierce and maim the man, while protecting the woman and her vagina, is also, perhaps, embedded in the fairy tale of Briar Rose, or, as she is better known, Sleeping Beauty. This young princess lies sleeping surrounded by a hedge of thorns, which spike and stab prospective suitors so much that they die miserably. However, when the right man comes along, the thorns vanish, becoming beautiful red and pink roses, and the hedge parts to allow the prince to waken Briar Rose with a kiss. The rose is, of course, a common European symbol for female genitalia.

Other apologia for FGM are more philosophical than physical. The Dogon of Mali believe that both sexes are born with two souls – one female and one male. For women, their male soul is situated in their clitoris, while a man's female soul is found in his foreskin. This idea of humans having an essentially dual or bisexual soul is one that is found in other mythologies and philosophies, perhaps most recently in the ideas of Carl Jung, with his theories of the anima and animus. For Jung, the integration of anima and animus (our female and male natures) is seen as essential to an individual's emotional, physical and spiritual well-being. However, for the Dogon, having a dual nature or soul is deemed to be dangerous in later life, as humans are said to be incapable of maintaining this double nature into adulthood. The Dogon argue that it's safer to be straightforward – a woman should be solely female and a man wholly male. Therefore their answer to this perceived problem is to cut off the contrary soul – via excision of a woman's clitoris and cutting off a man's foreskin (male circumcision).

The Dogon of Mali also credit the clitoris in their creation mythology. According to them, the world became populated after the great god Amma had sex with the female earth. In this version of creation, the earth's vagina is an anthill and her clitoris is a termite mound. However, when Amma attempted to have sex with the earth, the termite mound (her clitoris) rose up to block his way. Thwarted, he cut it down, and then had sex with the earth without any trouble. But the product of this intrinsically flawed first union was the evil and deceitful jackal – a symbol of all the problems of gods and humanity.

There seems to be a word of sexual warning in this story. The message appears to be that the clitoris, or female consent, is crucial in some way in the creation of balanced offspring. Why would this be? Is paying attention to the clitoris a critical factor in ensuring successful sexual reproduction?

A genital guardian angel?

The idea of the clitoris being the guardian of the vagina's best interests (and the woman's) is a common motif in a number of mythologies and fables, together with the idea of punishing women for having too much. Magically, in many of these folklore tales, the clitoris is given a life of its own. In the Trobiand Islanders' story of 'The White Cockatoo and the Clitoris', a woman called Karawata leaves her clitoris (her *kasesa*) to look after her earthbaking oven, while she goes into the garden. However, while she is away, a white cockatoo swoops down and strikes the clitoris, knocking it over. The bird then eats the contents of the oven. The following day, Karawata, hungry, again takes off her clitoris, leaving it to look after the oven while she goes to catch pigs and gather yams. And once again the cockatoo returns to strike the clitoris and consume the food in the oven. On the third day, the same thing happens again – and Karawata and her clitoris, deprived of food, die of hunger. One interpretation of this tale is that the earthbaking oven is a symbol for a woman's womb, with the contents offspring. Looked at in this light, 'The White Cockatoo and the Clitoris' appears to caution women about the perils of not paying attention to their sexuality, that is, dissociating themselves from their genitalia. The result is an empty oven – perhaps the loss of fertility – and eventually death from starvation.

Food and female genitals are core to another Trobiand Island tale, 'The Story of Digawina'. Digawina is a woman with a particular anatomical capacity – she is endowed with genitalia capacious enough to store large amounts of food inside herself. The name Digawina reflects this ability – *diga* means to fill out or pack into, while *wina* is an archaic form of *wila*, vagina. However, Digawina's vaginal talents – she can pack whole bunches of bananas inside herself, as well as large chunks of sugar cane, coconuts and yams – annoy her peers. Too much food disappears into her vagina at the local food distribution meetings, they think. And so the master of the distribution places a large black mangrove crab among the food. This crab cuts through Digawina's clitoris, killing her. The meaning of this tale? One suggestion is that it is a warning to women that if their sexual appetite is too voracious or too threatening to men, then they will be punished by the authorities – in this instance cutting the clitoris.

Controlling female sexuality, women and, ultimately, the paternity of offspring are undoubtedly some of the underlying reasons for practising female genital mutilation. Although many supporters of FGM attempt to deny the connection between cutting the clitoris and achieving sexual control over women, it is underlined in a number of ways. Many Muslim women have their clitoris excised, yet Muslims recognise, and indeed teach, that the clitoris is the source and wellspring of all female passion. Ethnographic evidence also points to FGM as an attempt to control female sexuality. Various African groups view the clitoris as an organ which enables women to enjoy sexual pleasure before marriage, and still remain virgins. However, one extrapolation of this concept is that the clitoris must be removed at puberty in order to concentrate female sexual desire in the vagina. If this is not done, no woman would want to get married, goes the thinking. Anthropologists record that among the Jivaro people of the upper Amazon River, clitoral excision was said to be carried out in order to lessen the extreme sexual passion of women, and give their husbands a much needed rest. Controlling female sexuality and paternity was also behind the practice in ancient Rome of putting one or more rings through the outer labia of female slaves. Today, it is hard to see how cutting a woman's external genitalia and then sewing them up when the husband goes away, only to open them again when he returns, is anything other than a crude and cruel attempt by men to subjugate and control the sex that produces new life.

The fear of women's vaginas wandering (and begetting unknown offspring) if they are not controlled (for example, by marriage) or purged in some way (say by FGM) appears to be a common fear in many male-dominated societies. The prevalence of laws controlling women's sexual and civil rights certainly suggests this. Some myths, like that of Digawina, also appear to function as cautionary tales for women about what will happen if they give full rein to their sexual appetites. The fear of the vagina that is out of male control appears to lie at the root of a genital myth of the Mehinaku people of Brazil. 'The Wandering Vagina' may serve as a reminder of what occurred in the past, as well as being a warning to women of what happens if they let their vaginas wander. It also revolves around sustenance again, and the vagina's search for it. According to Mehinaku mythology:

In ancient times, all the women's vaginas used to wander about. Today women's vaginas stay in one place. One woman of ancient times, Tukwi, had a vagina that was especially foolish. While Tukwi slept, her vagina would crawl about the floor of the house, thirsty and hungry, looking for manioc porridge and fish stew. Creeping about snail-like on the ground, it found the porridge pot and slid the top off. One of the men awoke and listened: 'Aah, nothing but a mouse,' he said, and he went back to sleep. But as the vagina slurped up the porridge, another man awoke and took a brand from the fire to see what was happening. 'What is this?' he said. To him it looked like a great frog, with a nose and an immense mouth. Moving closer, he scorched the vagina with his torch. Oh, it scurried back to its owner, slipping right inside her. She cried and cried, for she had been burned. Then Tukwi called all the women and lectured them: 'All you women, don't let your genitals wander about. If they do, they may get burned as mine were!' And so, today, women's genitals no longer go wandering about.

Prizing female genitalia

Although purging female genitalia is more common, its polar opposite, prizing female genitalia, is and has been practised by some societies. Many examples come from prehistory and ancient Greek and Turkish civilisations (as we've seen earlier). Ethnographic evidence from the last 150 years also highlights how female genitalia, in particular external genitalia, are prized, and women and girls given a sense of pride in their genital anatomy. Polynesia's Easter Island, in the South Pacific, is more generally known for gigantic stone figures; however, external female genitalia are also immortalised in stone here. In this society, a female's clitoris received particular attention from an early age, being deliberately manipulated and lengthened (and not, as far as is known, to emulate a phallus).

The culmination of this clitoral attention was the *te manu mo ta poki* or the 'bird child' ceremony, which was still part of living memory in 1919. This ritual was carried out at the clifftop ceremonial site of Orongo, where rocks depicting vulval and clitoral engravings still stand. During the ceremony, the girls straddled the engraved stones, displaying their enlarged clitorises to five priests. The longest were honoured by being carved in stone, and the girls possessing them got to choose the best men as partners. Genital qualities and genital pleasure are emphasised from an early age in other Polynesian societies. For example, the Marquesan people also performed ceremonies in which the beauty of a female's external genitalia was assessed. These rituals took place on large stones or boulders, known as the *ke'a vehine po'otu* ('beautiful girl stone') and the *ke'a vehine haka* ('dancing girl stone').

Elsewhere in Polynesia, anthropological studies from the first half of the twentieth century show Mangaian culture to have a healthy concern, respect and appreciation for female genitalia. This positive attitude is reflected in language. There are several synonyms for the clitoris (including *kaka'i, nini'i, tore, teo* and more), as well as for the vagina (*kawawa, mete kopapa, 'ika*). Moreover, Mangaian vocabulary also includes terms for features of female genitalia that are not expressed at all in English. The different shapes of clitorises are expressed using the modifying terms *keo* and *keokeo.* Clitorises are also described as being of a particular degree of sharpness, or as blunt. Other clitoral descriptor terms include projecting, erecting and protruding. I love this idea of considering the angles and curves of the clitoris and knowing and revelling in what you've got between your legs.

The fascination with female genitalia, not surprisingly, extends beyond language. Both Mangaian girls and boys are taught by elder women and men about sex, genitals and how to pleasure each other. This education includes means of achieving simultaneous orgasm, as well as, for men, how to bring women to multiple orgasms before their own orgasm, and how to hold back. For a Mangaian male, the ability to give a woman three orgasms to his one during sex is seen as an essential part of being male. If he cannot do this, he is being lazy, he's letting his penis go to waste, letting it 'get rusty'. Perhaps this education is the reason why it is said that for Mangaian men, the size, shape and consistency of a woman's mons Veneris is as important as the west's obsession with breasts. Particularly prominent mons are the most revered.

Vaginas with character

An appreciation of female genital beauty is expressed by other societies too – and in surprisingly varying ways. For the people of the Siriono tribe in Eastern Bolivia the concept of beauty itself – what makes a woman attractive – is focused on her genitalia. Here too prominent or plump external genitalia are prized. People on the Pacific atoll of Truk consider the vagina, as opposed to the phallus, to be the primary symbol of sexuality. For the Trukese, the vagina is said to be 'full of things'; these special things are the clitoris, inner lips and the urethra. For Trobiand Islanders, the clitoris, which as we've seen is a favourite subject for folklore, also features in cat's cradle – the game where intricate patterns are made with a loop of string held and twisted between the fingers. In 'The Clitoris of Ba'u', two large loops of string represent two vulvas, and two smaller loops sticking out at right angles to the main plane are clitorises. The game is to wriggle the fingers skilfully in such a way that the two clitorises jump and dance, as a rhyme to the clitoris is sung. Other cat's cradle games include depictions of adultery complete with genitals meeting, as well as enlarging testicles.

For Brazil's Mehinaku people, the role of the clitoris is taught in mythology. A myth that tells the tale of how the vagina came to be created speaks of how the clitoris 'is what makes sex sensual', and of how 'it makes the man's penis delicious for the woman'. The genital myths of Brazil's Mehinaku reveal the fascination with external female genitalia in other ways. They tell of how the ceremonial headdresses and earring feathers worn by Mehinaku men actually represent female genitalia. Mythology tells of how the first earrings were the pubic hair of the Sun's wife, and the headdress another character's labia. When fully adorned, the Mehinaku male is none other than an icon of female sexual anatomy.

Meanwhile, in Hawaii, the worship of genitalia was communicated in song and dance as well as mythology. Hawaiians have a whole song tradition called *mele mai*, or genital chanting. When royal babies were born, genital songs would be composed in their honour, describing and celebrating the sexual organ's beauty and future capacity. Queen Liliuokalani's genitals were said to be '*Anapau*, that is, frisky, vigorous, merry ones.' What a compliment! Frisky, vigorous and merry – you couldn't ask for anything more. Hawaiians also pampered the genitalia of infants, stretching and lengthening a girl's clitoris, and massaging a boy's penis, in moves that were seen as designed to enhance the genitals' beauty and prepare them for sexual enjoyment in later life. Not surprisingly, perhaps, the Hawaiian language has a large lexicon of words for sexual delight and gratification.

The long and the short of it

So far we've seen that the history of the clitoris is one of prizing or purging. So perhaps it's not so surprising that attitudes towards women's labia have been equally polarised too. For some societies, including Polynesia's Marquesan people, Easter Islanders and the Urua of central Africa, a sign of attractiveness was the possession of elongated dangling vulvar lips. For example, women in southern Africa, including the Khoi Khoi and Khoisan, were seen as more beautiful and powerful if they had inner labia extending beyond their outer lips (labia majora). Moreover, men were said to regard them as better lovers. And the longer the labia the better, it seems, as the projection of the inner or little lips (labia minora) beyond the outer ones was purposely manipulated. From an early age, a female's inner lips would be gently tugged, pulled and twisted to achieve the required length. Growth was also encouraged by delicately wrapping and twisting the labia around little sticks and twigs. This positive attitude towards labia can also be seen in the Trukese women's tradition of adorning their inner lips, by placing dangling jewellery and bells in labial piercings.

Since the seventeenth century, however, such differences in inner labial length have aroused the curiosity of the western world, in particular men of science. Amongst their targets were the women of hunter-gatherer societies of southern Africa, such as the Khoi Khoi and Khoisan. These women's delicately elongated inner labia appear to have fascinated, puzzled and terrified western men in equal measures. Science at this time, though, was inherently sexist, choosing to perceive women as lesser versions of men as we've seen. Female genitalia were typically studied to highlight the vast difference between women and men, and to underline the perceived lower nature of women. As a result, some seventeenth-century thinkers declared differences in labial length a deformity, while others put forward the idea that perhaps the women were hermaphrodites.

Science was also racist, and variations in the size of women's inner labia were viewed erroneously as evidence of one society's superiority over another. In the eighteenth century, the much-vaunted radical libertarian thinker Voltaire proposed that women with longer inner labia were so strange that they must belong to a separate species of human. Some even saw fit to suggest that here was the living missing link between apes and humans. Another racist notion that flourished was that just as the flowers of the African continent grew large and fleshy in the extreme temperatures, so too did female genitalia. The idea that women may have deliberately manipulated their genitalia to be as big and beautiful as possible does not appear to have been considered. It seems that western society, with its view of female genitalia being shameful, could not possibly perceive of a culture which could appreciate and admire a woman's genitals.

Not surprisingly, various demeaning names for elongated inner lips were mooted by western men. First the plain 'flap of skin', later the more serious Latin name, *sinus pudoris*, translated in various ways with its moralistic overtones as 'loincloth', 'veil of shame', or 'drape of decency'. Finally, 'apron', *tablier* in French and *Schürze* in German, was adopted. The genitals of many African women were also the subject of many photographic sessions in the late nineteenth and early twentieth centuries, and museums in South Africa and elsewhere have collections of plaster-cast genitalia. The subject of labial length was deemed worthy of medical investigation well into the twentieth century. The *Medical Journal of South Africa* of November 1926 reports on this disturbing piece of research amongst women in Sandfontein, south-west Africa: 'On asking a woman of these tribes to remove her linen cloth or apron, one could not, at first, detect any difference between her and an ordinary woman ... On separating the lips of the vulva it was easy to grasp the labia minora with a pair of forceps and pull them out for examination. This increased exposure gave rise to a distinct accession of shyness on the part of the women ... '

The Story of Saartjie Baartman

The story of one African woman, Saartjie Baartman, now famous as the Hottentot Venus (her original name remains unknown), represents the clash of two different cultures' beliefs regarding female genitalia – and the assumed superiority of one over another. For Saartjie's people (possibly the Khoi Khoi of southern Africa), long inner labia were considered to be a mark of beauty. However, for western society, they were viewed as problematic, representing sexual and racial difference. Believed to be born in 1790, Saartjie came to Europe in 1810, and lived and worked as an object of curiosity in both London and Paris. On her death, in her early twenties, in Paris in 1815, she was dissected by the renowned French anatomist Georges Cuvier, a man who was said to be fascinated by her genitalia. His sixteen-page manuscript describing her dissection focuses heavily on her genitalia. In it he describes her four-inch-long inner labia as being 'like two wrinkled fleshy petals'. He comments that if they are held apart, they create 'the figure of a heart', with the centre marked out by the opening of the vagina. His fascination with her genitalia is revealed in the fact that nine pages of his text are devoted, if that is the right word, to detailing them. In contrast, her brain merited one paragraph.

The rest of Cuvier's description of Saartjie is not as pleasant. The name he gives her – Hottentot Venus – is a derogatory one, a title which was also attached to other African women. Hottentot, deriving from a Dutch word meaning stammerer, is the name colonialists gave to the African people who speak an ancient language characterised by clicking sounds. The addition of Venus follows from the racist and sexist belief that women born in hotter climates had more sexual (implying bestial) natures than their colder-climate European sisters. This heightened sexuality was believed to be a result of the influence of the passionate planet Venus. The genitals of Saartjie Baartman are still arousing controversy today, and she has become a symbol of the racial and sexual prejudices of eighteenth- and nineteenth-century science. Her preserved labia were on display in a bell jar in Paris' Musée de l'Homme until 1985. In 1995 South Africa asked France for her remains to be returned to her country of birth. The initial response from the Museum of Man was that they couldn't find them. In 2002, however, they announced they had managed to track them down, and Saartjie Baartman was returned to her homeland at last.

There is a sad footnote to the story of the western world's attitude to differing labial lengths. As the photographs in this book show, the inner lips of women's vaginas are delightfully varied in design, size and hue, and are not by any means symmetrical. When not aroused, many women's inner labia are concealed by the fatty cushions or pads of their outer lips (the labia majora, literally 'big lips', although they don't look anything like lips). However, inner labial length does vary; some inner lips are longer than others and are visible beneath the outer lips – there is no labial standard. Despite this, though, many western women today feel the need to snip their labia surgically into a shape and size which they see as a semblance of normality. Apparently, the most common request is to trim the lips to the uniform and neutered look seen in most male-produced pornography. It seems that for some western women, taking pride in the unique shape of their genitalia is extremely difficult.

Hymen hysteria

There is another portion of a woman's external genitalia that has received considerable attention, although not always welcome. This is the hymen, the thin membrane of flesh which stretches across the opening of the vagina. And just as a woman's clitoris and labia have been repeatedly misconstrued and misunderstood, so too has the hymen. The existence of the hymen itself is a vexed issue and has been called into question countless times over the centuries. Numerous physicians and anatomists throughout history have professed their curiosity as to its existence. Many believed it to be a figment of other men's imaginations. Others saw it as one of the defining, and unique, features of womanhood. I myself have always been intrigued about this web or fold of flesh which I have never seen. I merely accept with blind faith that at one time I had one, but now it is no longer there. I did not witness its destruction.

The hymen appears to be an elusive creature for many. For example, early first-century medic Galen does not describe it in his otherwise detailed dissections of female genitalia. Instead, the word hymen, when he does use it, appears to refer to a much larger, all-encompassing membranous envelope of tissue beneath which the body's internal organs lie. The first text in Greek medical literature to mention the hymen focuses on denying the idea of it tearing during a female's first experience of sexual intercourse. In his influential second-century text, *Gynaecology*, Soranus writes:

The belief that there exists a slight membrane that occurs in the vagina and constitutes a transverse barrier, and that it is this that is torn either in painful deflorations or when the menstrual blood rushes out too quickly, and that this same membrane when it persists and thickens is the cause of the sickness called atresia [nonperforation] – all of these beliefs are erroneous.

Despite such shaky foundations, the hymen has, over the centuries, been invested with more social, moral and even legal significance than any other piece of human flesh. The issue it came to represent was that of virginity – the condition of never having had sexual intercourse. The importance of guaranteeing the virginity of a bride-to-be has its origins in the desire of men to ensure as far as possible that any offspring born to the woman they marry are their own. And from being an assurance of future paternity to the bridegroom, a female's virginity was subsequently imbued with moral significance, becoming an asset to be prized and fetishised. The hymen, because it was seen, wrongly, as the anatomical guarantee of female virginity, became both the sign and symbol of vaginal virtue. As a result, vaginal bleeding was seen as an essential part of a woman's first experience of sexual intercourse. In many cultures, if blood on the sheets was not forthcoming, a woman was in trouble – brides in biblical times could be stoned to death for failing the bloodied sheet test. Incredibly, in the sixteenth century, the hymen was viewed as constituting credible medical and legal proof of either virginity or childbirth.

The etymology of the word also reflects its supposed moral and physical significance. It is believed to be named after the Greek god of marriage, Hymen, who died on his wedding night, and who is said to reside in the curtain of vaginal tissue and hence is the first victim of the wedding night. *Membrana virginalis*, the 'veil of modesty', 'maidenhood', *integritas*, 'the guardian of their chastity' are some of the hymen's other moralistic monickers. The symbolism of the hymen was even extended to plants, with the hymen of plants being used to describe the fine, delicate husk surrounding a new bud, which bursts as the flower blooms.

The veneration of female virginity and the elevated importance of delicate tissue has led to some strange beliefs and sexual practices. Two of the central tenets of Christian faith focus on virginity – namely, the belief in Mary's Immaculate Conception of her son, Jesus, and his subsequent virgin birth. This double hymen miracle is highlighted in the Apocryphal Gospels, which has a suspicious Salome feeling with her fingers to ascertain the truth or not of Mary's virgin birth. But as Salome placed her fingers on Mary's vagina, she screamed with pain and withdrew them. Apparently, this divine intervention convinced her that Mary still had a hymen – a miracle had occurred. In terms of sexual practices, there persisted in the sixteenth century the horrific and erroneous belief that sexual intercourse with a virgin could cure a male infected with syphilis. A mutated form of this idea is still doing the rounds: in South Africa today it is said that as many as 36 per cent of the population believe that having sex with a virgin female will provide a cure for HIV and Aids. This idea has led to the appalling rapes of young girls and even babies.

The role of the hymen

The human hymen does exist. It is not a figment of imagination. However, its existence and appearance is highly variable, ranging from nonexistent to a fold of thin tissue lying to one side or stretched partially or completely across the vaginal opening. An intact hymen is a misnomer because every woman's hymenal tissue is different. Most importantly, a hymen is anything but a reliable indicator of whether or not a woman has had sexual intercourse. As an incredibly delicate and thin fold of membranous tissue, the structure and appearance of the hymen, if it appears in the first place, is all too easily altered; simply enjoying being a young girl – dancing, skipping, stretching – can be enough to do this.

The writings of one sixteenth-century Parisian anatomist, Ambroise Paré, reveal his awareness of the fragility and variability of the hymen: 'The vulgar (and even some learned men) believe that there is no virgin who does not have this hymen, which is the virginal gate. But they are mistaken, because one finds it only very rarely.' The early nineteenth-century French physician Jacques Moreau de la Sarthe had an alternative take on the delicacy of the hymen, warning in his work *Histoire Naturelle de la Femme* that girls who practised 'the habits of Lesbians' would destroy the thin tissue from too vigorous rubbing.

The extreme unreliability of the hymen to appear as society and religion demanded it should also spawned a novel market – hymen restorative services. Many techniques have been tried down the centuries. In the sixteenth century, the gallbladder of a fish is noted as a device to deceive a bridegroom. Other possibilities include herbs purporting to dry out and tighten the vagina. The medieval compendium on women's medicine, the *Trotula*, gives five 'constrictive' recipes for restoring a vagina to virginal status: these include the whites of eggs mixed with water and pennyroyal; and the newly grown bark of a holm oak. Shockingly, a sixth suggested 'virgin remedy' involved leeches. According to the *Trotula*: 'What is better is if the following is done one night before she is married: let her place leeches in the vagina (but take care that they do not go in too far) so that blood comes out and is converted into a little clot. And thus the man will be deceived by the effusion of blood.' Others advised tying a piece of string to the leech to avoid accidents involving lost leeches.

Doctors were often faced with the tricky ethical dilemma of whether to assist a woman in her quest for a new hymen. In his book advising students of medicine, the sixteenth-century Spanish doctor Juan-Alonso de los Ruyzes de Fontecha attempts to clarify the ethical debate. He suggests that if the doctor is confident that the woman wants to be married and wants to avoid causing herself and her family utter shame because she might appear spoiled to her bridegroom, then he is justified in helping her. However, if she appears to be merely attempting to pass herself off as a virgin without being one, then he should not help.

In the twenty-first century, some still view this membranous sliver as a suitable marker of virginity – and strive to resurrect it when it has gone. In Japan, such is the demand that there is now a booming market for the surgical speciality that is known as hymen rebirth. Tens of thousands of operations are estimated to be carried out in Japan every year. Clients are not just Japanese though. Many women are from wealthy Middle Eastern countries, where female lives can still depend on the existence or not of the hymen.

Two further questions hang over the hymen today – its existence in other species, and its biological function. Many texts teach that the hymen is unique to human females. It is not. However, its appearance in other species, as in humans, is highly variable. Hymens, or vaginal closure membranes or vaginal constrictions, as they are often referred to, are found in a number of mammals, including llamas, guinea-pigs, elephants, rats, toothed whales, seals, dugongs, and some primates, including some species of galagos, or bushbabies, and the ruffed lemur. And what about function? In the eighteenth century, the role ascribed to the hymen was a moral one. In the twenty-first century, however, one suggestion is that this fold of flesh across the vaginal opening has a reproductive function. For some mammals, this membranous fold has a relationship with their hormonal cycle: in guinea-pigs, the tissue dissolves during oestrus and then grows over again, remaining closed during the rest of the guinea-pig's 14–16 day cycle. In the case of the ruffed lemur, the vaginal opening is closed throughout most of the year and only opens during their restricted mating season.

The second suggestion is that the hymen may play a protective, or barrier role. This theory has particular resonance for aquatic mammals, some of which, significantly, have better developed hymens than land mammals. It is also thought to apply to those hymen-bearing mammals, such as elephants and, some say, humans, that spent part of their evolutionary past as marine mammals. The idea is that, for these mammals, the hymen could be an adaptation to a life spent in large part, at least, in the water. For example, the hymen would act to prevent water and water-borne particles, such as abrasive sand, from entering the vagina. In this sense, the hymen is understood as a marine modification, akin to a seal's sensitive nipples, which are retractable and covered by a flap of skin.

The clitoris is not a penile remnant

To return to the clitoris – which is always a good thing to do. Controversy still surrounds it, mainly because science is still at a loss to explain satisfactorily what its role is. Various theories have been put forward over the years in an attempt to give this precious wishbone of flesh a solid place in evolutionary history. All are speculative, and, to my mind, none are satisfying. One theory suggests that the clitoris is nothing more than the leftovers, as it were, from the sexes' common embryological origins in the womb. Because boys need a penis, girls are stuck with a penile remnant. This is known as the 'the clitoris is a vestigial penis' theory. A common analogy to it is that of men's nipples. Men have nipples, so the notion goes, because nipples are part of the body's blueprint for a human, so everybody has to have them, irrespective of whether they have a use for them. So, for these thinkers, the clitoris does not have an independent purpose, it is a by-product of the process of producing a penis, and merely a lucky accident for women.

A second clitoral theory purports that way back in the mists of time, there was a glorious period in history, a golden age of the clitoris, if you like. A time when the clitoris loomed large – both in physical structure and function. Sadly, because the clitoris subsequently fell out of favour (for some reason), and has now been out of action for so long, it has since shrunk both in stature and in the role it plays in sexual reproduction. What women are graced with today is a mere fraction of its former self, is the thinking. This is the 'the clitoris is a vestigial clitoris' theory. Its motto is: 'If you don't use it, you'll lose it.'

I do not agree with either of these two theories, for a number of reasons. First of all, the comparison of the clitoris with the penis is anatomically inaccurate. The human clitoris is not the homologue of the human penis, as we will soon see. It is therefore fallacious to suggest that the clitoris is a penile remnant. Neither is it a deformed or dud penis, and it is most definitely not biology's booby prize. Moreover, a second shortcoming of both of these theories is that they rely heavily on out-dated ideas of what constitutes a woman's clitoris – specifically the size and function that science has so far ascribed to it – which, as is noted here, have been misleading and/or incorrect many times in the past. Neither notion appears to have considered seriously other species' clitorises, or whether they can shed light on the role of a woman's.

Women are not alone in possessing and enjoying a clitoris. The erectile clitoris, in varying sizes, is a basic feature of female mammals' genital geography. It's also found in some reptiles, such as crocodiles and turtles, and in several flightless birds, like the ostrich, emu and cassowary. In elephants, the clitoris is well developed, and can measure up to 40 cm, and slightly longer when erect. In the past, though, some clitoral lengths have been exaggerated. In 1791, Johann Blumenbach, the German father of physical anthropology, reported the sighting of a fifty-two-foot long clitoris on a beached baleen whale. This certainly sounds like a fishy tale considering that the entire length of an adult whale typically measures only forty to fifty feet. Clitoral styles differ too. A sow's clitoral crown is conspicuously elongated and pointed, while marsupials possess a split, two-ended clitoris similar to the male marsupial's divided phallus. And just as some males possess a bone in their penis, the os penis, or baculum, so too do some females. An os clitoridis is found in raccoons, walruses, seals, bears, some rodent and carnivore species, and a number of prosimian primates. In female walruses, the clitoral bone measures over an inch long.

In primates, including humans, clitoral size varies. In some primates, such as mangabeys and mandrills, the clitoris is quite small, and appears embedded in the swollen labial and perineal skin. In contrast, other primates, including spider monkeys, woolly spider monkeys and two species of woolly monkey, have enlarged clitorises. The female spider monkey has the longest clitoris of any primate species. Extending away from the body, this primate colossus of a clitoris measures 47 mm, and, like the female spotted hyaena's clitoris, is often mistaken for a penis. Perhaps it is this gigantic clitoris that resulted in spider monkeys being seen as symbols of sexual excitement by the ancient Mayans, who painted pottery dishes representing them as such. Female squirrel monkeys use their erect clitorises to perform ritualised genital displays, which are thought to be important for communicating rank and affiliation. Primate clitoral structure can also differ markedly: in some species of prosimian primates – lorises, lemurs and bushbabies – the long pendulous clitoris is traversed by the urethra, as it is in the hyaena, the European mole, and some shrew species.

In monkeys and apes the clitoris is reported to be situated at or near the base of the vagina, a location which ensures it is subject to direct and regular stimulation during extra- and intravaginal thrusting. However, the enjoyment that primate females, and others, derive from touching their own clitorises is becoming more evident (see colour plate section). Free-ranging adolescent female chimpanzees sometimes finger and tickle their genitals, and have been heard laughing softly as they do so. In the olive baboon, young adult females are known to use the tip of their tail to stroke their perineum and clitoris. Female golden lion tamarins also use their coiled tail to stroke their genitalia, as do bonnet macaques while making pelvic thrusting movements. Japanese macaques will pleasure themselves by rubbing their clitoris back and forth between their index finger and their pelvis.

It seems that sex aids are not the sole province of humans either. Fascinatingly, many primate species have been observed using objects to assist them in stimulating their clitoris. For instance, chimpanzees have been seen using a mango or a piece of wood, while leaves and twigs were the tool of choice for one female orang-utan. A particularly inventive chimpanzee made her own vibrator by placing a carefully selected leaf under her vulva, and then flicking the stem, causing it to vibrate against her. And female self-stimulation is not confined to primates. Female porcupines have been observed to stimulate their clitoris in a particularly complex manner: their trick is to stand astride a stick, while holding it between their forepaws. The act of walking around while straddling the stick causes it to bump against the ground and vibrate, which in turn stimulates their clitoris. Meanwhile masturbation is a common pastime of female dolphins, with clitoral stimulation part of the play between dolphins of both sexes.

The enjoyment that female primates derive from their clitorises and external genitalia is evident in their behaviour towards primates of the opposite, and the same, sex. Sooty mangabeys sometimes reach down and manually manipulate their own genitalia during sexual intercourse. In one study, one young female orang-utan was seen to rub her genitalia against an adult male, and masturbate in front of him, in a move inviting sexual interaction with him. Meanwhile, female Japanese macaques often mount males, rubbing their genitals on the male's back, and during their oestrus period they mount females too. Same-sex stimulation is common among many female primates, including the bonobo, Japanese macaques, baboons, talapoins and rhesus and stumptail macaques. Typical female-female sexual interactions involve one partner mounting the other, in the traditionally male manner, and rubbing her genitalia against the back of her partner. Some primates, including chimpanzees and bonobos, mutually handle each others' genitals as well.

A purely for pleasure plaything?

The importance of the clitoris in providing pleasure is highlighted, in particular to my mind, by bonobo, or pygmy chimpanzee society. Bonobos, together with the common chimpanzee, are humankind's closest relative, and bonobos too enjoy a rich sexuality. Sexual interaction with both sexes, it seems, provides the glue to bonobo society, cementing friendships, sealing procreative relationships, and mending food disputes. Sex is also used to divert attention and change the tone of an encounter. All in all, bonobo sexual interactions work to reduce any tensions within the group. However, it's not just their sexual habits, their intelligence and their remarkably long legs (that stretch while walking) that make bonobos far more like humans than any other primate. In contrast to other primates (excluding humans), their external genitalia are situated more between their legs, or frontally (ventrally) oriented, than shifted back towards the anal area (see colour plate section). A bonobo's clitoris too is more frontally placed, as a woman's is. Their clitoris is also particularly prominent and erectile, with a full erection seeing it swell to nearly twice its unaroused size. Indeed, it is not unknown for one female to insert her erect clitoris into another female's swollen vulva.

In bonobo society, same-sex interactions are as frequent as those between the opposite sexes, and bonobos like to vary the sexual positions, as well as the partners, that they adopt. When two female bonobos sexually interact they rub their clitorises together, left and right for maybe fifteen seconds, in a move which has become known as the genito-genital, or G-G, rub (see colour plate section). They may do this with one female lying on her back and the other straddling her, or with one female standing and the other with her legs wrapped around her, being carried. The pace at which each female swings her pelvis from side to side is precisely timed so that each partner is always thrusting in opposite directions. Intriguingly, the rhythm that the females choose to G-G rub at has an average of 2.2 lateral moves per second, the same rhythm as that of a thrusting male during heterosexual sex. Eye contact between two females during a G-G rub can be maintained throughout.

Do female bonobos enjoy G-G rubbing so much because of the location of their clitoris? It certainly appears so. The prevalence of face-to-face sex between female and male bonobos would also seem to suggest this. Face-to-face sex (the ventro-ventral or belly-to-belly position, more commonly known among humans as the missionary position) was until recently thought to be unique to humans. However, it's now known that various species, including bonobos, gorillas, siamangs, orang-utans, and aquatic mammals such as dolphins, whales and porpoises, enjoy this style of sexual interaction. Indeed, in bonobo society, face-to-face copulation is almost as common as doggy style.

Primate genital antics, in particular, reveal that the clitoris is exquisitely sensitive in many species, with an important pleasure role to play. But why is this so? A third main clitoral theory suggests that the clitoris is a purely-for-pleasure plaything – it was designed with nothing more than pleasure in mind. Proponents of this theory vaunt its unique role in females, and laud its density of nerve fibres. However critics of the clitoris' role purely as an instrument of bliss and delight point to its extreme position from the site of sexual intercourse (in their eyes at least) as evidence to the contrary. Crucially, though, the nay-sayers' comments about design are, again, based predominantly on the idea of the clitoris as a small button, not a large wishbone structure astride the whole genital region, and sunk deep inside. Far from being too distant from the vaginal opening to be functional in providing sexual pleasure, the clitoris is, conversely, intimately associated with all other vaginal structures.

However, while I wholeheartedly support the role the clitoris plays in providing bliss, I disagree with the purely-for-pleasure theory for two reasons. Firstly, the clitoris has a purpose other than pleasure. Millions of years of evolution were not in vain. Yes, the clitoris is more than capable of producing extreme sensations of pleasure, but there is a physiological reason for this pleasure provision, it is not an end in itself. Secondly, the clitoris is not unique to females. Males have a clitoris too. And the role that a male's clitoris plays is the same role as performed by a female's.

Making genitals

To understand the true function of the clitoris a step back in time is necessary – to the first few weeks of an embryo's life, when the only difference between girls-to-be and boys-to-be resides solely in the chemical composition of their DNA. Each sex, typically, has twenty-three pairs of chromosomes. However, one sex has a heavier complement of chromosomes than the other because this sex has one chromosome that is far bigger than its counterpart in the opposite sex. The difference in weight lies with the human sex chromosomes, denoted X and Y. In women, the sex chromosomes consist of two large X chromosomes. In contrast, men have just one large X chromosome, paired with a Y. The Y chromosome is much smaller than the X, appearing stunted or shrivelled, with one of the arms of the Y shorter than the other. The fact that the Y chromosome carries far less genetic material than the X, making it weigh less, is a factor which is exploited in sperm sex-sorting techniques.

For humans, if the Y chromosome did not exist, it appears we would all be women, or at least all have ovaries, because the basic human blueprint is female. Both ovaries and testes have a common starting point – the genital or gonadal ridge, a nub of tissue which develops during the first three weeks of all embryos' lives. And for just over forty days and forty nights (forty-two to be precise), female and male embryos are indistinguishable from each other. However, after this period, embryos start to become obviously sexed. This happens in the following way. The destiny of the genital ridge – which is capable of becoming either ovaries or testes – depends on the chemical instructions that are conveyed to it, and these messages are relayed by genes residing on the embryo's sex chromosomes. If the embryo has a Y sex chromosome, then between days 43 and 49, it receives a set of genetic instructions that tells it to turn its genital ridge into testes. It's recently become clear that the X chromosome also gives out instructions to the genital ridge – these push it towards developing into ovaries and are also involved in kidney development. This happens between days 45 and 55. It is simply a difference in the genetic instructions received from chromosomes that is the prime mover in determining the type of gonads – ovaries or testes – that a human will possess. Not all species use chromosomes; reptiles, for instance, use temperature as the trigger for developing different gonads.

Possessing ovaries or testes is just the first step to having fully formed and distinctly different female or male genitalia. What happens next depends on the circulating levels of hormones which the foetus experiences in the womb. This hormonal milieu is a result of the hormones that the foetus' gonads and adrenals secrete, and also of the hormones produced by its mother. One hormone recipe will result in a foetus with the internal and external genitalia that we term female, while a different hormonal mix leads to the internal and external genitalia that we dub male. Only a delicate hormone balance exists between the two sexes, and it is not that unusual for internal and external genitalia not to fit the traditional patterns of female or male. The external genitalia of both females and males also has a common starting point – the genital tubercle, which can be seen by week four in the pelvic floor between an embryo's legs. Although when adult the two sexes' external genital arrangements may seem to be very different, this is not the case. They are just different styles or arrangements of this mound of genital tissue. The only difference is again in how that piece of flesh is sculpted by the cocktail of hormones it is exposed to *in utero*.

The creation of external female genitalia is thought to begin between days 63 and 77, while producing male external genitals starts a little later, around days 67 to 70. The process of sculpting differently shaped external genitalia is understood to be complete by days 84 to 98 (weeks 12 to 14). Figure 4.2 shows three different stages in the development of the external genitalia of females and males: the genital tubercle that is common to both females and males, the slightly divergent external genitalia at ten weeks, and, finally, the fully formed external genitalia, recognisable as female and male. Even at around ten weeks, faint traces of the different hormonal soups embryos are exposed to are visible in the more open, blossoming, curving form of the female-to-be's external genitals, while the male embryo shows a slight pulling in and focusing of the genital tissue destined to be a penis and scrotum.

These images also help to highlight which parts of a woman's external genitalia are analogous to those of a man. Figure 4.2 shows how a female's labia majora, or outer lips, correspond to a male's scrotum. The female's hormonal recipe sculpts the labio-scrotal swelling so that it spreads out and round, framing the genital area, while the male's hormonal instructions direct the same tissue to come together below to form the scrotal sac. It is not quite as straightforward to visualise the remaining matching bits of genital tissue, but they are there, and there does appear to be a pattern. In the female, genital tissue tends to open up, flowering or spreading, whereas in the male the equivalent structures tend to pull in or fuse. This can be seen with the female's inner lips, which unfurl and fan outwards, while in the male, the same tissue comes together, fusing in what is called the peno-scrotal raphe or midline. This is why men have what can appear

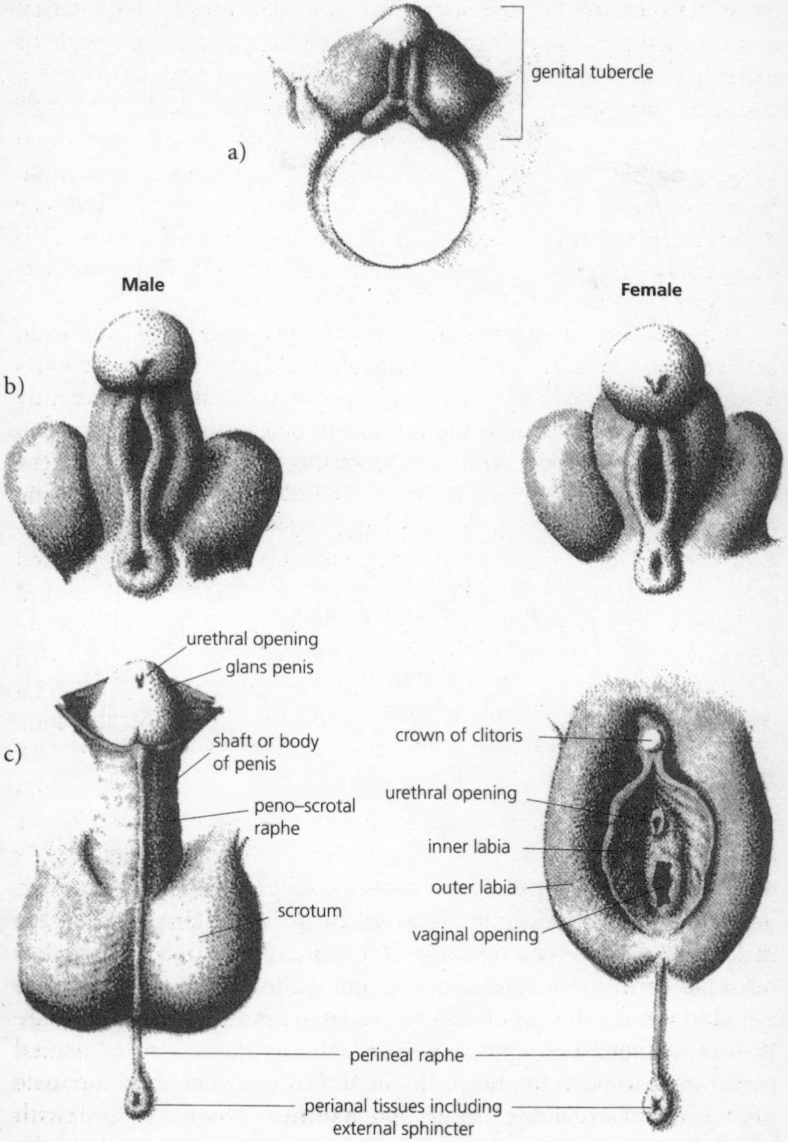

Figure 4.2 How female and male external genitalia form a) the common genital tubercle – this can be seen by week four; b) at ten weeks a difference in the two sexes' genitalia is just visible (at this point the length is between 45 to 50 mm) and c) after weeks 12–14 the sexes' genitalia are clearly distinguishable.

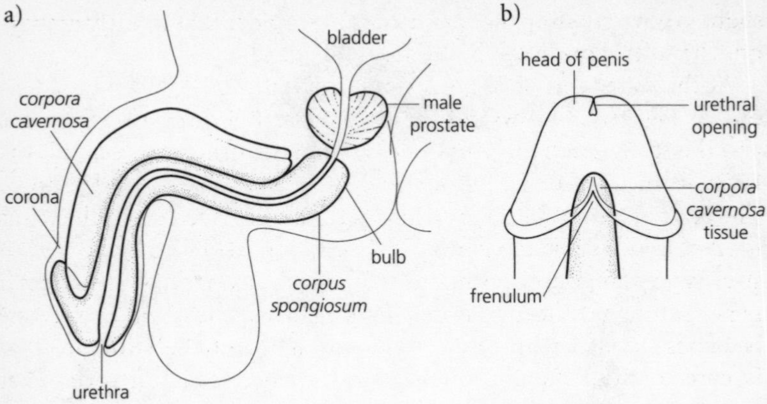

Figure 4.3 The penis a) note the three main structures – urethra, *corpora cavernosa* and *corpus spongiosum* and b) looking straight on and inside, you can see how the top of the *corpora cavernosa* tissue lies under the head of the penis (*corpus spongiosum* tissue).

to be a scar running the length of the underside of their penis and scrotal sac. The first time I saw an erect penis I was very confused by this penile line. I thought it must be a scar, but I was far too shy to ask the man in question about the terrible accident that he seemed to have suffered. I only realised my mistake on viewing another erect penis – two phallic tragedies was far too much of a coincidence. Genitalia are unique in showing this visible seam of creation.

What lies beneath

While depicting beautifully the common origins of female and male genitalia, the illustrations in Figure 4.2 do not highlight the full extent of female and male genital congruence. In order to do that, a look at what lies beneath the surface of the skin is necessary. First of all – the penis. Figure 4.3 shows how the penis consists of three main structures: the urethra, the *corpus spongiosum* and the *corpora cavernosa.* The first major structure is the urethra, the channel through which urine passes after leaving the bladder. The urethra is surrounded by a type of tissue known as the *corpus spongiosum* – which means literally 'spongy body'. The *spongiosum*, which runs the length of the penis, is about 14 cm long. At the base of the penis it appears as a pear-shaped bulb with a slight groove crossing the underside (a reminder that in early embryonic life two *spongiosum* bulbs fused together).

At the other end of the penis, the head, the *spongiosum* broadens out, as Figure 4.3 shows, becoming the glans of the penis (the glans and the *spongiosum* represent one continuous structure). *Glans* is the Latin word for acorn, and often refers to any small, rounded body. The edge or rim of the glans which faces the stomach when the penis is erect is known as the corona (whereas the frenulum is the fold of stretchy skin on the opposite side of the penis akin to the one under a person's tongue). During sexual arousal, the erectile *spongiosum* tissue becomes swollen with blood; however, it is not the structure that is core to the stiffening of the penis during sexual arousal. That honour goes to the third main part of the penis body – the *corpora cavernosa.*

It is the engorgement of the *corpora cavernosa* (literally, 'cavernous bodies') tissue that results in the stiffening of the penis – an erection. Surprisingly, man is unusual in that his *corpora cavernosa* lacks a penis bone, the os baculum, or os penis. In fact, the majority of primates possess a penis bone, which is formed by the ossification of the distal portion of the *corpora cavernosa.* Moreover, the following mammalian orders all have penis bones, with the first letters of the five names spelling out a particularly apt mnemonic: *Primates, Rodentia, Insectivora, Carnivora* and *Chiroptera* (bats).

In males, the endpoint, the tip or crown, of the *corpora cavernosa* is not visible, as it lies beneath the surface of the glans. However, due to the large number of nerve fibres in this tissue, it is incredibly sensitive, and indirect touch, that is, applying pressure, is capable of providing men with exquisite sensations of pleasure. From its starting point, the *corpora cavernosa* runs the length of the penis, and measures typically about 12 cm. It consists of the crown (approximately 6 mm long) and a long body or corpus (10 cm), and finally, at its root, the *corpora cavernosa* splits slightly, ending in two short, separated legs or crura, each about 2.5 cm long. Crown, corpus and crura: this is the three-part structure of a man's *corpora cavernosa.* Does anything sound familiar? This is the male clitoris. Together the urethra, the *corpus spongiosum* and the *corpora cavernosa* make up the main components of the external genital apparatus known as the penis.

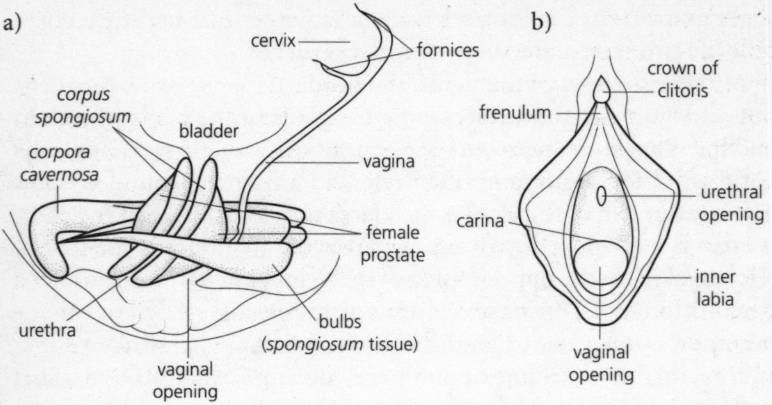

Figure 4.4 The vulva a) note the three main structures – urethra, *corpora cavernosa* and *corpus spongiosum* and b) the frontal view, with the clitoris (*corpora cavernosa* tissue) above the urethra (which is surrounded by *spongiosum* tissue).

The triune vulva

How does a woman's vulva compare? External female genitalia, too, have three main structures (excluding the vagina itself). These are: the urethra, the genital tissue surrounding the urethra, and the clitoris. A close look at female genitalia illustrates this more clearly (see Figure 4.4). A point to stress here when visualising the analogous female and male genitalic parts is that female genital structures tend to pull apart as they develop, whereas the corresponding male parts come closer together. First off, the urethra. A woman's urethra, like that of a man, is the route via which urine leaves the body. In women, the urethral opening is situated just above the vaginal opening, and just below the crown of the clitoris. However, just like a man's, a woman's urethra is surrounded by *spongiosum* tissue, as the cross-section figure shows. This is why it is sometimes referred to as the urethral sponge.

This urethral *spongiosum* tissue is also intimately related to a bulbous structure which in females is split into two bulbs (compared to the male's singular fused *spongiosum* bulb). In women these are called the vestibular bulbs (or the urethral bulbs), and are also composed of *spongiosum* tissue. These bulbs extend backwards for between

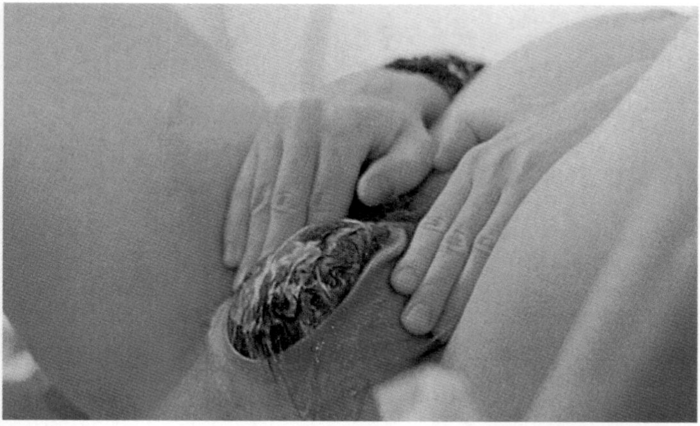

a)

b)

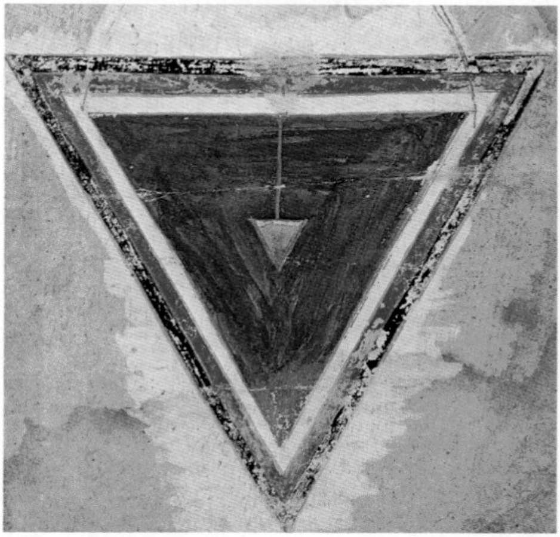

c)

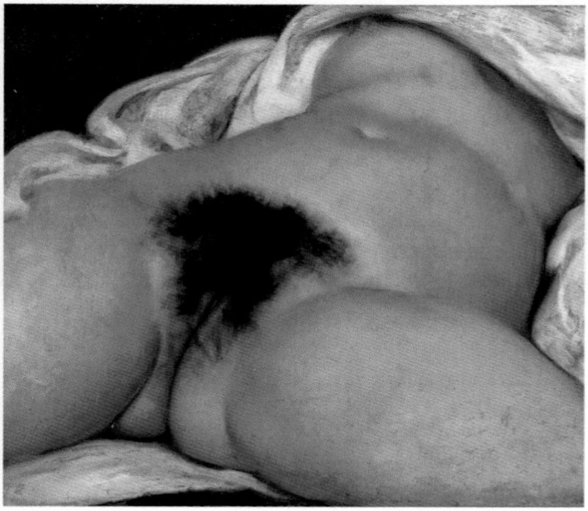

Vaginal views: a) the vagina giving birth; b) the yoni as yantra – the primordial triangle, symbol of the supreme goddess (Rajasthan, c. seventeenth century); and c) 'The Origin of the World', Gustave Courbet, 1866.

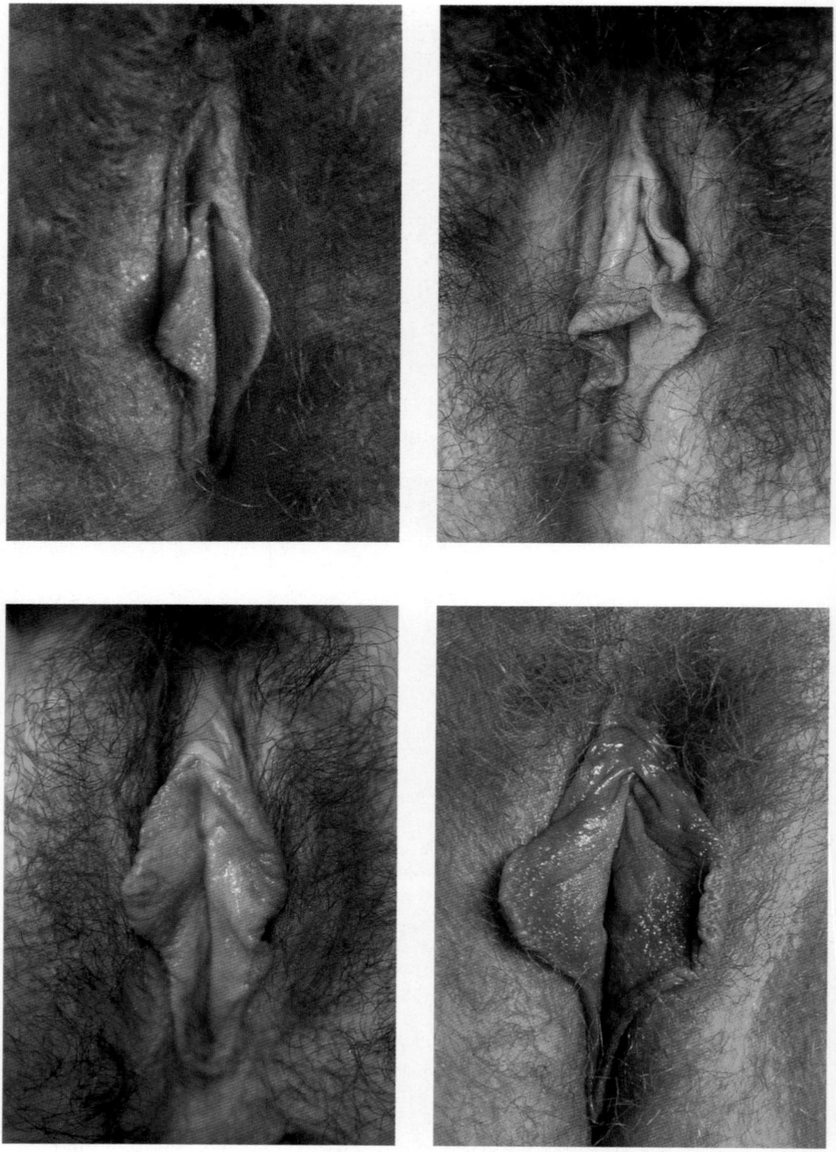

Vulvas, vaginas, yonis: the variety and beauty of external female genitalia is stunning – every woman is unique.

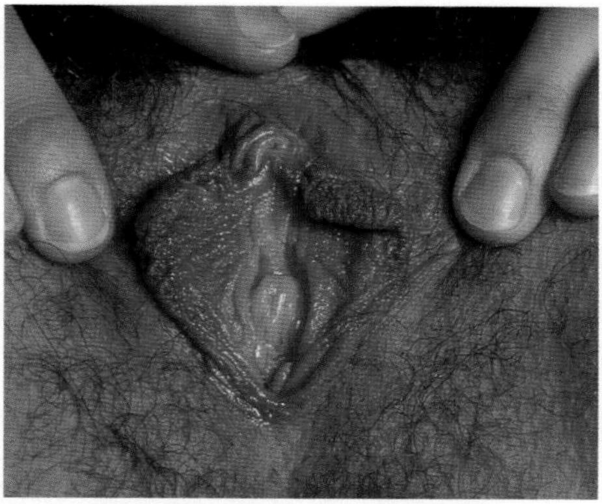

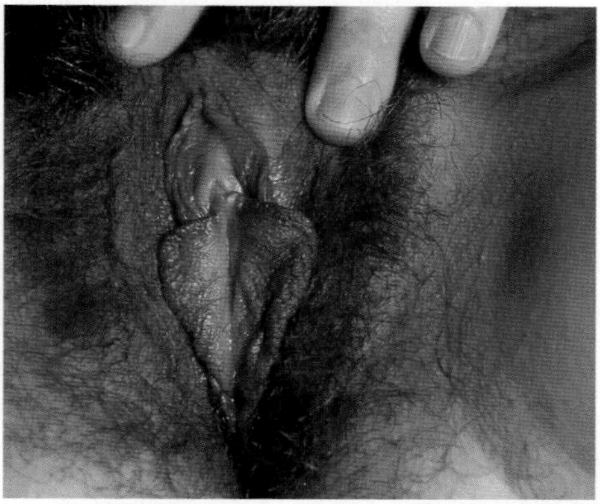

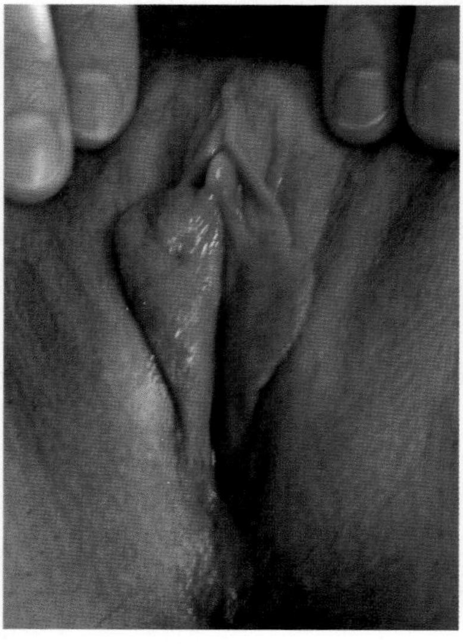

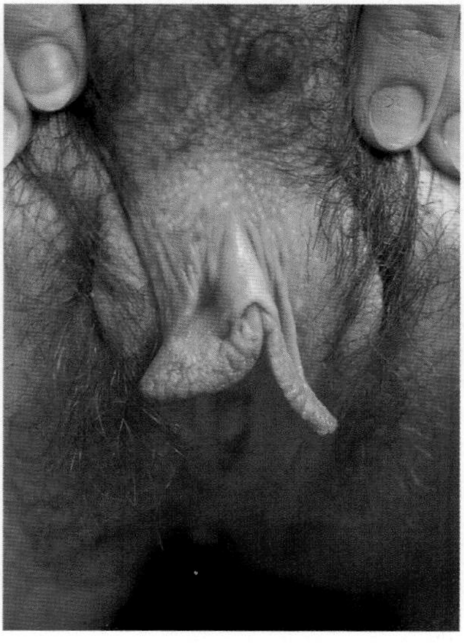

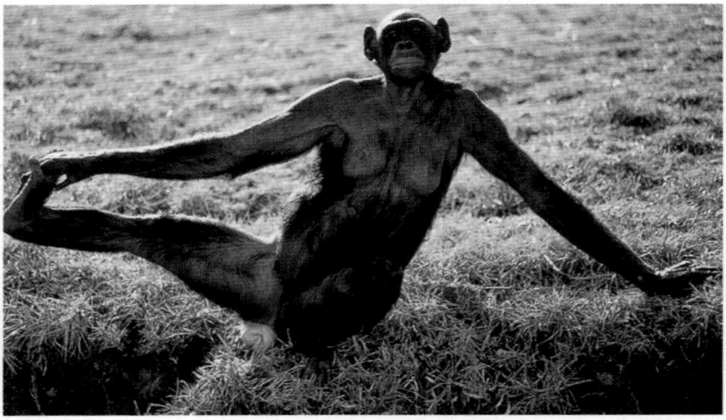

a)

b)

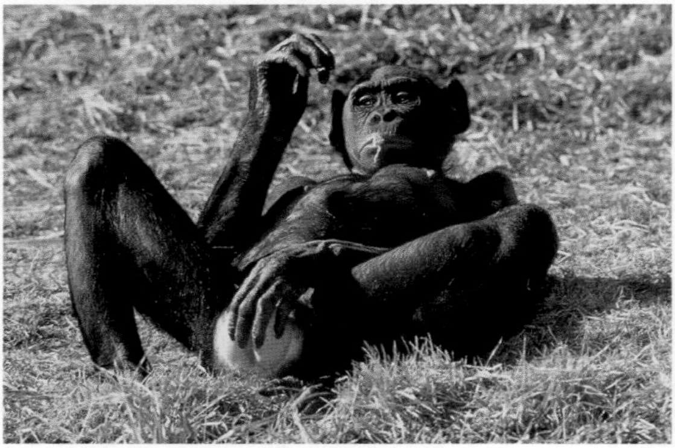

c)

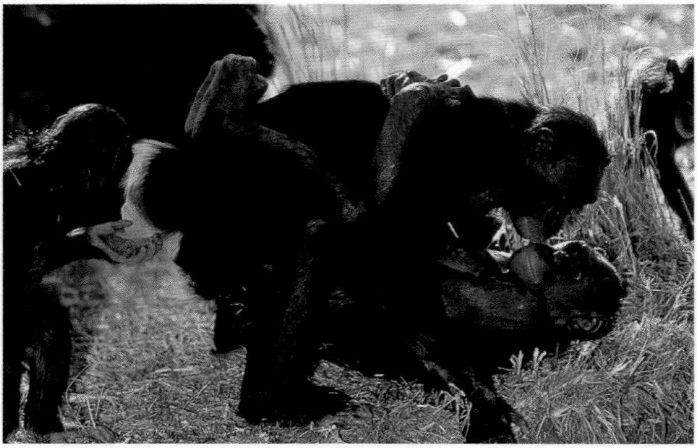

Female bonobos enjoy their genitalia: a) a bonobo's vulva has a frontal orientation with a particularly prominent clitoris; b) pleasuring yourself is appreciated by bonobos too; and c) two bonobos indulge in a spot of genito-genital, G-G rubbing, and gaze into each other's eyes, while youngsters try to get in on the act.

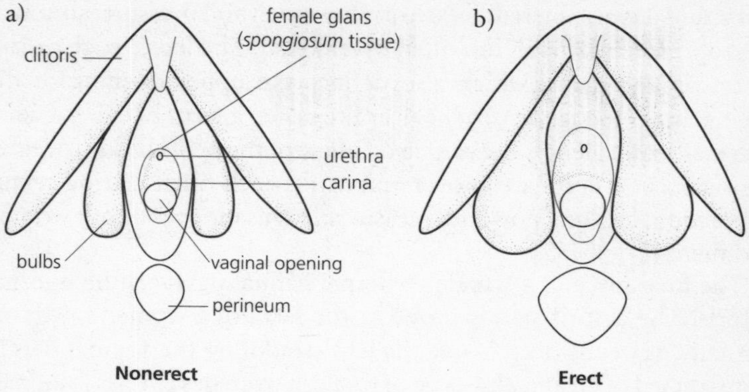

Figure 4.5 How a woman's clitoral and *spongiosum* tissue respond to arousal: a) non-erect and non-aroused and b) when sexually excited these tissues plump up with blood producing deliciously pleasurable sensations.

3 and 7 cm either side of the urethral opening. From the front, the bulbs, which form two crescent-like arcs, taper upwards to begin in a point, the commissure, situated above the urethra and below the crown of the clitoris.

In fact, it's now realised that a woman's *spongiosum* tissue is analagous to that of a man – the difference is merely that a woman's is more spatially diffused. And just as a man's *spongiosum* tissue become spongy and swollen during sexual arousal, so too does a woman's. The *spongiosum* tissue surrounding her urethra swells, as the aubergine-shaped pair of *spongiosum* bulbs plump up with blood. Significantly, these vestibular bulbs swell so much during sexual arousal that they in effect form an enlarged ring-shaped collar or cuff around the vaginal entrance (see Figure 4.5). The fact that these erectile bulbs are highly sensitive to touch, pressure and vibration, helps to explain the delicious sensations produced by stimulation of this region. 'This ring-shaped padding now grips the neck and body of the penis the way a horse collar grips the neck of the horse' was how German anatomist Georg Ludwig Kobelt described it in 1844.

The visible external tip of the *spongiosum* tissue (the glans penis in men) can also be seen in women. Indeed, just as a man's glans has the distinctive shape of an acorn, so too does the area surrounding a woman's urethral opening, especially when aroused. This is a woman's glans, and it is also incredibly sensitive to touch and pressure, although its erotic potential is all too often overlooked. The lower edge or rim of a woman's glans, which also defines the upper opening of the vagina, bears the name *carina*, 'dear little one', a term of endearment. The male equivalent is the *corona* or *sulcus* of the penis head. Together the carina and corona rub over and caress each other during sexual interaction, creating powerful pleasurable sensations for both women and men.

The final piece of a female's external genital jigsaw is the queenly clitoris. The clitoris stands proud at the head of a woman's external genitalia, yet runs deep inside, its legs straddling the vaginal barrel. Constructed of an amazing type of tissue, a woman's clitoris is incredibly sensitive to touch – both directly on its visible and protruding head or crown, and indirectly, via stimulation of the skin and tissue surrounding its body and legs. Viewed from the side, as Figure 4.4 shows, a woman's clitoris has a kink in it, akin to a bent knee, around where the corpus (body) becomes the crown. When a woman is not sexually aroused this portion of the clitoris points downwards. However, during sexual arousal a woman's clitoris floods with blood and becomes erect (see Figure 4.6). Erection results in the clitoris expanding and enlarging, together with a noticeable lifting of the clitoral crown to a more upwards-facing direction. Indeed, it is quite easy to see this erection occurring as the crown of the clitoris raises up and in doing so retracts slightly underneath the hood of skin above it. At this point of sexual arousal the exposed part of the clitoris can be far too sensitive to appreciate too much direct contact.

A woman's clitoris is, in fact, made up of exactly the same type of tissue that a man's *corpora cavernosa* is. That is, the structure that is called a clitoris in women is found in men too, but in men it is called the *corpora cavernosa.* Men have a clitoris. This is why it is inaccurate to say that a woman's clitoris is a penile remnant, or a homologue of the penis. A woman's clitoris (her *corpora cavernosa*) is analagous to a man's *corpora cavernosa* (his clitoris). This fact has been recognised before, but was not appreciated and did not become common knowledge. It is spelt out very clearly in the 1987 book *Eve's Secrets: A New Theory of Female Sexuality* by Josephine Lowndes Sevely. Indeed, this fact is also indicated in anatomical texts where the male structure is referred to as the *corpora cavernosa clitoridis.*

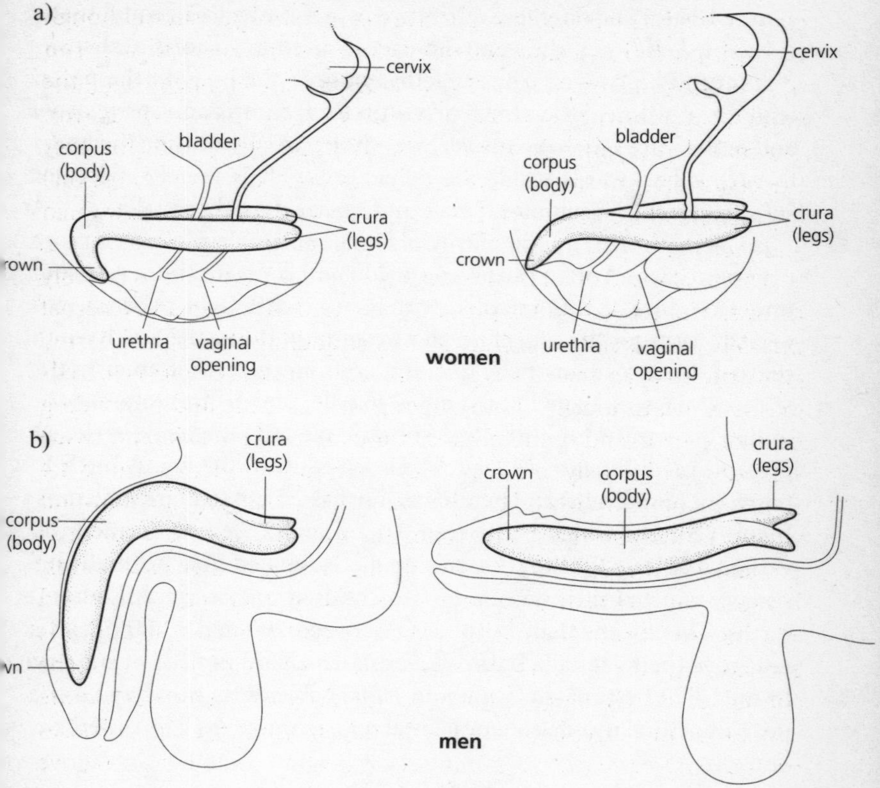

Figure 4.6 A comparison of the sexes' clitorises a) the non-erect and erect female clitoris; and b) the non-erect and erect male clitoris.

The two analagous clitoral structures are shown side by side in Figure 4.6 and, as the illustration reveals, are strikingly similar. The main difference is that the female clitoris is more spread apart or bifurcated – its legs are longer, while its body is shorter. In contrast, the male clitoris comes together more – its legs are shorter, while its body is longer. Both sexes' clitorises are remarkably similar in size, occurring typically in a 5:4 ratio. This ratio is, in fact, the common weight ratio for men and women (160 lbs to 128 lbs). Overall, the external genitalia of women and men are far more alike than they are dissimilar, and they do, of course, share the same starting point of genital tissue. The only real difference is in the way this genital tissue is sculpted. In men, the genitalic parts – urethra, clitoris and *spongiosum* and bulbs – all come together outside the body in the penis, whereas in women, the same parts – urethra, clitoris and *spongiosum* and bulbs – are more expansive, extending partially outside the body, as well as backwards inside the pelvic cavity. It is merely style, not substance, which separates female and male external genitalia.

At birth, the extreme similarity of female and male genitalia is more pronounced, and often causes confusion and consternation. A lack of understanding of this, coupled with a somewhat rigid adherence to what constitutes the 'norm' in the western world in the twenty-first century, leads to many baby girls undergoing clitoridectomies in the first few days of their lives. This is female genital mutilation done under the banner of corrective surgery, western medicine-style. At present, medical standards allow clitorises up to 0.9 cm at birth to represent femaleness, and penises as short as 2.5 cm to mark maleness. Infant genitalia which is between 0.9 cm and 2.5 cm is deemed too variant and is up for the chop or snip. It's estimated that 'normalising' surgery is performed on one or two children out of every thousand births. This means that, in the UK, between 700 and 1,400 babies a year have their genitalia branded as abnormal and in need of surgery. In the US, it's estimated that about 2,000 babies a year undergo some form of clitoral mutilation, or genital reassignment, as it is sometimes known.

Why the clitoris is crucial

The clitoris in its entirety, from its ultrasensitive majestic crown, through its glorious body, down to the tips of its elegant legs, is an organ crying out for a greater appreciation and understanding of what it does. To my mind, the clitoris' function is two-fold, encompassing sexual pleasure and sexual reproduction, with these two roles inseparable from each other, and crucial – in both sexes. A comparison of the two illustrates how this is the case. Firstly, sexual pleasure. Female sexual arousal, just like male sexual arousal, can be triggered by a seemingly infinite variety of sources. The sight or smell of a particular partner, the memory of an erotic encounter, all types of touch, either directly on the genitalia or anywhere else on the body, tastes and sounds, all these can kick-start the rush of blood to the clitoris that heralds the onset of genital arousal.

Moreover, the way in which a woman's clitoris, or *corpora cavernosa* tissue, becomes engorged and erect with blood mirrors the mechanism followed in men (this is why Viagra works for women too). When a woman is not sexually aroused, the smooth muscle cells of her clitoral tissue are in a contracted state and blood flows freely in and out of the surrounding blood vessels (sinusoids). However, all that is needed to make them relax is a signal, or chemical messenger, in the shape of a neurotransmitter or two, released by a female's nerves in response to sexual excitement. As the smooth muscle cells relax, they dilate and expand, trapping any incoming blood in the sinusoidal cavities between the smooth cells. The result is an erection – a clitoris plumped full of blood, engorged, lengthened and exquisitively sensitive.

This mechanism of arousal is also at play when women are not conscious of it. During sleep, in particular during periods of REM sleep, which occur in approximately 90–100–minute cycles four or five times a night, woman experience nocturnal erections affecting their clitoris, labia and vagina (as well as an increase in uterine contractions). These tumescent episodes, which result from increased genital blood flow, parallel men's nocturnal erections of their *corpora cavernosa*, and are evident from early infancy and throughout adult life. The reasons why this should happen so routinely during sleep remain unclear. One suggestion is that these nocturnal erections function as a 'battery-recharging mechanism', increasing blood flow, which in turn brings in fresh oxygen to energise the erectile organ. The importance of a healthy blood supply to erectile organs is well documented. Any substance, drug, disease or habit that damages or impedes blood flow will also have a negative effect on a person's ultimate erectile ability. However, whatever the biological purpose of nocturnal erections, they seem to have one beautiful side-effect – very sweet and satisfying dreams.

In order to enhance erotic sensitivity and act as a sensory trigger for arousal and orgasm, external female genitalia, just like a man's external genitalia, are densely populated with multiple sensory receptors and richly endowed, or innervated, with sensory nerves. The clitoral crown alone is credited with containing a higher concentration of nerve fibres than any other part of the human body. The clitoris and labia, in particular, are densely packed with specialised sensory cells called Meissner and Pacinian corpuscles. The job of Pacinian corpuscles, which are also found in the subcutaneous layer of the fingers, breasts and bladder, is to detect changes in pressure. Pacinian corpuscles can respond very rapidly, which makes them exquisitely tuned to varying or vibrating sensations. The corpuscles consist of concentric membranes of connective tissue, like the layers of an onion, with the gaps between filled with a viscous gel. Any movement or vibration deforms the layers, sending a nerve signal to the brain (essentially they convert mechanical energy into electrical energy).

Meissner's corpuscles are much smaller and are found closer to the surface of the skin. Their role is to respond to the lightest of touches, and, not surprisingly, they are also to be found on the palms of hands and the soles of feet, as well as tongue and nipples. Adept at picking up low-frequency vibrations, these sensory cells are of an ovoid or egg-like structure within which the nerve ending branches and orients itself parallel to the surface of the skin. Other clitoral nerve structures include Krause's end-bulbs and Ruffini corpuscles. Working together, this multitude of sensory cells contribute to an extremely sensitive external genital system, tuned to respond instantly to touch, vibration and pressure, whether it comes in the form of kisses, caresses or stroking.

The clitoris and sexual reproduction

As we saw earlier in this chapter, the female clitoris was once ascribed a role in ensuring successful reproduction, before it was realised that women can conceive without experiencing orgasm. What I would like to suggest is that this early theory was correct, the female clitoris is crucial in ensuring successful sexual reproduction. Consider the role of a man's clitoris or *corpora cavernosa*: without an incredibly sensitive clitoris, a man's penis would never get, and remain, stiff enough to gain safe, non-damaging access to a woman's vagina. In precisely the same way, a woman's clitoris prepares her genitalia to accept and maintain the presence of a penis inside her, safely. That is, both sexes' clitorises prepare their genitals for the amazing feat of transferring and accepting gametes without physical injury or infection occurring. For sexual intercourse – the intimate act of enveloping one organ inside another – is, at heart, potentially a very risky and dangerous business.

For a female, the clitoris is the guardian of the internal recesses of the vagina, standing sentinel without and within. An actual genital guardian angel. As any woman who has ever had sexual intercourse when she is not aroused knows, it hurts. You're rubbed raw. You invariably bleed. And then comes the urinary infection. And, potentially, the sexually transmitted infection. Sex without arousal, without the intimate involvement of the clitoris, leaves a wound (literally) between your legs, and an open route to frequent infections, disease and, yes, death. And yet sexual intercourse when aroused is so vastly different. Then there is no pain, no blood, no follow-up infections. Just smooth, sliding, gliding, expansion and bliss. And the clitoris is the key to this dramatic change of affairs.

This is because increased blood flow, as a result of clitoral arousal, also results in increased blood flow to the vagina, and it too swells. This vaginal engorgement causes droplets, called transudate, to appear on the surface of the mucosal vaginal lining. And this increased vaginal lubrication, as a result of increased blood flow (courtesy of the clitoris), means the delicate lining of the vagina is far less likely to become damaged or torn during sexual intercourse. Why is it so important not to damage the vagina during sex? The very serious answer is that infections, such as with HIV, only occur when there are abrasions to the membrane lining the vagina. And the most common cause of vaginal abrasions? Sex without a woman being sexually aroused and lubricated. That is, sex without the clitoris being erect. This is why the female clitoris is as important as the male clitoris in ensuring successful sexual reproduction. And this is why the clitoris' roles in both sexual pleasure and reproduction are crucial and inseparable.

Recent research by scientists investigating the size and structure of the clitoris has also revealed another role for the female clitoris in preparing the vagina for pleasurable and non-traumatic sexual intercourse. As previously pointed out, dissections show that the clitoris has a far more intimate relationship with the urethra and vagina than previously thought. The size of the clitoris is such that its legs wrap round the vaginal barrel, while together the clitoral body and legs surround the urethra on three sides (the other side of the urethra is embedded in the upper, or front wall of the vagina). This close connection between the structures means that they work together as a unit, as does the penis. Significantly, during sexual arousal, one effect of clitoral engorgement or erection is to put pressure on the urethra, squeezing it shut. This move is thought to prevent bacteria entering the urethra and then causing bladder or urinary tract infections, again highlighting the clitoris' protective and preparative role.

Significantly, the need to prepare genitalia via arousal for successful (i.e. safe) sexual reproduction is not confined to humans. Animals practise the techniques too. Typically this involves the male stimulating the female externally, and not just genitally, before she is ready to receive him internally. Singing, tapping, thrusting, rubbing, vibrating, licking, feeding: males have multiple manoeuvres and call into play many parts of their anatomy – mouthparts, vocal cords, fake phalluses and the real thing – in their bid to persuade the female to desire sexual interaction and hence to have the best shot at making sex an evolutionary success. As highlighted in the previous chapter, male mites and ticks must perform many minutes, sometimes hours of oral stimulation of the female's genitals. Moving their mouthparts against her genitalia causes them to swell, allowing the male to insert his spermatophore. Likewise the sine qua non for many male insects, including beetle and wasps, involves innervating a female's genitalia by tapping her near her genital orifice. Song is the innervation stimulus for the female Caribbean fruit fly – but it has to be composed of the correct sound pressure levels.

Mammals too have to stimulate external female genitalia prior to penetration. Female rabbits, as has been revealed before, require up to seventy rhythmic constant-amplitude, high-frequency extra-vaginal thrusts from the buck if they are to assume the lordosis position necessary for intercourse to occur. Similarly, tactile stimulation of the female is a key component in female rats assuming lordosis. Here, the male rat must palpate the female's flanks with his paws, together with making pelvic thrusting movements against her perineum. When in oestrus, such sensory input fired off to the female's brain stem results in the lordotic response. Male primates too routinely make a series of rapid and shallow extravaginal thrusts before the vagina envelopes the penis. They also use their fingers, mouths and whatever else comes to hand to stimulate external female genitalia.

The necessity of clitoral stimulation is also underlined by the peculiar genitalia of a particular species of bird – the buffalo weaver (*Bubalornis niger*). And this time, it's very clear how essential clitoral stimulation is to both females and males. Like other birds, both female and male buffalo weavers urinate, defecate and reproduce via a cloaca. For females, the cloaca also serves as an oviduct for the expulsion of eggs, while for the male, it is the channel through which sperm is ejected (the male does not have a penis). However, somewhat startlingly, both sexes of this weaver bird possess a clitoris – in essence, a projection of erectile tissue. In males this organ measures 15.7 mm, while the female's is 6.1 mm.

Mesmerisingly, weaver bird copulation is characterised by lengthy mutual clitoral rubbing – with the male buffalo weaver mounting from behind and rubbing his clitoris up against the female's clitoris. These mounting bouts can last up to twenty-nine minutes, and at the end the male experiences what has been described as an orgasm, with his wing beat slowing to a quiver, his feet clenched and his leg muscles in spasm. It is only then that the male ejaculates semen from his cloaca (not his clitoris) on to the female's everted cloaca. Significantly, studies have shown that it is stimulation of the male's clitoris that is responsible for ejaculation. Whether or not stimulation of the female's clitoris is a factor in whether she everts her cloaca or accepts his sperm for fertilisation has not been looked at. However, the behaviour of these birds does underline the importance of clitoral stimulation for both sexes if successful sexual reproduction is to occur.

The way ahead

What this chapter has, I hope, shown is the importance of the clitoris in ensuring sex is pleasurable – and hence more likely to be successful, rather than deadly, in terms of sexual reproduction. There is still, however, a lot that needs to be learnt about female genitalia, both outside and in. One area that has not received much attention at all is the innervation of female genitalia, presumably because sexual arousal has until now not been seen as being important in terms of successful sexual reproduction. Female genitalia are understood to be well supplied with sensory nerves. It's known, for instance, that stimulation around the clitoris, labia, vaginal opening, lower vagina and perineum is picked up primarily by the pudendal nerve, while the pelvic nerve transmits sensations from the vagina, urethra, prostate and cervix. The hypogastric and vagus nerves are also involved in triggering and maintaining female sexual arousal, and ultimately orgasm (as we'll see later).

The precise nature and location of all branches of these essential sensory genital nerves, though, is not known. This means that these arousal-promoting nerves cannot be spared if a woman has to undergo any form of pelvic surgery. In contrast, nerve- and hence erection- and arousal-sparing surgery is a routine part of any pelvic operation on men. In this respect, as in many others, knowledge of female sexual anatomy and function still lags far behind that of male sexual anatomy and function. It is hoped that increased awareness of the importance of the clitoris in supporting female sexual arousal and non-traumatic (i.e. successful) sexual intercourse will change this in the near future.

One remaining controversy hanging over the clitoris in the twenty-first century is its name – and what it represents. Some groups are pushing to redefine the clitoris so that this one word encompasses many other parts of female sexual anatomy. Their desire is to see the clitoris as being composed of eighteen parts – including the inner labia, hymen, vestibular bulbs and pelvic floor muscles. Considering that female genitalia have been reduced so much in terms of stature and function in the past, I am loath to call these eighteen parts a clitoris. It is also, I believe, misleading and confusing to do this. It would be a step back, rather than forwards. The understanding of female genitalia needs to be expanded by words and images, not reduced in order to fulfil some idea of what is politically correct.

I also feel uneasy that the desire to rename objects – such as insisting on the Fallopian tubes being the egg tubes, because Fallopius was a man, and the tubes are women's property – smacks of previous cultures' attempts to rewrite history to their liking. The Egyptians chiselled out hieroglyphs in an attempt to force their people to forget prior religions or ideas – today we try to alter language. Yet acknowledging history is essential, whether it is the history of anatomy or the history of language. What is important regarding the clitoris is appreciating its actual structure; understanding how the clitoris works in glorious concert with the rest of a woman's genitalia – outside and in; and realising that female and male genitalia are more similar than not – and that extends to their core role in sexual reproduction and pleasure.

Note

All the measurements given in this chapter relate to the handful of cadaver clitorises dissected in the name of research. They refer to the averages from both pre- and post-menopausal women. Importantly, these measurements should not be read as being set in stone, or as absolutes, or norms. Not enough research has yet been done to give any such lengths with certainty. All women vary, as do all men.

5

OPENING PANDORA'S BOX

A hungering maw. A gluttonous gullet. A toothed, voracious, ravenous, greedy chasm. *Vagina dentata* – the vagina with teeth – is an ancient anxious image that flows through folklore, mythology, literature, art and humankind's dreamworld. For many the most powerful of all vaginal myths and superstitions, the *vagina dentata* is also, perhaps, the most common. Its prevalence around the globe is stunning. Snapping and snarling, emasculating and mutilating men, the *vagina dentata* is to be found from North to South America, across Africa, and in India and Europe too. The omnipotence of this motif of the devouring vagina has also survived millennia, with many cultures' creation mythology imbued with castrating and deadly images. The first women of the Chaco Indians were said to have teeth in their vaginas with which they ate, and men could not approach them until the Chaco hero, Caroucho, broke the teeth out.

The Yanomamo of South America say that one of the first beings on earth was a woman whose vagina became a toothed mouth and cut off her partner's penis. In Polynesia, Hine-nui-te-po, the goddess of the underworld and the first female on earth, from whose womb all others fell, uses her vagina to slay Maui, the Polynesian hero. Maui crawls into Hine-nui-te-po's vagina in the hope of returning to her womb, thus cheating death and winning immortality. Instead, he is bitten in two by her vagina's snapping, lightning-generating flint edges, and so, because of his defeat by the goddess' vagina, all other mortals must die.

Psychology suggests that sexual folklore seethes with stories of snapping vaginal teeth because of male fears about what lies within the dark, unknowable, unseeable mysterious space that is the interior of the vagina. Others view *vagina dentata* images as the embodiment of masculine angst before the insatiable vortex of female sexual energy.

In the stories themselves, the origin of female genital fangs and the reasons underlying their sometimes deadly behaviour are not always explained. In some, sources both material and spiritual are blamed. One North American Indian myth tells of how a meat-eating fish inhabits the vagina of the Terrible Mother. In the Middle Ages, Christian authorities pointed the finger at the moon and magic when trying to find an explanation for the so-called fact of witches stealing men's penises with their vaginal teeth.

The following fable from the Mehinaku, a tropical-forest-dwelling tribe of Brazil, intimates a male role in vaginal dentition:

> In ancient times, there was an angry man who constantly berated others. One evening, a woman took many shells – they looked just like teeth – and put them in her inner labia. Later, when it got dark, the man wanted to have sex. 'Oh, she is beautiful,' he thought. The woman was pretending to sleep. 'Let's have sex,' he said. Oh, but his penis was big. In it went . . . it went all the way in . . . Tsyuu! The vagina cut his penis right off, and he died right there, in the hammock.

This story, like many others, ends in the castration and death of the male.

In some folk legends, notably those of the Navajo and Apache, deadly toothed vaginas go one step further, and are described as detached organs, walking around independently and biting as they go. Just like the Baubo figurines described earlier, this is the vagina personified, but this time more terrifying – with teeth. For instance, New Mexico Jicarilla Apaches tell of a time when only four women in the world possessed vaginas. These women, known as the 'vagina girls', had the form of women, but were in essence vaginas. They were also the daughters of a murderous monster called Kicking Monster.

Picture the scene. According to the legend, the house that the four vagina girls lived in was full of other vaginas, all hanging around on the walls. And understandably perhaps, rumours about the vagina girls and their house brought many men along the road to their door. But once there the men would be met by Kicking Monster, kicked into the house, never to return. This continued, so the story goes, with man after man disappearing, apparently swallowed up in the house of the four vagina girls with vaginas hanging from the walls. Enter Killer-of-Enemies, the marvellous boy hero:

> Outwitting Kicking Monster, Killer-of-Enemies entered the house, and the four vagina girls approached him, craving intercourse. But he asked: 'Where have all the men gone who were kicked into this place?' 'We ate them up,' they said, 'because we like to do that'; and they attempted to embrace him. But he held them off, shouting, 'Keep away. This is no way to use the vagina.' And he told them, 'First I must give you some medicine, which you have never tasted before, medicine made of sour berries; and then I'll do what you ask.' Whereupon he gave them sour berries of four kinds to eat. 'The vagina,' he said, 'is always sweet when you do like this.' The berries puckered their mouths, so that finally they could not chew at all, but only swallowed. They liked it very much, though ... When Killer-of-Enemies had come to them, they had had strong teeth with which they had eaten their victims. But this medicine destroyed their teeth entirely.

The removal of vaginal teeth (symbolising the devouring aspect of female sexuality) by brave male heroes is a core component of many *dentata* stories. Pincers, flints, a piece of string, the berry medicine of Killer-of-Enemies, iron tongs, rocks and rods that are as thick or long as a penis, are all used as excision tools in a bid to tame the toothed vagina and create a compliant woman. In some telling instances it is only after a woman has had her teeth pulled – that is, she is tamed by having her spirit and insatiable threatening sexuality broken – that a man will marry her. In this sense, pulling vaginal teeth is a metaphor for how some men would like to make women meek and biddable, remoulded in a shape defined by them. In these stories, instead of shaming her into submission, physical means are used to tame her sexuality. The following depiction of dental extraction comes from India:

> There was a Rakshasa's [demon's] daughter who had teeth in her vagina. When she saw a man, she would turn into a pretty girl, seduce him, cut off his penis, eat it herself and give the rest of his body to her tigers. One day she met seven brothers in the jungle and married the eldest so that she could sleep with them all. After some time she took the eldest boy to where the tigers lived, made him lie with her, cut off his penis, ate it and gave his body to the tigers. In the same way she killed six of the brothers till only the youngest one was left. When his turn came, the god who helped him sent him a dream. 'If you go with the girl,' said the god, 'make an iron tube, put it into her vagina and break her teeth.' The boy did this ...

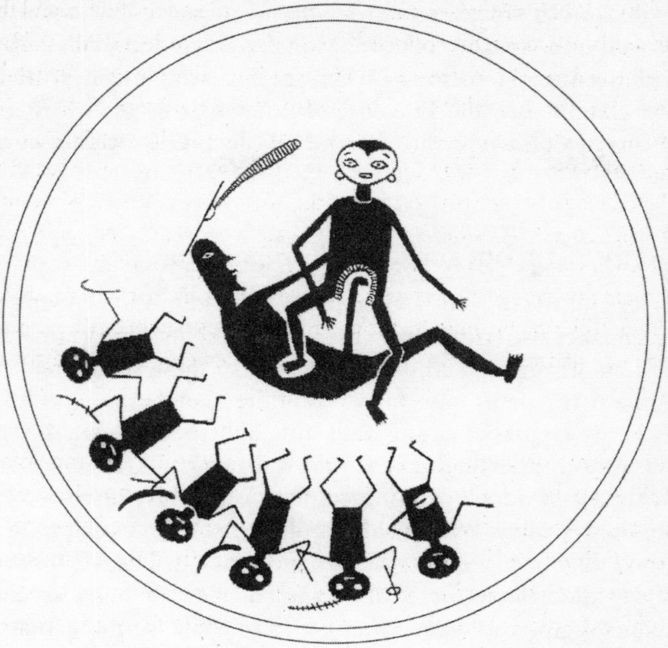

Figure 5.1 The *vagina dentata*: round the world, art and myth tell of how men may meet their end if they dare to venture inside the deadly toothed vagina.

Fashioning hard phallic weapons that will never be flaccid in the face of female genitalia is also a common thread in these *vagina dentata* myths. Presumably this relates to male fears of women's seemingly insatiable sexual nature, their ability to enjoy orgasm after orgasm with their genitalia when men may only be able to manage one before becoming limp. I'm sure it's no coincidence that sharp-edged devouring teeth are the female weapon of choice – they stand in stark opposition to male fears of a soft, impotent penis. Creating an alternative tool is at the heart of another story of seven siblings and their efforts to remove a woman's vaginal teeth. This is one of the Pre-Columbian myths of North American Indians, and is depicted in explicit eleventh-century ceramic Pueblo artwork (see Figure 5.1). This Mimbres myth bowl illustrates the final brother's efforts to remove a woman's vaginal teeth with a false penis made out of oak and hickory. Re-enactments of vagina tooth smashing can be found in some cultures' rituals. In Navajo and Apache folklore, Monster-Slayer kills Filled Vagina, one of the more ferocious of her species, who mates with cacti, with a club. Today, the Pueblo and other native North Americans use a carved wooden phallus to symbolically break a vagina woman's teeth.

Not only teeth, but snakes and dragons too

Teeth are not the only terrifying object to be found in woman's extra orifice. Snakes also stream from the deep, dark, invisible vaginal interior in folklore and legend. Vagina snakes, so these stories relate, can bite off a man's penis, poison it, or kill the man. Some serpents lurk solely in the vaginas of virgins, and sting only the first man to venture inside. Among the Tembu it is said that women who crave sexual excitement may attract demonic serpents called Inyoka, who come to live in their vaginas and give them pleasure. Women can then send out their vagina snakes to bite any men they dislike, or those who don't pay attention to them. In Polynesia, where there are no snakes, voracious vagina eels come into play. In one tale from the Tuamotos Islands, the eels in a woman called Faumea's vagina kill all men. However, she teaches the hero, Tagaroa, how to entice them outside, and so he sleeps with her in safety.

It seems that fears of what lies inside the vagina have allowed men's imaginations to run riot over the centuries. Men of Malekula talk mysteriously of a vagina spirit, called 'that which draws us to it so that it may devour us'. Hungry dragons too are often to be found inside the vagina of folklore and myth, and some have speculated that the many legends of brave heroes killing dragons with sharp-edged teeth are spin-offs from the original dragons in the vagina idea. If this is the case, good old St George, for killing England's symbolic vagina/female spirit. Vaginal teeth can also be metaphoric, as revealed by the Muslim belief that the vagina can 'bite off' a man's eye-beam, resulting in blindness for the man who is brave enough to look deep into its depths. It is said that a sultan of Damascus lost his sight in this manner, and had to travel to Sardinia to be cured by a miracle-working statue of the Virgin Mary – whose vagina is, of course, safely veiled by her ever-permanent hymen.

Apparently not content with arming the vagina with all things devouring and venomous, many cultures fill their mythology with stories of gruesome creatures that are women above, but hell-beasts below. The Greeks told of lustful she-demons born of the Libyan snake-goddess Lamia. Their name – *laminae* – means either 'lecherous vaginas' or 'gluttonous gullets'. Or how about the Naginis, Indian figures which are cobras from the waist down and goddesses from the waist up, or the Echidna, which appear as pretty nymphs on top and slithering snakes beneath. Even William Shakespeare had his King Lear fulminating in this way about women, suggesting that what is below is bad, and revealing his deepest fears about females. Lear, in his madness, cries:

> Down from the waist they are Centaurs,
> Though women all above:
> But to the girdle do the Gods inherit,
> Beneath is all the fiends':
> There's hell, there's darkness, there is the
> sulphurous pit,
> Burning, scalding . . .

This angry, terrified view of women, what is below their waists and between their legs, is deeply disturbing and yet it is one that is painted over and over again. It also pops up in interpretations of one of the classic Greek myths, the story of Pandora, whose name means 'the all-giving' or 'gift to all'. According to Greek mythology, Pandora was the world's first woman and the one to blame for all the 'ills that beset men'. Her crime? It's said that she opened a box or vessel that contained all the evils of the world, letting them out and leaving only hope remaining inside. Does Pandora's box have genitalic connections? Some have certainly read it as a symbol of female genitalia. The artist Abraham van Diepenbeeck placed Pandora's vessel suggestively over her vagina, and, of course, box is slang for the vagina. Paul Klee's twentieth-century response to the centuries-old myth is more vaginally overt. Facing straight on, he painted Pandora's box as female genitalia, as a casket with oval carvings, complete with evil vulval

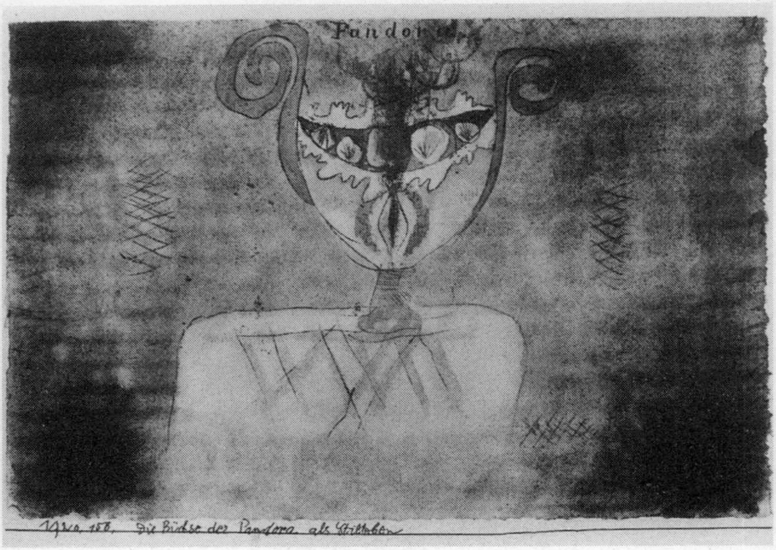

Figure 5.2 Pandora's box as envisaged by Paul Klee.

vapours being emitted from the genital cleft (see Figure 5.2). This extraordinary drawing also depicts Pandora's vessel with handles resembling Fallopian tubes, and a base ridged like the muscular interior of the vagina.

The inside view

So what is the inside story? Although myth may tell of a mouth with sharp dentition, ready to snap up and spit out unwelcome intruders, or a male vision of fear and hell, science has something else to say about what lies within the vaginal walls. After centuries of misunderstanding the vagina, of either ignoring it or calling it variously a royal highway, a passive vessel, and even essentially devoid of sensitivity, a new view is emerging: there are no teeth, snakes or dragons and, unlike the empty, dead space envisaged by early thinkers, the interior of the vagina is anything but a passive black hole. Instead, science reveals an amazing, expanding, contracting, sensitive muscular organ, where multiple erogenous zones rub shoulders with a remarkably robust pathogen defence system. In fact, flexibility or fluidity, not unyielding dentition, is the vagina's key design concept.

Have you ever considered that a woman's vagina is teeming and overflowing with life? Or that a veritable biological soup thrives here in this exquisitely balanced environment? Maybe not, but this is, in fact, the case. Why should this be? The answer lies in what the vagina represents. Just like the mouth, or any open orifice, the vagina provides potential pathogens (disease-causing agents) with an avenue to the interior of the body. Moreover, the vaginal gateway heads the route to the rest of a female's reproductive organs, the crown jewels of a species' survival. It's not surprising, therefore, that like the mouth, with its super salival defence system, backed up by mucous membranes and tonsils and teeth, the vagina too has a very potent protection structure in place. But that is not all. The vagina is not just about defending against disease. It has another crucial and yet distinct role – enabling access to some, but not all, intruders. Depending on the situation, a woman's vagina needs to be capable of acting as both bodyguard and bouncer. To be able to perform in this perfectly poised, polar manner, the vaginal interior, or *lumen*, needs a wondrous environment. Snakes or sharp teeth are not the answer. On the contrary, the vaginal solution is a wet, moist and fluid one.

The joys of mucus

Mucus is the vagina's major medium. Defined as a protective secretion, mucus is the means by which the vaginal interior maintains its integrity in the face of all comers. Without the never-ending exuding of fluids, the vagina would not able to function effectively. For not only does mucus provide lubrication during sexual activity, it also acts as a selective barrier against pathogens, and supports a cornucopia of essential organisms. Yet despite its indispensability, mucus, more often than not, gets a bad name. Slimy, gloopy, gummy, oozing from clefts and crevices, the nasal brand is tarred with the slang word 'snot' while the vaginal variety suffers with the useless, demeaning designation of 'discharge'. In many cultures, vaginal discharge equals dirt, often translating as such in language. Moist, wet, well-lubricated genitals are viewed by some as disgusting, polluting and to be avoided.

In some central and southern African countries, a dry vagina is promoted as the genitalic gold standard – as rated by men. Women use concoctions of salts and herbs in a bid to fulfil this strange male desire for an arid vagina. One study of intravaginal practices in Zimbabwe revealed that more than 85 per cent of women have used drying salts at least once. Horrifically, however, the dry sex that men are said to crave leads inevitably to chafing and cracking of the vaginal walls, leaving women at risk of infection. As previously noted, it is now recognised that it is only when there are abrasions or damage to the mucosal lining of the vagina that viruses, such as HIV, can infect a woman. That is, if there is no damage to the vaginal wall, infection cannot occur as immune cells are not exposed to the virus. Zimbabwe, frighteningly, has one of the world's highest rates of HIV infection, a fact which is without doubt in part explained by the craze for moistureless sex.

There is another very disturbing aspect here. Many, if not all, vaginal contraceptives actually contain chemicals, such as nonoxynol-9, that damage the mucosal layer of the vagina, leaving it open to infection. It seems astoundingly bad science to me that this situation exists, that a chemical that damages female genitalia can be used as a common vaginal contraceptive. What's more, nonoxynol-9 is the major ingredient of such contraceptives as contraceptive jelly. When used in conjunction with a diaphragm, nonoxynol-9 is placed in direct contact with the cervix, which is even more easily damaged than the vagina. This is because cervical cells are extremely thin (only one cell thick), fragile and easily damaged. If nonoxynol-9 damages the vaginal cell wall, which is far more dense, sturdy and resilient than the cervix (the surface layer of squamous epithelium vaginal cells is up to 16–30 cells deep), then what level of damage is nonoxynol-9 doing to the cervix? In my own experience, using a diaphragm and contraceptive jelly with the major ingredient nonoxynol-9 led to regular cervical bleeding and severe abrasion to the cervix. When I stopped placing nonoxynol-9 in direct regular contact with my cervix, the bleeding stopped and the abrasions healed.

There is no one fount of female mucus. Instead, female fluids well up and flow from a variety of vaginal sources, coming together to form a cocktail of secretions. Both external and internal genitalia contribute. In the mix are fluids from the Bartholin's (or major vestibular) glands, which sit at five and seven o'clock to the entrance to the vagina, as well as those from the nearby minor vestibular glands. A woman's prostate gland (sometimes called Skene's or paraurethral glands) also furnishes fluids, as do the vaginal walls, both as a result of sexual arousal and as vaginal wall cells are shed. Mucus cascading cyclically from a woman's cervix coalesces with fluids from the uterus and Fallopian tubes above. Cervical mucus comes in columnar flows and together with uterine or endometrial secretions, is the major ingredient of female mucus. However, secretions from the sweat glands and oil-producing sebaceous glands situated in the smooth, glossy skin of a woman's inner labia also blend in, as does mucus from newly discovered interlabial glands, about which very little is yet known. The end result is a potent, heady and dynamic brew.

One of the reasons why the precise number and nature of the constituents of vaginal mucus is as yet unclear is the lack of research done in this area. However, there are thousands of micro-organisms thriving in this flora. Mucus is plump full of them. Among them are sugars, proteins, acids of all sorts, simple and complex alcohols, bacteria and antibodies. All these molecules and many more as yet unidentified flow into and are supported by the vagina's mucoid environment. This bountiful fluid is also in continual flux, depending on a woman's menstrual cycle, her sexual arousal and activity, her physical and mental well-being, even the food she eats. In many ways, a woman's vaginal mucus is a barometer of herself and her lifestyle.

For many mucosal compounds, the major role appears to be one of defence, of making sure that this warm, moist ecosystem does not become a haven for disease. Indeed, it is argued that female genitals have their own separate immune system, courtesy of mucosal secretions. Mucus protects in a variety of manners, not least by lubricating vaginal tissues. This viscous moving fluid acts as a physical barrier as its continual slow flow down and out of the vagina prevents micro-organisms from attaching to the cell walls of a woman's vagina. It can also block indirectly, by providing bacteria with a false receptor or target to bind to.

Female genital mucus also supports an ace team of defensive agents. This mucosal posse includes molecules such as lysozyme, which punctures bacterial cell walls; lactoferrin, which mops up the iron that some micro-organisms need to grow; several classes of virus-neutralising antibodies; defensins or antimicrobial peptides; and phagocytic cells, which can engulf and swallow all intruders, including sperm. One cervically produced antibody, secretory immunoglobulin A (IgA), works like a killer sheepdog – rounding bacterial particles up into one coherent mass, and then preparing them for ingestion and digestion by phagocytic cells. Another cervical fluid constituent – a protein called secretory leukocyte protease inhibitor (SLPI) – has been shown to play a critical role in wound healing by reversing tissue damage and hastening healing. Its uses seem manifold – with evidence suggesting that it has anti-inflammatory, anti-fungal, anti-bacterial and anti-viral properties.

The need for a tart vagina

Centuries ago, vaginal pH was thought to be important in determining the sex of any child conceived – acid (low pH) for a boy, alkaline (high pH) for a girl. This is an ancient scientific theory that has yet to be proven. Vaginal pH, however, is of vital importance for women, but its significance lies in ensuring a healthy vagina. In fact, maintaining vaginal pH is an important way in which some organisms within vaginal mucus keep potential pathogens at bay. In the healthy pre-menopausal woman, vaginal pH should remain low, hovering around pH 4.0. That is, it's best to be acidic, or tart, but not as tart as a lemon (pH 2.0). More like a glass of good red wine. Keeping to this level of acidity is key because it determines a 'healthy' balance of vaginal micro-organisms, or flora, in vaginal mucus. That is, an acidic vagina keeps numbers or ratios of micro-organisms in check. In contrast, a too alkaline environment tends to result in an overabundance of some micro-organisms, which can then become pathogenic (disease-causing) agents. Low pH is also good for the cervix, as it protects the extremely thin and fragile cervical cells from damage.

The guardians of low vaginal pH are a particular type of bacteria, lactobacilli, which occur naturally in the vagina. This may seem surprising, as bacteria are a type of micro-organism that often get a bad name. In fact, when first discovered at the end of the nineteenth century, the many varieties of vaginal bacteria were incorrectly viewed as unclean, disease-causing agents. But bacteria, be they the vaginal variety or not, do not deserve their negative press. As with many things in life, striking the right balance is what is important, and this is true for all types of bacteria too. Too few vaginal lactobacilli can result in a rise in pH to alkaline levels, and the flourishing of microorganisms (with their increased numbers making them potentially pathogenic). The best way for a woman to keep her lactobacilli at the healthiest levels is to lead as healthy a life-style as possible – that's all you have to do, and your vagina will do the rest naturally. Dousing the vagina in man-made chemicals, such as those contained in so-called vaginal douches, deodorants and wipes, is not recommended ever, as this removes the vagina's natural defences.

Sperm bodyguard and bouncer

The story of what happens to sperm inside female genitalia highlights how vital a woman's vaginal environment is. This is because having an acidic vagina is critical in removing unwanted or surplus sperm. For human sperm, the vagina represents an extremely hostile and lethal environment, and prolonged sperm survival is not possible under these selectively acidic conditions (twenty minutes is the maximum). Out of the sixty million or more sperm contained in one human ejaculate, most will die in the vagina. The buffering or balancing effects of seminal plasma (the medium in which ejaculated sperm are suspended) offers some protection to sperm against the acidic conditions in which they find themselves. However, its effects are limited – following sperm ejaculation in the vagina, vaginal pH rises to between pH 5.5 and pH 7.0, but this shift to a more sperm-friendly flora is transient. Within at least two hours, a legion of lactobacilli will have tipped vaginal pH back in the female's favour.

Once deposited in the vagina, if human sperm are not killed by the acidic conditions, engulfed and eaten by marauding phagocytic cells or simply ejected by the woman, they face another challenge – cervical mucus. Produced primarily by glands in the top half of the cervix, cervical mucus creates a dense mucoid plug which essentially fills the uterine cervix. And from there columns of mucus cascade ceaselessly down into the vagina, averaging around 20–60 mg a day. This cervical mucus has a crucial reproductive role – namely, acting as a very effective biological barrier, or sperm bouncer.

When faced with this mucus, sperm have a problem. It seems they are incapable of passing through, round, over or under this formidable mucoid material. They have met their match, and the next stage underlines this. Unable to overcome this viscous hurdle, sperm are then swept out of the vagina, escorted off the premises by the slow, unstoppable flow of bouncer cervical mucus. There is, however, one sticking point in this scenario. Cervical mucus is mercurial, and does not always act as a sperm bouncer. In fact, on some days of the month, cervical mucus undergoes a compete role reversal, metamorphosing, dramatically, into a sperm bodyguard.

For just a few days every month – typically from about two to three days prior to ovulation, and up to twenty-four hours post-ovulation – cervical mucus becomes sperm's major ally in its fertilisation quest. While other elements of the vaginal environment rush to repel the newcomers, bodyguard mucus moves to embrace them. The difference between bouncer mucus and mid-cycle bodyguard mucus is immediately apparent in other ways too. Visually the change in consistency, sheen and colour is stunning. What was an opaque milky-white glutinous fluid mass of limited elasticity (maximum extended length about 2.5 cm) transforms into a glistening, translucent, silky and seemingly endlessly stretchy amorphous substance (some say it's like egg white). Mucus columns of between 7 and 10 cm in length are not uncommon.

This extreme stretchiness of mid-cycle mucus is one of its key characteristics, and, indeed, has given rise to the term 'spinnbarkeit' – that is, the capacity of cervical mucus to elongate. Another feature (noted by scientists) is that this fertile mucus forms a fern pattern when dried. This is because of its high salt content. For women monitoring their fertility, the point to remember is that the more stretchy and akin to egg white the mucus, the closer you are to ovulating. Another thing to look out for is that production is scaled up too. At mid-cycle, ten times more mucus – 600 mg – streams forth daily. This increased mucus flow preceding egg release is also accompanied by changes in a woman's cervix. The external os (mouth) opens up to around 4 mm in diameter between twenty-four and forty-eight hours before ovulation – a move that is believed to enhance the likelihood of conception occurring.

Research shows that mid-cycle bodyguard mucus can both shepherd and shelter sperm, offering a safe passage out of the vagina through the cervix and into the uterus, as well as a safe alkaline harbour. If sperm are lucky enough to land near a column of mid-cycle mucus, they appear to be sucked inside the mucus structure. And when enveloped in these mucus arms, genital contractions are believed to draw sperm nestled in their mucus environment up into the cervix and uterus. Incredibly, it seems that cervical mucus can support human sperm for prolonged periods of time, as research shows that sperm sequestered in folds of cervical mucus, or cervical crypts, can survive, remaining motile, for between five and eight days (uterine fluids may also play a role in this support).

It's now appreciated that fluctuations in the levels of circulating hormones are the driving force behind the physical changes in mucus which make bouncer mucus impenetrable to sperm, and result in bodyguard mucus drawing sperm passively in. Increasing levels of oestrogen in the days preceding ovulation result in the structure of cervical mucus becoming one of parallel filaments of long mucin molecules, with canals in between along which sperm can travel. However, post-ovulation, increasing levels of progesterone disrupt this ordered structure, and the filaments form a criss-cross matrix through which sperm cannot traverse.

Mid-cycle bodyguard mucus also has another vital reproduction role to play, and this time it's a selective one. The microstructure of mucus reveals how this selection could function. The canals or channels separating one parallel mucus section from another are extremely thin. At between 0.5 and 0.8 μm they are smaller than a sperm head, making any movement through this mucus a very tight squeeze for sperm. Indeed, experiments with human mucus show it bulging and stretching around sperm. The precise importance of forcing sperm to be in such close proximity to cervical mucus is as yet uncertain.

One intriguing idea is that this extreme proximity forces necessary interactions between mucus and sperm, perhaps preparing sperm for fertilisation by shearing certain seminal components from their surfaces. Recognition is another exciting suggestion, as it is known that this enforced closeness does play a sperm-screening role, with mid-cycle cervical mucus acting as a biological filter, sorting the normally shaped sperm from the morphologically abnormal ones. However, recognition may involve far more than just sorting shapes; selecting a complementary genetic partner may also form part of cervical mucus' multiple functions. Scientists are just at the start of understanding how the female genital tract as a whole, including mucus, selects a female's Mr Right Sperm.

Reading the vagina

Penis size, it is said, is a prime concern for many, if not all, men. However, this male obsession with genital size is not, it seems, confined to the phallus. Around the world, estimating and classifying vaginal size and attempting to map out the internal contours of the vagina has proved to be irresistible to men, often with eye-opening and entertaining results. In the west, the desire to put a name to a woman's genital landmarks has led to some wonderful medical monickers. There's 'the fold of Shaw', 'the pouch of Douglas', 'the column rugarum', 'the hollow of modesty', 'the canal of Nuck' and 'the elastic sac of Sappey'. These titles were, of course, all bestowed and imposed by men. Today they seem ridiculous, and are, in the main, obsolete.

Outside the west, Arabic, Indian, Japanese and Chinese cultures provide beautifully detailed and inventive information on the interior of the vagina, and how it has been perceived. For example, the Arabic erotic manual, *The Perfumed Garden*, written by Sheikh Nefzaoui, details thirty-eight varieties of vagina, and thirty-five types of penis. Vaginal descriptions include, *el aride*, 'the large one' – a thick and fleshy vagina; *el harrab*, 'the fugitive' – a small and tight vagina that is also short; and *el mokaour*, 'the bottomless', a name referring to a deep vagina, one that is lengthier than usual. The possessor of this larger vagina, *The Perfumed Garden* points out, needs a particular partner or position to truly arouse and satisfy her fully.

Ancient Japanese culture, in the sacred text *The Sutra of Secret Bliss*, also describes differently sized vaginas, associating them with one of the recognised five elements of life – earth, water, fire, air and ether (heaven). The *Daikoku* is the dark earth vagina, one that envelops and holds the penis; the *Mizu-tembo* is the moist water vagina, with a small opening and a wide interior, while the *Bon-tembo* is the celestial vagina – most beautiful and fragrant. This variety of vagina is also known as the Dragon's Pearl, because its tight opening and narrow passage lead to a pearl-like womb. Poetically, it is said that anyone fortunate enough to enter a vagina like this cries out in ecstasy.

India's famous sex manual, the *Kama Sutra*, provides a particularly detailed look at both sexes' genitals. This book, depicting the erotic science of ancient Indian culture, arranged women and men in terms of their sexual characteristics. That is, classifying them by the size of their genitalia, their force of passion or carnal desire and 'their moment of sexual impulse' (the time factor). For women, this classification, which was written by men, results in four orders, three temperaments and three kinds. Each of these ten categories describes the characteristics of the particular vagina, and the *Kama Sutra* also gives advice on the sexual compatibility of women and men in terms of their sexual characteristics. Vaginal length or depth is revealed by the three kinds of women, and is as follows:

1) The *migri* (female gazelle) or *harini* (doe) is the woman with a deep-set vagina (six fingers deep) that is cool as the moon and has the pleasant scent of a lotus flower.
2) The *vadama* or *ashvini* (mare) is the woman with a vagina nine fingers deep, with freely flowing yellow juices and the scent of sesame.
3) The *karini* (she-elephant) is the woman with a vagina twelve fingers deep with abundant juices that smell like elephant's musk.

Many other methods of describing or classifying the vagina exist. Tantric texts divide the vagina into six regions governed by different Indian goddesses – Kali, Tara, Chinnamasta, Matangi, Lakshmi and Sodasi. Meanwhile some eastern texts describe the lower vulval portion of a woman's vagina as having the following four properties: 'First, it looks like the tip of an elephant's trunk; second, it is twisted, like the turns on a shell; third, it is closed up, as if by something soft; and fourth, it opens and closes like a lotus flower.'

If you want to read the vagina, there is also the option of using the ancient Chinese art of reflexology. Using this viewpoint, the lower third of the vagina and the vaginal opening correspond to the kidneys, the central third the liver, and the uppermost third of the vaginal chamber the spleen and pancreas. The cervix, meanwhile, corresponds to the heart and lungs. This way of looking at the vagina also stresses the importance of stimulating each portion of female genitalia – from the kidneys up to the heart and lungs – shallowly and deeply and circling from side to side if a woman is to be truly satisfied and sexually energised. It sounds good to me.

The Palace of Delight

Looking at the various systems employed over the centuries to classify and understand the interior of the vagina, it's hard not to get the feeling that genital measurement isn't perhaps a particular male métier, as some vaginal dimensions are somewhat startling. Chinese sexual manuals, such as the Taoist text *The Wondrous Discourse of Su Nü*, detail how vaginas come in eight different varieties – each determined by the depth of the vaginal interior, and each 2.5 cm longer than the previous. However, some, such as the Zither String, seem surprisingly short, while others, like the North Pole, are somewhat on the lengthy side. In ascending size, the Eight Valleys, as they are known, are:

1) The Zither String or Lute String (*ch'in-hsien*), 0–2.5 cm
2) The Water-caltrop Teeth or Water-chestnut Teeth (*ling-ch'ih*), 5 cm
3) The Peaceful Valley or Little Stream (*t'o-hsi*), 7.5 cm
4) The Dark Pearl or Mysterious Pearl (*hsüan-chu*), 10 cm
5) The Valley Seed or Valley Proper (*ku-shih*), 12.5 cm
6) The Palace of Delight or Deep Chamber (*yü-ch'üeh*), 15 cm
7) The Inner Door or Gate of Prosperity (*k'un-hu*), 17.5 cm
8) The North Pole (*pei-chi*), 20 cm

Chinese sexual manuals also classified the relative position of the vulva – be it high (in a forward/upward location), that is, placed more ventrally or towards the belly, to the middle, or low (lower on the perineum).

So what is the average length of the vagina? Importantly, what the above ancient measurements do not articulate is that the interior of the vagina cannot be calibrated in this way – with just one length. For every woman, the ventral or anterior wall of her vagina – the belly side – is shorter than the opposing, posterior, wall (adjacent to the rectum). This is because the cervix, which sits at the apex of the vagina, projects down into the vagina, making the ventral vaginal wall shorter than the other. (The twin arch-like spaces that are created between the vagina wall and the curving cervix are known as the anterior and posterior fornices – singular, fornix – a word that is said to derive from the habit in Roman times of prostitutes renting vaulted or arched basements for them and their clients to fornicate in – the Latin word for arch being *fornix*).

And the average length from vaginal entrance to fornix and cervix? Most recently, average vaginal length (when not sexually aroused) has been placed anywhere between 7 and 12.5 cm, with the posterior length of the vagina from 1.5 to 3.5 cm longer than the ventral vaginal wall. Importantly, just as all penises vary enormously in size, so too do all vaginas. There is no standard. And just as all penises lengthen when aroused and erect, so too do all vaginas, as we shall see.

The fabulous shape-shifter

While all women have an intrinsic vaginal size, vaginal structure and volume can be altered. The key characteristic of the vagina is, after all, flexibility, and this flexibility in shape derives from the fact that the vagina is, in essence, a fibromuscular tube. Strategically placed muscles encircle and form its length and breadth. Hence the vagina can constrict or be constricted, dilate and change internal pressure. In fact, courtesy of her richly innervated and sensitive genital musculature, a woman's vagina is anything but a passive, unresponsive organ. This fact is demonstrated remarkably eloquently by the miracle of childbirth.

The vagina expands to at least an eye-watering ten times its normal size during the delivery of a typical bouncing baby. The cervix, too, must dilate to a great degree, becoming as wide as the vagina is long. For the cervix, this amazing feat of distension can only be achieved by the prior softening of cervical tissue, and results in a permanent visual record of childbirth. In a woman who has not experienced childbirth via vaginal delivery, the os, the extremely slim opening of the cervix to the uterus, appears as a small dimple in the middle of the circular cervix. After vaginal delivery, this indentation takes on a special character, like the upward curve of a smile, or the wink of an eye, if you will. A smiling, winking cervix is the sure sign of a woman who has brought a child into the world vaginally.

The fantastic flexible nature of the vagina is also immediately obvious during sexual arousal and intercourse – a fact that was recognised and appreciated by western men of science over three hundred years ago. While Reinier de Graaf reckoned the vagina to be '6, 7, 8 or

9 finger-breadths long', he also observed in his pioneering work *The Generative Organs of Women* that: 'During coitus it applies itself everywhere to the penis and accommodates itself along every dimension in such a way that its concave shape becomes one with the convex shape of the penis ... During childbirth it adopts yet another shape ...' De Graaf was also quite astute in noting that it was sexual arousal that had a strong effect, commenting how 'during coitus it shortens, lengthens, constricts and dilates more or less according to the degree of the woman's excitement'. Delightfully, under the chapter heading ' Concerning the Vagina of the Uterus', the Dutchman enthuses, rhapsodises even, how:

> The woman's vagina in fact is so cleverly constructed that it will accommodate itself to each and every penis; it will go out to meet a short one, retire before a long one, dilate for a fat one, and constrict for a thin one. Nature has taken account of every variety of penis and so there is no need solicitously to seek a scabbard the same size as your knife ... Every man can thus come together with every woman and every woman with every man, if there is compatibility in other respects ...

The importance of females possessing powerful shape-changing genitalic musculature is highlighted by the ways in which a vast array of other species use their vaginal muscles, in particular to improve their reproductive success. Female hyaenas, as we've seen, need pelvic muscles robust enough to retract their elongated clitoris back to create an internal vagina. Many insects have vaginal (bursa) muscles steely enough that they can prevent copulation occurring or force out an unwanted member. The vaginal muscles of honey bees are thought to be responsible for triggering the male's ejaculation, while the male marsh-dwelling bug, *Hebrus pusillus*, must rely on the strong milking action of the female's genital muscles to suck sperm from his phallus. Genital musculature also underlies the routeing of sperm to storage or disposal sites, or ovaries, in many insect species.

Muscles, muscles, muscles

The effects of possessing strong vaginal muscles can be just as stunning in humans. Today, fine vaginal muscle control is most directly in evidence within the shows of the sex industry. Smoking cigarettes, firing ping pong balls, writing messages, opening bottles, even picking up sushi with chopsticks – vaginas can perform all these feats and more. However, while these cunning stunts may be financially rewarding for women and titillating for men, the human vagina's impressive muscularity was not designed with bottles, balls and cigarettes in mind.

It is in the ancient teachings of eastern cultures that another, more sensual and mutually pleasure-oriented role is seen for a woman's vaginal muscles. *Pompoir* (a Tamil term) or *bhaga asana* (from the Sanskrit) are two of the names given to the vaginal technique of embracing and locking the penis and keeping it in a prolonged erection by means of the vaginal musculature alone. For men, *pompoir* is an exercise in penile passivity, as all that moves are the vaginal muscles. Using the pelvic floor muscles in this way has been seen for centuries as a way of enhancing sexual pleasure for both partners and controlling sexual timing. It is also enjoyed as an intensely pleasurable means of self-stimulation by women, and it is in this particular pose that a famous statue of the Indian goddess Kameshvari is thought to be sitting in the town of Bheraghat.

In the sixteenth-century Indian erotic manual the *Ananga Ranga*, written by Kalyanamalla, a woman who has mastered the sexual and pleasure potential of her pelvic muscles is known as a *kabbazah*, which is an Arabic word meaning 'holder' or 'clasp'. The 1885 translation of the *Ananga Ranga*, by Richard Burton, describes the muscular art of the *kabbazah* and *pompoir* as follows:

> This is the most sought-after feminine response of all. She must close and constrict the yoni (vagina) until it holds the lingam (penis), as with a finger, opening and shutting at her pleasure, and finally acting as the hand of the Indian Gopala-girl, who milks the cow. This can be learned only by long practice, and especially by throwing the will into the part affected. Her husband will then value her above all women, nor would he exchange her for the most beautiful queen in the Three Worlds.

Even Islam's Muhammad is reported to have said: 'Allah made intercourse so pleasurable and attractive that it is imperative to enjoy sex fully with every nerve and muscle.'

The contractile vaginal talents of many women are described throughout history and literature. Ancient Greece's famous courtesans, the *hetaira*, are famed for being able to split a clay phallus with their vaginal muscles. This was a test of their genital strength and skill. Such talents are also among those ascribed to Diane de Poitiers (1499–1566), the mistress of King Henry II of France, to explain the fact that she was, shockingly to some, twenty years older than her royal partner. French author Gustave Flaubert enthuses about his encounters with the professional prostitutes exiled in the Egyptian town of Esneh: 'her cunt milking me was just like rolls of velvet – I felt ferocious'. Across the globe, Shilihong was a Shanghai sex worker famed for her exceptional control of her vaginal muscles. She is said to have been able to move a man's penis in and out of her simply by contracting and relaxing her muscles, a movement that bestowed a sucking-like sensation. The 'Shanghai squeeze' of Wallis Simpson is said to be one of the reasons why Britain lost a king in 1936. Mrs Simpson, it was noted, 'had the ability to make a matchstick feel like a Havana cigar'.

The importance of education

The erotic and sexual techniques of this muscular vaginal artistry are still to be found today – but only in those women who choose to train their vaginal muscles. In India, vaginal exercises are known as *Sahajolî*, and for some girls they are taught from childhood, first by their mother and later by a Tantric guru. *Sahajolî* also form part of the training of Devadasîs, Indian temple dancers. Such vaginal exercises are practised by devotees of Tantric or sexual yoga, and are designed to enhance sexual pleasure. They include abdominal and pelvic flexes (*mudra*) as well as muscle locks (*bandhas*), and some, such as the *Mula Bandha*, can work for men too.

The ability to exercise vaginal muscle control is viewed as a key vaginal quality in Polynesia's Marquesan society. The Marquesans refer to vaginal contractions as *naninani*, and women who have the strength and staying power to retain control over multiple squeezes during repeated sex sessions are, not surprisingly, revered. Moreover, great emphasis is also placed on particular pelvic movements during sex, which, it is said, play a major part in the mutual pleasures of sexual intercourse. The Marquesan term for this sensual pelvic motion is *tamure*, named for the Tahitian dance of the same name, which features movements resembling those of sexual intercourse.

Significantly, the capacity to move the pelvis in a particular way during sex is not the sole province of women. Marquesan men are expected to be able to roll with it too, and perhaps this is why sex commonly ends with the orgasms of both parties. Marquesan women apparently have no problems reaching orgasm, be it simultaneous or not. It's obvious that vaginal muscle control is one key to this orgasmic art (as is male participation), but sex education is also a vital factor. On reaching puberty, Marquesan girls and boys receive sexual instruction – girls from their grandmothers or women of their grandmothers' generation, and boys from an older woman. Their education involves positions, techniques of sexual stimulation and general sexual hygiene. Sadly, though, this way of educating appears to be on the decline.

The sexual heart

Considering the potential strength and dexterity of her vaginal embrace, it is not surprising to find that a woman's genital musculature is complex. Criss-crossing, encircling, embedding, pulling, grasping, tugging and pushing, together this muscular network enables all a female's internal pelvic organs – urethra, vagina, uterus and rectum – to remain in the right place, and perform all their functions. These muscles surround and penetrate the vaginal walls, tying the vagina into the pelvic structures. Three groups of muscles are today recognised as enclosing and surrounding the length of the vagina (see Figure 5.3 and Table 5.1). They are – in ascending order – the muscles of the perineal body (the small muscular mass that fits between the floor of the vagina and the rectum), the muscles of the urogenital diaphragm, and the muscles of the pelvic floor, or diaphragm.

These muscular groups effectively divide the vagina into three compartments – the upper, the area above the pelvic floor; the middle, which is encircled by muscles from both the pelvic floor and the urogenital diaphragm; and the lower, associated with the perineal body musculature. This division of the vagina into three areas as defined by muscle groups tallies with Taoist teachings on vaginal muscular control. When able to isolate and flex these groups of

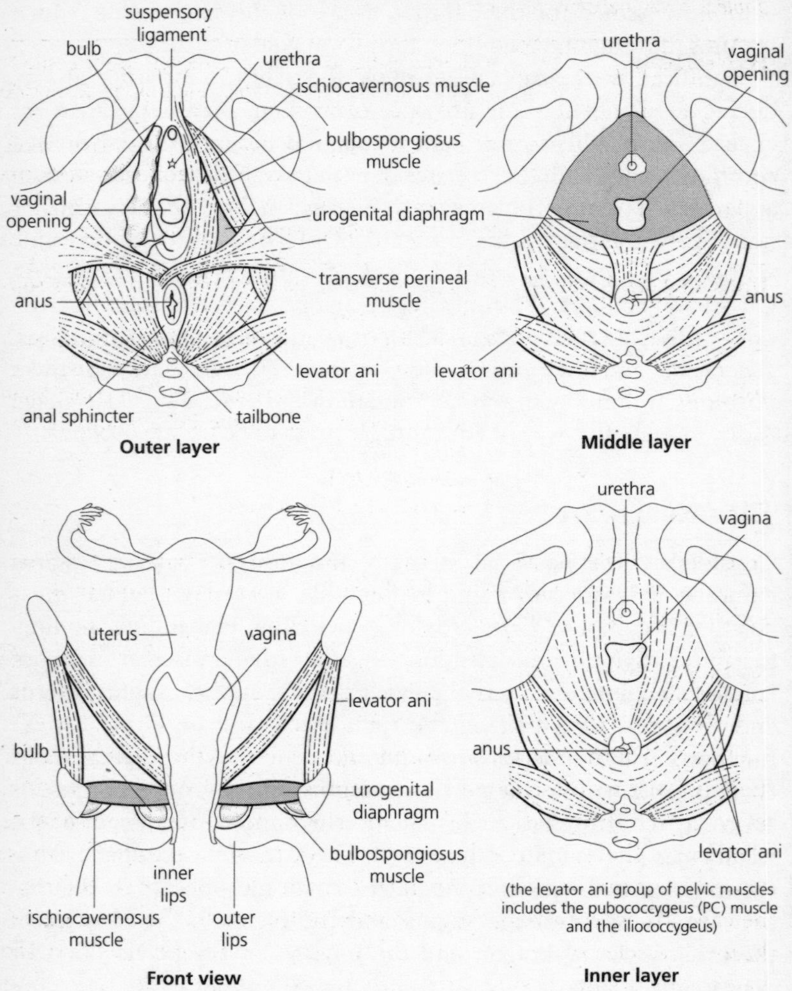

Figure 5.3 A woman's vaginal musculature is impressive, complex and powerful, and comes in three distinct groups or layers. Use them, don't lose them.

muscles at will, as a result of mastering Taoist sexual techniques, women are then able to move two small mineral eggs (2.5 cm in diameter) within their vagina in different directions, or bring them together with a bang.

Table 5.1 Vaginal Musculature

Perineal body	• anal constrictors ('the gatekeepers of the castle') • superficial transverse (provide support from side to side) • *bulbospongiosus* or *musculus constrictor cunni*, covers the vestibular bulbs and surrounds the vaginal opening • *ischiocavernosus* – the clitoral muscles
Urogenital diaphragm	• deep transverse perineal muscle (provides support from side to side) • constrictor of the urethra (sphincter urethrae)
Pelvic floor	• *pubococcygeus* (PC), runs from the pubic bone to the coccyx. Part of the PC is known as the *puborectalis.* • *iliococcygeus* (IC) • *coccygeus* (*ischiococcygeus*)

Together the PC, the IC and the urethral and rectal muscles are known as the levator ani group (meaning literally 'to raise the anus'). The bulbospongiosus muscle is sometimes referred to as the bulbocavernosus.
Adapted from Lowndes Sevely, Josephine, *Eve's Secrets: A New Theory of Female Sexuality*, New York: Random House, 1987.

Looking at the drawings of Leonardo da Vinci, you can see that the Italian artist was fascinated by the musculature of the lower vagina, in particular the muscles of the perineal area. Amongst his numerous sketches of the human body are ones of the muscles around the anus, which focus on their circular petal-like external appearance. Tellingly, he called these muscles 'the gatekeeper of the castle'. Da Vinci's gatekeeper muscles of the perineal body include ones that support the vagina from side to side, others that constrict the anus, as well as muscles that cover the crura or legs of the clitoris and one that covers the vestibular bulbs. This latter muscle also loops round and surrounds the vaginal opening, and when contracted, constricts the lower vagina, in particular making the opening of the vagina smaller. It is now known as the *bulbospongiosus* muscle, but was previously called the *musculus constrictor cunni*, for obvious reasons. The clitoral muscles (the *ischiocavernosus* muscles) also alter on arousal, contracting as the clitoris fills with blood and becomes erect. This movement pulls the clitoris into closer contact with the vagina, and is seen as the crown of the clitoris raises, typically arching back under the clitoral hood. Above the perineal body are the muscles of the urogenital diaphragm – which again support the vagina from side to side, and also constrict the urethra.

The group of muscles known as the pelvic floor, or diaphragm, is the set that has received the most public attention. This is the muscle group that women are recommended to exercise post-childbirth or to help with sexual arousal or incontinence problems. As a group, the pelvic floor forms a sheet of muscle slung intimately round the middle section of the pelvic organs. A side view reveals the funnel or cone-shaped structure. The most famous pelvic floor muscle is the *pubococcygeus* muscle, PC for short. Its name reveals where it runs from – the pubic bone – and where it runs to – the coccyx, the tail end of the spine. In animals, the PC muscle is the one that wags the tail. The PC muscle, together with the other pelvic muscles in this group, act to support the pelvic organs (the urethra, vagina and rectum in women), and also assist in maintaining continence when bouts of coughing, sneezing or muscular activity raise intra-abdominal pressure. During pregnancy, the pelvic floor group must also support the combined weight of the uterus and the unborn child.

While the PC muscle is a principal player in the pelvic floor grouping, it does not act alone. Rather it works in glorious concert with its surrounding group of muscles and those adjoining. Together a woman's genital muscles orchestrate the delicate caressing or harder grasping action of the vaginal chamber. The rhythm goes something like this. As the PC muscle contracts, another portion of the pelvic floor muscle, the closely related *puborectalis*, contracts too. Together the effect is to narrow, elongate and partially straighten the lower two thirds of the vagina. As this happens the upper part of the vagina, including the fornices (arches) around the cervix, widens and balloons, with a resultant lowering of pressure. Closer to the vaginal entrance, the *bulbospongiosus* muscle also contracts. Because this muscle encircles the vaginal entrance, vaginal pressure in the lower third is higher than in the middle third – and the pressure in the middle third is higher than that of the upper. Taken as a muscular whole, with its three distinct groupings of muscles clasping, contracting and expanding, it is not too difficult to understand why the vagina has been described as a sexual heart. Or to envisage the vagina effectively milking the phallus with a grasping, pulsing grip.

Use it, don't lose it

Disappointingly, though, decades of leading a sedentary lifestyle, sitting and slouching on the closest easy chair or sofa, instead of squatting on your haunches, means that for many people – women and men alike, and not just post-childbirth – their pelvic muscles are slack. Like any other muscle, if you don't use it, you'll lose it. Just as the muscle mass of an individual's biceps or pectorals can be strengthened and sculpted as a result of regular exercise, so too can a person's pelvic muscles. The result of such exercise is an organ with exquisite muscle control.

There are also health benefits. In both sexes improved strength and control of the pelvic floor muscles results in improved urinary and faecal continence. Levels of sexual arousal and performance are enhanced too. Indeed, for many women, simply contracting and relaxing their vaginal muscles if they are strong enough is sufficient to trigger orgasm. In men, improving pelvic muscle strength has been shown to reverse a diagnosis of impotence. In women, research shows that the strength of a woman's pelvic muscles ranges from 2 or 3 microvolts to 20 or 30. On average, women can produce a 9–10 microvolt contraction; however, below the average stress and urge incontinence are increasingly more likely. But above the average, women can look forward to an increasing likelihood of multiple orgasms in proportion to muscle strength.

A word of caution should be sounded, though, regarding the practice of exercising pelvic muscles. Learning to work a muscular group can be tricky, not least because most women are unable to see their own muscles move. Kegel exercises are often recommended for women. However, the original pelvic floor exercises, as devised by Californian gynaecologist Dr Arnold Kegel in 1951, are markedly different from those typically promoted today. Kegel's original workout involved the insertion of a resistive and compressible device inside the vagina. Contraction of the pelvic floor muscles resulted in a reduction in volume of the resistive device which was shown as a pressure reading on an external handheld meter. This was the Kegel perineometer. Only in this way, Kegel reasoned – by providing resistance to work against and some form of feedback about what was happening internally – could women increase their awareness of their pelvic floor muscles, and appreciate and enjoy the muscles' gain in strength. Kegel even made casts of vaginas, called mulages, to illustrate the effects of diligent use of his perineometer. This Kegel perineometer, it is argued, was the world's first biofeedback device.

Today, electronic biofeedback instruments or a specialised physiotherapist can help those with particularly weak pelvic muscles. Regular exercise with a readable resistive device is also recommended – or try a partner's penis. However, the simple squeeze against nothing routines that bear Kegel's name are not as effective. They provide neither resistance to work against or any feedback on what is happening, i.e., is it working and am I improving? All too often a different muscle group is flexed too, or the right muscle group is contracted but not relaxed properly, which can lead to chronic pelvic tension and persistent pain.

The shape of things to come

Flexing the vagina's muscles is integral to sexual arousal because this simple action can reroute circulating blood, pulling it rapidly into the capillaries of the surrounding vaginal walls. This increase in blood flow causes the walls to billow with blood, and their blood volume increases too. This is vasocongestion (vaso – denoting blood) of the vaginal walls. Vaginal vasocongestion then has two knock-on effects on a woman's vaginal walls – they lubricate and they lengthen. Lubrication first. Associations between the vagina, sexual arousal and wetness have existed for many years – the inner lips of the vagina were known since the first century as *nymphae* – water goddesses in Greek – while in ancient Greek comedies, male actors playing female roles wore bags of fluid to denote genital excitement. In Japan, the word for sexual intercourse is *nure*, meaning to grow wet.

However, despite this history, in particular an accurate description by Reinier de Graaf in 1672, the idea that the walls of a woman's vagina exuded fluid during sexual arousal was not widely accepted until over three hundred years later. Viewpoints only began to change when

William Masters wrote his seminal paper, 'The Sexual Response of the Human Female: Vaginal Lubrication' in 1959. Masters noted that as sexual excitement rose, as a result of either physical or mental activity, a 'sweating' reaction occurred on the surface of the vaginal walls.

> Individual droplets of a lubricating material suddenly appear scattered over the rugal folds of the normal vaginal architecture. These individual droplets present a picture somewhat akin to that of a perspiration-beaded forehead. With continued increase of sexual tension the droplets coalesce to form a smooth, glistening coating for the entire vaginal wall. This sweating reaction progresses to establish complete vaginal lubrication early in the excitement phase of the human female's sexual response cycle.

Significantly, the vaginal wall lubrication reaction is an incredibly rapid one. The lubricating fluid, or transudate, can appear between ten and thirty seconds after the initial perception of sexual excitement, but can disappear as rapidly if excitement does too. It's now recognised that the production of this lubricating fluid is a result of the vaginal walls becoming thickened and engorged with blood. However, it should be said that sexual arousal is not the only method of production. Many kinds of muscular activity, if they bring the pelvic muscles into play, have this lubricating effect. I know that a Saturday morning wake-up work-out at the gym will always result in increased levels of vaginal lubrication. At the end of such a session, I am most definitely not sexually excited, but I am very physically aroused and wet – from both sweat and vagina juices.

How a woman's vaginal walls lengthen during sexual arousal and intercourse is a topic that has also only recently been fully appreciated – visually, that is. Experiments in the 1960s by Masters and Virginia Johnson suggested that the walls of the vagina enlarged during sexual excitement. Unfortunately, the fact that they used an artificial penis to achieve this effect was said to mar the legitimacy of their observations. Ultrasound experiments in the early 1990s also pointed to the vaginal walls growing in size, in particular the anterior (stomach-side) wall. However, it wasn't until the turn of the twentieth century that Magnetic Resonance Imaging (MRI) provided the first clear pictures of the shape-changing nature of the vagina. MRI gives a snapshot, or dynamic image, of a person's insides, including their soft tissues, and as it is also non-invasive, to the extent that probes and monitors are not placed inside the vagina, it can be said to be the truest representation to date of how sexual arousal and intercourse affects the vagina. Only a handful of studies have so far been conducted, but these highlight the vagina's extreme flexibility and erectile capacity. One experiment recorded anterior vaginal length leaping from 7.5 cm in the non-excited state to 15 cm when aroused, a 50 per cent increase – quite impressive. Posterior vaginal length grew too, expanding from 11 cm to between 13 and 15 cm. In comparison, vaginal length in chimpanzees is estimated to be around 12.6 cm when unaroused, but leaps to 16.9 cm during arousal, and with external sexual skin fully swollen.

Increased vaginal lubrication and length are not the only internal changes that can be felt in female genital tissue during sexual arousal. The erectile tissue surrounding the urethra – the *spongiosum* – transforms too, becoming engorged with blood at heightened levels of sexual excitement (this is the same type of erectile tissue that surrounds a male's urethra). In a woman, the urethra is typically between 3 and 4 cm long, and runs from the neck of the bladder to the urethral glans – the point where the urethra exits the body, below the clitoris and just above the vaginal opening. The erectile spongiosum or urethral tissue completely encircles the urinary passageway and runs its entire length. In breadth, it measures between 2.5 and 3.5 cm, and is slightly thicker towards the neck of the bladder, and thinner towards the glans.

When a woman is aroused, the swelling of the *spongiosum* can be felt through the anterior or ventral (stomach) wall of the vagina. This is possible because of the very close relationship between the erectile urethral tissue and the ventral vaginal wall. The lower edge of the urethral glans defines the upper opening of the vagina, while the base of the urethral tissue comprises part of the ventral vaginal wall. Indeed, it could be said that the urethra and its surrounding spongy erectile tissue and musculature are inseparable from the vagina because the floor of the urethra is the ceiling of the vagina.

Hair pins for girls, bullets for boys

Just as the *spongiosum* tissue surrounding a man's urethra is erotically sensitive to pressure changes (such as those of a clasping hand or vagina), so too is a female's corresponding urethral tissue. Many women experience intense pleasure from stimulation of their urethra – either indirectly, via the ventral vaginal wall, or directly, by touching the urethral glans. A woman's glans and carina (the lower edge of the glans) is incredibly sensitive, and careful caressing can be just as arousing for women as it can for men. The rubbing of a man's corona over a woman's carina, as part of very shallow gentle thrusting, is a particularly intense and erotic sensation for many women. Some women also enjoy the sensations of internal urethral stimulation – although it should be said that extreme caution is advised here. Items such as hair pins have been lost in the ecstasy of orgasm, ending up in the bladder, with possible serious health consequences. Medical history also records the case of a man who chose to indulge in urethral stimulation with a rifle bullet – which ended up in his bladder.

Although the erotic potential of female urethral tissue was understood by many individuals as an integral part of their sexual geography, it wasn't until the middle of the twentieth century that such sensations were noted by the academic community. The person who pointed this out – Ernst Gräfenberg – was a very forward- and free-thinking gynaecologist. Born in 1881, Gräfenberg was a pioneer of research into female sexual reproduction and pleasure. A German gynaecologist, he covered in his work a multitude of aspects of the physiology of reproduction. He was the first to describe the physical connection between the stimulation of the growth of an ovarian follicle and that of the lining of the uterus, the endometrium. (However, it is not his name that forms the term Graafian follicle, but that of Reinier de Graaf, who also studied the developing follicle.) Gräfenberg was also the first to describe the cyclical variation of the acidity of vaginal secretions, and published in 1918, a twenty-nine page paper on vaginal secretions. Some credit him with developing the first test for ovulation. To add to this, he was a leader in the production of birth control methods, developing the interuterine device (IUD), the Gräfenberg ring in 1928, and later collaborating on the plastic cervical cap.

However, it wasn't until the last decade of his life that Gräfenberg started a revolution in how the female urethra and its surrounding structures are viewed. In 1950, in the *International Journal of Sexology*, he published a ground-breaking article entitled 'The Role of the Urethra in Female Orgasm'. In this, he pointed out the pleasure women derive from stimulation of this organ: 'Analogous to the male urethra, the female urethra also seems to be surrounded by erectile tissues ... In the course of sexual stimulation, the female urethra begins to enlarge and can be felt easily. It swells out greatly at the end of orgasm.' Gräfenberg also noted how the 'floor' of the urethra is the 'ceiling' of the ventral vaginal wall and how: 'An erotic zone could always be demonstrated on the anterior wall of the vagina along the course of the urethra. Even when there was a good response in the entire vagina, this particular area was more easily stimulated by the finger than the other areas of the vagina.'

Gräfenberg found that the most sensitive part of the anterior vaginal wall for the women in his study lay 3–4 cm inside the vagina – in the vicinity of the posterior urethra, just around where the urethra becomes the neck of the bladder. This is the area that over thirty years later was renamed the Gräfenberg spot, or G spot, and is celebrated in the best-selling book *The G Spot and Other Discoveries About Human Sexuality.*

The vexing question of vaginal sensitivity

Gräfenberg's work was viewed as highly controversial for two main reasons. First of all, he pointed out that the urethra was surrounded by erectile tissue, just as the male urethra is. Second, he highlighted how sensitive the interior of the vagina is. These comments on vaginal sensitivity went against the thinking of the time – which had tended to underline the supposed insensitivity of the vagina and the urethra. Indeed, many people today still claim that the interior of the vagina is insensitive. They are incorrect in their assumptions and, as we shall see, their claims are based on biased theories and flawed science. First of all, the idea of the vagina as insensitive has its roots in eighteenth- and nineteenth-century misogynistic and hypocritical notions of females being creatures devoid of all sexual sensitivities. Women, the great minds of these times opined, were not much bothered by sexual feelings. This view was promoted despite plenty of evidence to the contrary.

The idea of the unresponsive, insensitive vagina was also, unfortunately, given some credence by twentieth-century studies. This research proclaimed that on the crazy basis of the Q-tip test, or cotton wool bud test, the vagina was not very sensitive. It may be true that touching the tip of a cotton wool bud to the vagina's walls won't elicit much sensation, but that's hardly surprising or a robust touch test. Sex consists of far more than the touch of a Q-tip. What these studies did show, but failed for some reason to highlight, was the vagina's sensitivity to vibration and pressure.

In fact Gräfenberg was correct about the sensitivity of the urethra and the interior of the vagina. Recent research has shown that female genitalia are profoundly innervated (by the pudendal, pelvic, hypogastric and vagus nerves) and capable of detecting vibration, touch and pressure changes, in particular deep pressure. Tactile stimulation of the extremely sensitive external genital skin produces one type of sensation, while deep-pressure proprioceptive receptors within the perineal and vaginal musculature produce exquisite sensations too – either as a result of contraction of muscles or their distension by a penis, fingers, vibrator or whatever. Visceral sensory receptors are also thought to convey arousal and orgasm sensations to the brain. This means the vagina is deliciously responsive to the low throb of slow strokes, the hard, persistent pressure of deep thrusts, or just simply squeezing the vaginal muscles.

Gräfenberg was also correct about the particular sensitivity of the anterior vaginal wall. Recent studies into its microstructure and sensitivity have pointed to geographical differences in the innervation of the vaginal chamber. The deeper you go inside the vagina the more nerve fibres there are in the walls, with the anterior wall much more densely packed with vaginal nerves than the posterior one. There are also specific differences in the number and nature of nerve fibres found in the area of the anterior vaginal wall adjacent to the bladder neck. These include an extreme number of richly innervated vessels, plus the presence of yet-to-be-explained giant coiled corpuscle-like structures.

The revelation that the microstructure of a woman's vaginal walls suggests that they are far more sensitive than previously recognised is not surprising to me. I know the ability of my vagina to feel the merest flicker of movement when I am joyously and deeply aroused. One of the sweetest sensations of life is the delicate, pulsatile, tickling feeling of my man orgasming inside me. I don't know whether it's the ejaculatory spurt of semen or the contractile quiver of orgasm that I feel, but whichever it is, it's divine.

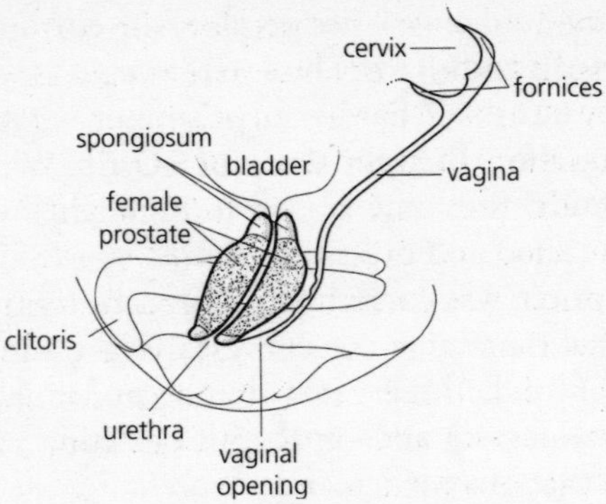

Figure 5.4 The female prostate: the sprawling complex of glands and connecting ducts that is the female prostate extends along the urethra.

The female prostate

Some things, it seems, never change. For instance, the tissue surrounding the female urethra is still a subject of enormous controversy, more than fifty years after Gräfenberg published his pioneering article. Today, though, the furore is focused on the fact that the tissue surrounding a woman's urethra is more than just erotically sensitive and erectile. Surprisingly, it is also secretory as a result of numerous glandular structures traversing its length and embedded in it. These glands and their connecting ducts empty their contents into the urethral passageway, and together the complex of secreting structures and its associated smooth musculature are known as the female prostate (see Figure 5.4). At the start of the twenty-first century, however, the above sentence is not accepted by all scientists. The tale of the female prostate is one that, in part, parallels that of its sister, the clitoris. It is a story of anatomical parts found and lost and found again. And, like the clitoris, despite a wealth of evidence to the contrary, the idea that the female prostate may be a functioning part of a female's reproductive anatomy is doubted.

The presence of a female prostate, however, has not always been denied. In fact, the existence of the female prostate was accepted for nearly two millennia – and only became a matter of dispute at the end of the nineteenth century. Greek anatomist Galen (130–200 CE) was one of the first western scientists to explore the attributes of the female prostate, writing in Book 14 of his work *On the Usefulness of the Parts* that women as well as men have '*prostatae*'. Galen also commented on the possible function of the female prostate and its secretions in relation to reproduction, saying: 'the fluid in her [the female's] *prostatae* is unconcocted and thin. This contributes nothing to the generation of offspring.' Over 1,500 years later, in his ground-breaking manuscript *The Generative Organs of Women*, Reinier de Graaf recorded the first detailed dissection and description of a woman's prostate, and agrees with Galen's suggestion that a woman's prostate is analogous to that of a man.

In fact, it wasn't until 1880 that medical opinion on the set of glands and ducts that make up the female prostate began to alter. Prior to this, it was generally accepted that women had a prostate too. The description of an American gynaecologist, Alexander Skene, was the catalyst for the volte-face, which changed the female prostate's terminology as well. Skene, for some reason, chose to focus on just two of the many glands of the female prostate. The two glands he picked are typically larger than others, and are depicted clearly in the drawings by de Graaf in 1672. However, Skene chose to ignore this, and instead claimed the discovery for his own, naming the glands, in a very original manner, as Skene's glands.

From then on in, the idea that the female possessed a prostate fell out of fashion. Subsequent discoveries of other glands and ducts surrounding the urethra were dubbed paraurethral glands (*para* – meaning beside or near). Moreover, this demoting of the female prostate to Skene's or paraurethral glands coincided with the female prostate being labelled as a vestigial, or non-functioning remnant of an organ. The result – women had Skene's glands, not prostates, and if they did have prostates this was a non-functioning remnant. Today the term 'urethral sponge' is also used to describe the erectile *spongiosum* tissue surrounding the urethra and its intertwined set of secretory glands and ducts.

Spot the difference

Women, however, do have a prostate and it is a functioning reproductive organ. Significantly, women are not the only females to possess functioning, secreting prostates. Well-developed prostates can be found in females from at least four different mammalian orders: *Insectivora* (including shrews, moles and hedgehogs), *Chiroptera* (bats), *Rodentia* (including rats, mice and squirrels) and *Lagomorpha* (hares and rabbits). The size of the prostate in these species varies, but all produce secretions, although the function of these female prostatic fluids in reproduction remains unknown.

At the end of the 1990s, the debate over whether the female prostate was merely a vestigial or non-functioning organ was squashed when research on its ultrastructure revealed that just as in the post-pubertal male, the prostatic glands in the adult female display mature secretory and basal cells, which are hormone-dependent. Studies have also recently pointed to the female prostate's neuroendocrine function, as it produces, like the male prostate, the neurotransmitter serotonin. There is also evidence showing the cyclical nature of urethral and prostate tissue. This cycle, with a rhythm of 30±5 days, reveals that during the luteal or secretory phase of a woman's menstrual cycle (the fourteen or so days post-ovulation up to the start of the next period), the thickness of urethral tissue decreases, an effect which can weaken the mechanism by which the urethra closes. However, despite such structural, histological, animal and endocrine evidence to the contrary, many scientists continue to refute that women have a functioning prostate.

So what does the male prostate have that the female prostate doesn't? Why does its existence get to be acknowledged, and the female's is challenged? The male prostate is, in essence, a small walnut- or chestnut-shaped structure that surrounds the urethra at the bladder neck. Unlike the female prostate, which can be felt and stimulated through the roof of the vagina, the male prostate can only be directly felt through the rectum, as it nestles between the bladder and the rectum. Stimulation of the prostate through the rectum is an essential part of sexual pleasure for many men. The male prostate is also indirectly stimulated as a result of the pressures involved in thrusting in sexual activity, and can be felt throbbing at the base of the penis during ejaculatory orgasm. Stimulation of the male prostate causes both emission and ejaculation of prostatic fluids. Like the female prostate it is comprised of glands, ducts and smooth muscle. These structural similarities are not surprising because both organs develop from the same portion of embryonic tissue – the urogenital sinus.

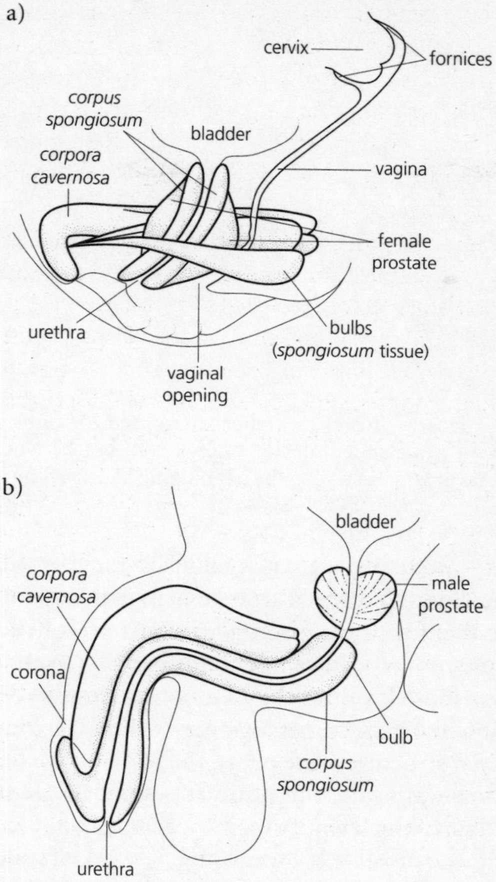

Figure 5.5 The female and male prostate compared: a) the female prostate is more diffuse while b) the male prostate is more concentrated in one area. Both surround the urethra.

The differences between the two sexes' prostates can be seen in the number and style of dispersion of glands and connecting ducts. While the female prostate has fewer glands than the male's, it has far more ducts, forty or more, which are spread along the length of the urethra (see Figure 5.5a). The male prostate's glands and ducts (between ten to twenty) are concentrated together and interlaced with smooth

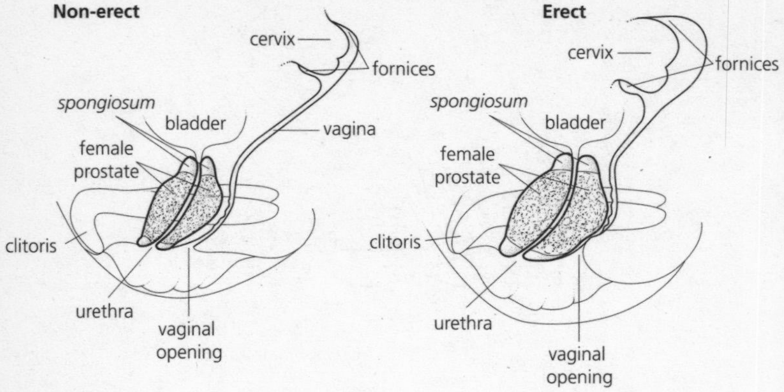

Figure 5.6 The female prostate: a) when unaroused it can be difficult to feel prostatic tissue through the anterior vaginal wall but b) when aroused, the engorged female prostate can often be felt bulging and swelling into the vagina.

muscle tissue, producing a greater expulsive force on ejaculation (see Figure 5.5b). This difference in arrangement parallels the development of the tissue that forms the external genitalia of women and men (as previously mentioned). In females, this genital tissue tends to open out as it develops, forming the clitoris, urethra, vagina and labia, whereas that of the male comes together, with all the component parts in one external structure – the penis.

For the male prostate, the result is a small, 2.5 cm structure of glands and ducts, which empty their contents in one area. Conversely, in the female, the prostate is a sprawling network of glands and ducts, traversing and embedded in the length of the erectile and erotically sensitive urethral *spongiosum* tissue, and opening into the urethra at different points. And when some women are aroused, this grouping of glands and ducts can be felt swelling and pushing against the anterior vaginal wall (see Figure 5.6b). For some individuals this prostate protrusion is small, say bean-sized; in others it is larger, and, over time, is suggested to increase in size the more stimulation it receives.

Research shows that some women have a higher concentration of glands and ducts at the bladder neck; some a higher concentration adjacent to the urethral glans, while others have tissue distributed fairly equally along the length of the urethra (see Figure 5.7). It is this

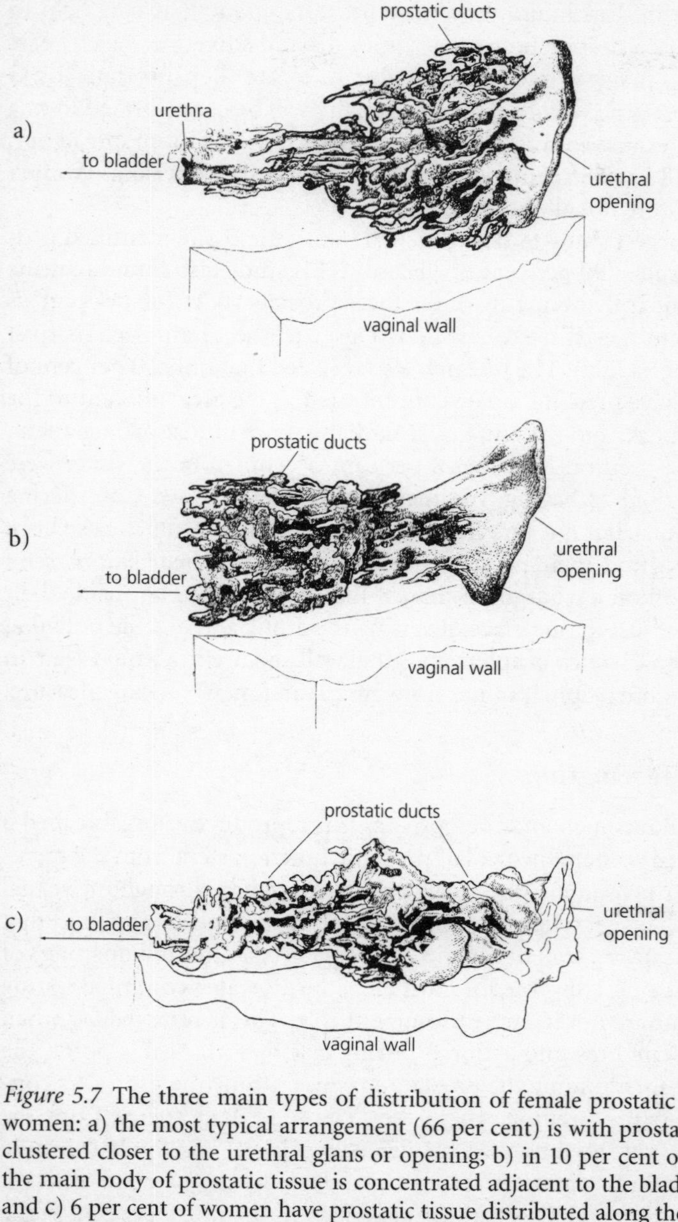

Figure 5.7 The three main types of distribution of female prostatic tissue in women: a) the most typical arrangement (66 per cent) is with prostatic tissue clustered closer to the urethral glans or opening; b) in 10 per cent of women the main body of prostatic tissue is concentrated adjacent to the bladder neck and c) 6 per cent of women have prostatic tissue distributed along the urethra (Adapted from drawings of wax models of the human female prostate by Huffman, J.W., 1948).

variation in distribution of female prostatic tissue that may help to explain why, despite hours, days, months and sometimes even years of trying, many women are not able to locate their prostate (or G spot). For some women, erotic sensitivity will be concentrated in one zone of the anterior vaginal wall; for others it will be more spread out. Some will have little prostatic tissue. This is not surprising. Women differ. We are not all the same.

The largest study to date of female prostatic tissue identified prostatic tissue in 90 per cent of all cases. This study also found that the most frequently occurring of the three prostate styles (66 per cent) is that where the cluster of tissue is closer to the urethral glans (just inside the vagina). The research also revealed that only 10 per cent of women have prostatic tissue concentrated in the area adjacent to the bladder neck, and the remainder have the more diffuse arrangement, along the urethra. A further 8 per cent of women in the study were characterised as having 'rudimentary' prostatic tissue. Considering these results, it is not surprising that the majority of women have been unable to find their prostate or G spot, as most instructions send women off on a wild-goose chase – looking for it too far inside their vagina, or just in one place. Realising the erotic and erectile potential of the whole stretch of anterior vaginal wall and urethra would seem to be a far more helpful pointer for women (and men) seeking pleasure.

A fluid fascination

So why do women and men possess this reproductive organ called a prostate? For men, theories of prostatic function stem from the secretion that prostatic tissue oozes into the urethra throughout sexual arousal. This secretion forms part of the drop of glistening fluid that can typically be seen on the tip of the glans (the urethral opening) of an erect penis. However, for most men, the prostate's continual resting secretions are not its most prominent role. This is reserved for when the prostate fires into action – during ejaculation. At this point, the muscles surrounding the prostate spasm, pushing the prostate's contents into the urethra, where they combine with sperm from the testicles (via the muscular vas deferens tubes), plus fluids from the bulbourethral glands (Cowper's glands) and the seminal vesicles. Together these fluids constitute male semen – about 70 per cent of the total volume comes from the seminal vesicles, and roughly 30 per cent from the prostate. Tests show that prostatic fluid contains a rich mixture of molecules, including zinc, magnesium, citric acid, amino acids, enzymes and prostaglandins.

This fluid from a man's chestnut-shaped prostate gland is said to be responsible for giving semen its characteristic smell. And coincidentally, the smell of chestnuts has a semen-like odour, a fact which has been recognised and commented on through the centuries, and which inspired the story, 'La Fleur de Châtaignier', by the Marquis de Sade. This sweet chestnut smell is attributed to the presence of the chemical l-pyrroline, which is also found in male pubic sweat. One speculation regarding the role of prostatic fluid is that it may serve to buffer, or protect, sperm from the toxic effects of urine in the urethra, or the harshly acidic conditions when deposited within the vagina. Another suggestion is that ingredients of prostatic fluid may serve to improve sperm motility by making sure sperm don't remain stuck, clogged up in the urethra. In the male mole rat, the prostate is known to have sex-attractant properties. However, the precise function of male prostatic fluid in human reproduction remains unknown.

How does a woman's prostatic fluid compare? Visually, female prostatic fluid is a clear or opalescent liquid. Drops of female fluid can be seen glistening on a woman's urethral glans during sexual arousal, just as the male variety can be viewed on a man's glans. The chemical make-up of the two prostatic fluids is similar too. Like male prostatic fluid, its components include large amounts of the enzyme prostate-specific phosphatase (PSAP), plus other enzymes and some urea and creatinine. The precise composition is as yet undefined, although it has recently been recognised that female prostatic fluid also contains the sugar, fructose, which a man's seminal vesicles produce. The recognition in the 1980s of the female prostate as a rich source of PSAP has had important ramifications for the forensic and medicolegal professions. Prior to this, alleged cases of male rape or sexual assault were bolstered by the presence of PSAP in vaginal fluids or on a female's clothing, as it was believed that females did not produce this enzyme. Today, the presence of PSAP cannot be used as evidence in this way.

Another product of both male and female prostates – prostate-specific antigen (PSA) – has been found to be key in the diagnosis of disease. Since the discovery that raised levels of PSA can indicate cancers of the male prostate at an early stage, PSA testing has become a crucial part of cancer screening programmes for men. Raised PSA levels can also be indicative of tumours of the female prostate, although this cancer is far rarer than male prostate cancer. It is also now suggested that recurrent urinary tract infections or cystitis may well be inflammation of the prostate, or prostatitis – the name for inflammation of the male prostate.

When women gush

Although arguments about the existence of the female prostate have in the main been quelled by recent research investigating the organ's ultrastructure, there remains one major area of controversy highlighted by Gräfenberg's 1950 paper on the role of the urethra in female orgasm. This polemic is the ability of the female prostate to expel pleasurably and often orgasmically, in large gushes or spurts, quantities of prostatic fluid via the urethra. Gräfenberg described the phenomenon as follows:

> Occasionally the production of fluids is so profuse that a large towel has to be spread under the woman to prevent the bedsheets getting soiled ... If there is the opportunity to observe the orgasm of such women, one can see large quantities of a clear, transparent fluid are expelled not from the vulva, but out of the urethra in gushes ... In the cases observed by us, the fluid was examined and it had no urinary character. I am inclined to believe that urine reported to be expelled during female orgasm is not urine, but only secretions of the interurethral glands correlated with the erotogenic zone along the urethra in the anterior vaginal wall.

He adds that sometimes the production of fluid is so abundant that 'the female partner is inclined to compare it with the ejaculation of the male'.

At the start of the twenty-first century, the idea of female ejaculation – the emission of prostatic fluids under pressure from the urethra – is still highly controversial. On one side are the scientists who have published scientific papers in support of female ejaculation. On the other are those who deny the existence of female ejaculation, and usually of the female prostate too. There are also advocates in film and literature. For example, in 2002, a Japanese film entitled *Warm Water under a Red Bridge* had at its centre a woman who 'gushes more water than Moby Dick' every time she has an orgasm.

Then there are the women and men who have direct and enjoyable experiences of female ejaculation in all its glory. I am one of them. The first time I was fortunate enough to see a fellow female ejaculate was an eye- and mind-opener for me. The spurting force of the fluid, its abundance, its musky aroma, its very appearance and existence – these all made me marvel and wonder. I am most definitely not the first to have been amazed in this way. The idea that women can, and do, expel prostatic fluids forcefully when sexually aroused is an age-old one – with written evidence flowing back over two millennia and more.

In the east, descriptions of female ejaculation can be found in the ancient sex manuals of China, Japan and India. In many cases, a clear distinction is highlighted between the wetness or slipperiness of lubrication, and the fluids of ejaculation. The book *Secret Instructions Concerning the Jade Chamber*, which provides advice on flirting, the selection of sexual partners, and pretty much every aspect of sexual contact, has this to say:

> [The yellow emperor asked] 'How can I become aware of the joyfulness of the woman?' Replied the Immaculate Girl: there are five signs, five desires, and ten movements. By looking at these changes you will become aware of what is happening in her body. The first of the five signs is called 'reddened face'; if you see this you slowly unite with her. The second is called 'breasts hard and nose perspiring'; then slowly insert the jade stalk [penis]. The third is called 'throat dry and saliva blocked'; then slowly agitate her. The fourth is called 'slippery vagina'; then slowly go in more deeply. The fifth is called 'the genitals transmit fluid' [female ejaculation]; then slowly withdraw from her.

A similar passage is to be found in the book *Secret Methods of the Plain Girl*, which teaches that 'Her 'jade gate' becomes moist and slippery; then the man should plunge into her very deeply. Finally copious emissions from her 'inner heart' begin to exude outwards.' It is believed that the areas within the vagina that the Chinese called 'the little stream' or 'the black pearl' refer to the female prostate, while it was known as 'the skin of the earthworm' to the Japanese. Other

Chinese terms include 'palace of yin', which refers to the place where the orgasmic secretion known as 'moon flower medicine' is situated.

Indian sexological texts dating from the eleventh century onwards also refer to the female prostate and its ejaculatory role. The *Ananga Ranga* describes in some detail female genital anatomy, and refers to the especially erotically sensitive area of the vagina, the *saspanda nadi*, which when stimulated results in the production of copious quantities of 'love juice'. One earlier description of female ejaculation can be found in the seventh-century Kamasastra text, in a work of the poet Amaru called the *Amarusataka*. Other descriptions can be found in the *Pancasayaka* (eleventh century), *Jayamangala* (Yasodhara's commentary on the *Kama Sutra* from the thirteenth century), the *Ratirahasya* (thirteenth century), as well as the late Kamasastra work *Smaradipika*. Tantric texts also talk of a third erotic emission from female genitalia, as well as vaginal lubrication and cervical secretions.

The problem of female seed

The western world, too, has had a long and deep fascination with the emission of vaginal fluids. Major medical works from Aristotle onwards (4 BCE) refer to the female emission of copious quantities of seed. In Aristotle's time, physical evidence taught that both women and men produced genital fluids during sexual arousal. The question was how to interpret this. The answer arrived at was that emitting fluids, be it semen, sweat, breast milk or blood, maintained balance within the body. Sexual intercourse, therefore, with its many fluid by-products, was a very good way of achieving harmony or equilibrium.

Ancient thinking also held that body fluids could be converted, and tried to pin down their source and nature. Aristotle talks of women and men with fair complexions ejaculating more copiously than their darker peers. This, he said, was because those with darker complexions are typically hairier. He notes that a dry, bland diet leaves one deficient in ejaculate, compared with anyone enjoying watery, pungent victuals. He also talks of women emitting violently (*proiesthai*) into the vagina during orgasm. While observing the differences in ejaculate, Aristotle adds that both women and men are tired after ejaculation. Galen comments that the semen of a man is always thicker and hotter than a woman's because women are intrinsically less hot or perfect than men; for instance, they do not have sufficient 'heat' to unfurl their internal penis.

One of the main arguments against the accuracy of historical descriptions of female ejaculation is that descriptions of female seed, semen or sperm (*sperma muliebris*) could refer to any of the many aspects of female genital secretions – cervical, vaginal wall, etc. However, some texts by western writers describe ejaculation and the source of this female semen in such detail that there is little room for doubt as to what they are referring to. Take Aristotle, for example:

The path along which the semen passes in women is of the following nature: they [women] possess a tube (*kaulos*) – like the penis of the male, but inside the body – and they breathe through this by a small duct which is placed above the place through which women urinate. This is why, when they are eager to make love, this place is not in the same state as it was before they were excited.

Galen too makes the distinction between the increased secretion of vaginal fluids as a result of sexual excitement, and the ejection of fluid at orgasm or heightened levels of arousal. In *On the Usefulness of the Parts* he comments:

The fluid in her 'parastatae' is unconcocted and thin. This contributes nothing to the generation of offspring. Properly, then, it is poured outside when it has done its service ... This liquid not only stimulates to the sexual act but also is able to give pleasure and moisten the passageway as it escapes. It manifestly flows from women as they experience the greatest pleasure in coitus, when it is perceptibly shed upon the male pudendum; indeed, such an outflow seems to give a certain pleasure even to eunuchs.

Reinier de Graaf provides the clearest insight. He devotes a whole chapter, 'Concerning the "Semen" of Women', to the issue of female seed, describing how 'women are beset by nocturnal pollutions just as much as men, and both in widows and maidens who suffer from hysterical fits, thick and copious quantities of semen pour from the genital parts if these are tickled'. However, de Graaf also describes the urethra and the prostate and, critically, recognises and details *all* the possible different sources of vaginal fluids, as well as depicting the particular way in which fluid is emitted from the prostate via the urethra.

He describes the prostatic fluid as coming 'in one gush so to speak', and answers his critics as to where this fluid is from, explaining: 'The first-mentioned ducts [rediscovered as Skene's glands] ... and the outlet of the urinary passage receive their fluid from the female "parastatae", or rather the thick membranous body around the urinary passage.' De Graaf also strives to find a function for female ejaculation, suggesting that:

> The function of the 'prostatae' is to generate a pituito-serous juice which makes women more libidinous with its pungency and saltiness and lubricates their sexual parts in agreeable fashion during intercourse. This liquid was not designed by Nature to moisten the urethra (as some people think). The ducts are so placed at the outlet of the urethra that the liquid does not touch it as it rushes out.

He adds that 'the discharge from the female "prostatae" causes as much pleasure as does that from the male "prostatae".'

The ethics of expelling seed

The issue of female seed raised an interesting debate within the western medical profession, and one that would rage for years, from Hippocrates onwards. It would eventually result in the invention of the vibrator, as we'll see. Because wisdom held that emission of fluids was beneficial for health, the opposite stood too – retention of fluids could induce ill health in both women and men. This belief was accepted until well into the nineteenth century, and its long history means that medical literature is full of references to female seed – and the best way to release it. Treatments for the afflictions caused by retained female seed – called in various centuries *suffocation ex semine retento*, suffocation of the womb or mother, hysteria and green sickness – typically involved a midwife rubbing inside the vagina with scented oil, the insertion into the vagina of penis-shaped objects, or prescribed sexual intercourse (there is an urban legend from the seventeenth century relating to an attractive young doctor).

Texts record that young widows, and virgins of marriageable age, were those most likely to suffer from semen retention. One ballad,

'The Maid's Complaint for Want of a Dildoul', has the sixteen-year-old virgin narrator singing of how she will do anything 'for a dil doul, dil doul, dil doul doul'. Another late-seventeenth-century ballad, 'A Remedy for the Green Sickness', relates how:

> A handsome buxom lass
> Lay panting on her bed.
> She look't as green as grass
> And mournfully she said
> Unless I have some lusty lad to ease me of my pain
> I cannot live
> I sigh and grieve
> My life I now disdain.

This medical practice of female-pleasuring raised serious questions of ethics. Were the doctors of the day acting morally or not in removing seed from young, unmarried women, especially when sexual pleasure or orgasm accompanied the expulsion? Or was it simply their medical duty because retained semen, according to seventeenth-century thinking, degenerated into a poison of considerable strength – equivalent to the venom of a mad dog, serpent or scorpion? To practise female expulsion of seed or not became the focus of animated debate in medical circles at the start of the 1600s. In 1627, one doctor, the French physician Francois Ranchin, wrote that the debate of 'Whether One Is Allowed to Rub the Vulva of Women in Hysterical Paroxysm' was one that was 'very serious and extremely important'. However, while he acknowledged that there were good arguments to show that it 'is a well proven therapy', and that 'it is inhuman to recommend against the use of that salutary method', Ranchin came down on the moral side of the fence. 'We, however, following the teaching of the theologians, hold friction of this kind to be abominable and damnable, particularly in virgins, since such pollution may spoil virginity,' he declared.

Do all women ejaculate?

Another argument that the nay-sayers of female ejaculation like to bandy about is the question of why the phenomenon is one that only some women experience. However, while every woman's sexual response is unique, there are some compelling explanations for why this may be. First of all, statistics vary as to the percentage of women who experience female ejaculation. Some American studies estimate 10 per cent of the population, others 40 or 68 per cent. Numbers also fluctuate when it comes to estimating the amount of fluid excreted – values range from 3 ml to 5 ml, with 10 to 15 ml appearing to be typical. These sorts of variances, in particular the fact that not all women visibly expel fluid under pressure from their urethra during sexual arousal and/or orgasm, provide the major arguments against the possibility of female ejaculation occurring. However, as every scientist knows, just because a process does not occur in all people equally does not mean it cannot exist at all.

It is not just medical, historical and sexual texts that point to the occurrence of female ejaculation. An awareness of the role of the female's urethra and prostate in sexual arousal is found in many cultures. Tradition dictates that the eligible women of the Batoro of Uganda are taught by the older women of the village to ejaculate. This custom is known as *kachapati*, or 'spray the wall'. The Mohave Indians of the American West believe that women ejaculate, as do Trobiand Islanders and the Trukese people of the South Pacific. One study of the sexual behaviour of the Trukese reported: 'Coitus is phrased by several of our informants as a contest between the man and the woman, a matter of the man restraining his orgasm until the woman has achieved hers. Female orgasm is commonly signalled by urination, although failing this a woman still gives adequate indication of its onset.'

For the Trukese and other Micronesians, female sexual arousal is characterised by 'urination before and during the climax' (it is not uncommon for female ejeculation to be confused initially with urination). Mangaian men differentiate between a woman's orgasms and the point during intensely pleasurable sex sessions during which 'a woman thinks she's urinating – but that's not urine', it is 'another type' of sensation. The Ponapese people of the South Pacific gave this advice about conception: 'If a Ponapese man wishes to impregnate his principal wife, he first stimulates her to the point where she urinates and only then proceeds to have intercourse with her.'

One explanation for why not all women visibly ejaculate hinges on the strength of a woman's pelvic muscles. Women with strong pelvic muscles, it is suggested, experience more forceful muscle contractions during sexual arousal and orgasm, and it is this muscular force that pressures the prostate glands to give up their fluid. Studies have backed this up, showing that the PC muscle contractions of female ejaculators were significantly stronger than (almost double) those who did not expel fluid forcefully. Those women with stronger pelvic muscles also experienced significantly stronger voluntary uterine contractions. The strength of a man's pelvic muscles may also play a role. Strong male pelvic muscles, so the theory goes, result in a penis which, when erect, angles right up against the man's stomach, at an angle which is more effective for anterior wall stimulation.

Getting the angle right

The sexual position adopted by women and men is also mooted as playing a part in who ejaculates and who doesn't. It is argued, by some, that there are disadvantages for humans in face-to-face sexual positions – namely, that the anterior wall of the vagina is not as stimulated as in a rear entry position, that typically used by quadrupeds. For the majority of quadrupeds, the opening of the vagina is just under the tail, making doggy style the easiest option. This is not the case, though, for all mammals, as we have seen. Some, including elephants, bonobos and humans, have vaginas that have shifted position. Instead of lying approximately parallel with the spine (as in cats and dogs), the vagina has swung forwards towards the stomach side, changing the angle of entry. For a woman standing up, the first two fifths of her vagina angles back at approximately 30 degrees to the vertical (when unaroused), the middle two fifths at 55 degrees and the final fifth at 10 degrees, tracing an approximate S shape. This change in angles can sometimes make it difficult for a woman inserting a tampon. One trick is to insert the tip with the index finger, and then push the rest of the tampon in with the thumb. This thumb technique works better because it fortuitously provides the particular vaginal angle needed. Try it.

The changed angle of vaginal entry may be one reason why humans and bonobos can and do enjoy sexual intercourse in a variety of positions – female on top, male on top, as well as rear entry and many more. Curiously, bonobos seem to prefer face-to-face sex. Female bonobos have been seen manoeuvring their male partners into their favourite position, and astonishingly, bonobos have developed a gestural sign language to communicate the sexual positioning desired. However, for large lumbering elephants, changing sexual position is not as easy. A female elephant's perineum is half a metre long, and this awkward entry angle results in sex being a delicate and risky business for elephants. Perhaps this is why they often take to the water to enjoy sex.

Lack of stimulation of the anterior wall could certainly be a factor in suppressing female ejaculation; however, the length of stimulation time rather than an absence of stimulation due to position is likely to be the culprit with face-to-face sex. Recent MRI pictures of sexual intercourse reveal that, contrary to previous expectations, face-to-face sex can result in the anterior wall being preferentially stimulated. Indeed face-to-face sex could be said to provide a circular kind of stimulation. As both (and it's important that it's both) women and men thrust towards each other, their thrusts are felt and transmitted through their genitals, as both pressure and touch sensations. Men feel the thrust and clasp of the vagina through their clitoral tissue, and urethra and *spongiosum* tissue, with the deep-pressure sensations of thrusting reverberating all the way through to the prostate. For women, tactile and pressure stimulation is felt as the penis presses up against both the cervix and the anterior vaginal wall, in turn pushing against the prostate, *spongiosum*, urethra and through to the clitoris, which is stimulated from both inside and outside, in face-to-face sex, as the clitoral crown rubs against the man's body. These MRI studies also illustrate beautifully how, with increased stimulation, the anterior vaginal wall swells, lengthening and bulging into the vaginal interior.

Finally, a new and radical theory of female ejaculation is that most, if not all, women do ejaculate prostatic fluid, but that in many women this fluid, or part of it, is not expelled outside the body. Rather it is pushed back down the urethra the other way – into the bladder. In other words, it is ejaculated, but in a retrograde manner. This change of ejaculation direction, retrograde ejaculation, is not uncommon in men, and is directly related to lax or ineffective pelvic musculature. This results in a lack of closure of the internal bladder valve and ejected semen is forced backward into the bladder. Could this be occurring in women too?

In an effort to find out whether female retrograde ejaculation was a possibility, female urine – both pre-orgasm and post-orgasm – was analysed to see whether it contained the prostatic marker prostate-specific antigen (PSA). Twenty-four women were involved in the study, and six of these women had their ejaculate analysed too. The women involved in the study masturbated to orgasm and had not had any sexual contact with men for at least two days. The results were startling. PSA was not detected in pre-orgasmic urine; however, it was detected in significant amounts in post-orgasmic urine in 75 per cent of the women, suggesting that the female prostate actively secretes fluids during sexual arousal and/or orgasm, and that retrograde ejaculation of prostatic secretions is not uncommon. Out of the six women who provided ejaculation samples, PSA was present in all of them, the average value being 6.06 ng/ml (nanogram/millilitre). The mean PSA value in post-orgasmic retrograde ejaculation samples was 0.09 ng/ml.

Spurting the sperm away

The big question that remains to be answered about female ejaculation of prostatic fluid revolves around what its evolutionary purpose could be. Female prostatic fluid seems too saline to have a vaginal lubrication function, plus its production tends to peak and spurt with or approaching orgasm, not at the onset of arousal. Female ejaculation, however, does not necessarily coincide with orgasm. Some women ejaculate before orgasm, some during and some after. While there is no general pattern regarding timing of expulsion, one characteristic of female ejaculatory behaviour is the 'bearing down' or pushing out muscular motion associated with it, where the cervix and vagina push downwards and forwards sometimes with enough force to eject not only prostatic fluid, but probing penises or fingers too.

There is also consensus on the stimulation required to produce female ejaculation of prostatic fluids. A rhythmic deep-pressure stimulation is needed – provided either by rhythmic thrusting or rubbing against the anterior vaginal wall. Tentative strokes are out. This stimulation picture is consistent with the stimulation required by the male prostate – which is provided either by the stimulus of thrusting movements during sexual intercourse, or by direct pressure applied in the rectum via fingers, penises or whatever takes your fancy.

Important hints as to the female prostate's role come from the nature of semen itself – which in all species is a complex viscous mix of chemicals and sperm. A male's prostate is just one of a number of accessory glands which add their contents to the ejaculated semen and sperm package. In men, these accessory glands are the prostate, the seminal vesicles and Cowper's glands. In other species there can be more or fewer. It's now known that the products of these accessory glands perform a variety of functions designed to improve the male's reproductive success. Some seminal ingredients protect sperm on their passage out of the urethra; for example, pre-ejaculate serves to neutralise the acidity of the urethra, after urine has passed down it. Others in the seminal mix, such as the sugar fructose, are thought to make sperm more motile, ensuring a smooth exit out of male genitalia, while some ingredients can trigger female genital muscle contractions, or even increase female fecundity by stimulating ovulation.

From an evolutionary perspective, male accessory gland products represent different attempts by males to persuade females to keep and use their sperm after they have deposited it. They are biological adaptations for survival of the species through sexual reproduction. However, females of all species have many tricks up their sleeves when it comes to getting rid of unwanted sperm, as detailed earlier. In this context, could the female prostate provide a co-evolutionary response to the male's accessory gland products? Could the female's prostatic fluid improve her prospects of removing surplus or unwanted sperm?

It is not just women who eject a fluid from their genitalia during and after sexual activity. Many females of other species do too. Indeed, the female's initial response to insemination by the male in the majority of mammals, insects, spiders and birds is to spurt back seminal material, utilising her strong genital musculature. However, there is a question mark hanging over what precisely it is that the female is ejecting. Typically female ejection studies comment that the material is apparently semen or presumably semen. The vast majority of studies that have analysed the material have looked only for the presence of sperm. It is possible that female prostatic fluids are present; however, detailed analyses of all the components of ejected fluid, and who contributed them, have not yet been performed. Fascinatingly, though, one study that has investigated the role of the female in contributing genital fluids found that females do add to ejected material. This study of the fruit fly, *Drosophila mettleri*, found that females make a significant contribution to ejected sperm (in this case sperm sacs). This is also the case with female rats, who shed their vaginal lining in order to aid in the removal of sperm plugs.

If female genital fluids (perhaps prostatic) are typically present in the ejected material from females of many species, what role are they playing? One strong possibility is that female prostatic fluid may help to wash away sperm. Sperm, as anybody who has come in close contact with it knows, is typically thick and sticky, especially in mammals and birds, and is perfect for clinging in the crevices and folds of female reproductive tracts. Indeed, it is speculated that the very viscous nature of some species' sperm is an adaptation to make it difficult for females to eject and reject it. If this is the case, a co-evolutionary response from the female to produce some 'lubricant' to ease sperm ejection would make perfect evolutionary sense. The saline nature of female prostatic fluid could help to remove this stubborn spermatic substance, especially if produced under pressure, and in combination with a muscular bearing down of the genitalia. Other ingredients of female prostatic fluid, such as fructose and PSA, suggest such a sperm removal role. In males, fructose is thought to aid the smooth passage of sperm out of male genitalia, while PSA is known to participate in the liquefaction of sperm.

The idea that females use prostatic or genital fluids to help rid themselves of unwanted sperm, be it from the immediate or previous partner, has important implications for sexual reproduction strategies. Humans are one of the very few species which attempt to practise serial monogamy; other mammals enjoy the pleasures of multiple partners. While for monogamous women today prostatic fluid expulsions may not perform a reproductive function, for females with multiple sexual partners, whether or not they ejaculate and wash away a current or previous partner's sperm could have a direct influence on whose sperm they retain and ultimately use to fertilise their eggs. If this is the case, then males could attempt to swing the balance back in their favour by persuading (i.e. stimulating) females to eject previous males' sperm prior to depositing their own. Curiously, this is what the males of some species have been found to do – they copulate with or sexually stimulate the female until she ejects any previously stored sperm.

Dunnocks and damselflies provide two examples of how this can occur. Female dunnocks, a species of bird, typically copulate up to several hundred times per clutch, when just a couple of copulations would do, so for a male to have a chance at being a father he must be able to persuade her to get rid of any other male's sperm. Consequently, the male's approach focuses on performing sufficient foreplay dunnock-style, before sperm transferral. For dunnocks, foreplay means poking and pecking at the ruddy tumescent exterior of the female's cloaca – her combined urethra, vagina and anus. As the male continues to stimulate her externally, the female's cloaca becomes pinker and more distended, and from time to time can be seen making strong pumping movements. It is during these pumping movements that small droplets of what is presumed to be sperm only emerge. When the male sees these droplets appear he inspects them closely, and only after this inspection will he transfer his sperm. Elsewhere, detailed work on one species of damselfly has shown that part of the intricate internal architecture of the female genitalia comprises a cuticular plate bearing mechanoreceptive sensilla. If, and only if, the male can distort this genital plate with his aedeagus (insect phallus) during copulation, will the female eject previously stored sperm. Is this the damselfly's equivalent of a G spot?

The behaviour of the male dunnock and damselfly in their attempts to be the ones to fertilise their respective females' eggs recalls the previously noted conception advice of the South Pacific Ponapese people, who practise polygamy: 'If a Ponapese man wishes to impregnate his principal wife, he first stimulates her to the point where she urinates and only then proceeds to have intercourse with her.'

Perhaps the Ponapese wisdom is correct. Confirmation of the female prostate's role in sexual reproduction will only come if further research into the prostatic secretions of females of many species is carried out, including analysing the significance of its rich and heady musky aroma. It would also be helpful to understand more about the make-up of vaginal mucus and fluids in relation to sexual health and reproduction. Sadly, the current status of such research lags far behind equivalent studies of male seminal fluids. However, despite the lack of scientific focus on female sexual fluids, one thing is certain. With not a tooth, a sharp edge or a snake in sight, the nature of the vagina is fluid in every sense of the word – flexible, flowing, mutable, mercurial, sinuous, shape-shifting, protean and wet.

6

THE PERFUMED GARDEN

Adultery, the art of misbehaving genitally, has been frowned upon by human societies throughout history. The punishments typically meted out for this sexual malpractice range from the obvious and straight-to-the-point practice of chopping off the offending genitalia, to the seemingly more subtle act of mutilating or amputating an adulterer's nose. However, nasal dismemberment, which on first sight may not appear to be a punishment that fits the crime, is, historians and anthropologists record, a surprisingly common penalty for enjoying the pleasures of sex with someone other than your spouse.

Roman poet Virgil (70–19 BCE), in his epic poem the *Aeneid*, describes how female and male adulterers were castigated by nasal castration. Anthropology texts from the early twentieth century detail how among the Ashanti of Ghana, and in Afghanistan, an adulteress was chastised by the severing of her nose, whereas in Samoa, an insulted and jealous husband would bite his wife's nose off. Not just nasal amputation, but ears, lips and scalp too were taken as part of the tribal customs of indigenous North Americans. For women of the Baiga tribe of northern India, both the nose and the clitoris were lopped off by wrathful husbands. Meanwhile, such was the prevalence of nasal dismemberment in ancient India (it was the official punishment for adultery) that Indian physicians developed surgical methods for reconstructing the nose. Early Indian medical texts detail how the technique was to use a skin flap from the forehead to form a new nose.

Intriguingly, associations between the nose and a person's genitals are not restricted to adultery and amputation in antiquity. On the contrary, naso-genital connections span centuries of art, literature and science too. In his *Physiognomica*, Aristotle alleges a link between lechery and the shape of the nose. During Roman times, the nose was read as a symbol for the genitals in a number of ways. For men, a large nose was seen to signify an equally ample penis, a correlation that still has resonance for some today. For these individuals, the phallic cast of a man's nose coupled with the scrotal aspect of a man's cleft chin is not viewed as a coincidence. The licentious Roman emperor Heliogabalus (218–22 CE) reportedly welcomed into his sex club only those men who were deemed to be *nasuti*. By this he apparently meant those men whose nose suggested their penis would be acceptable to women – those whose nose made the grade, genitally speaking, Not surprisingly, ancient caricatures often depict male noses with a distinctly phallic appearance. By the Middle Ages and for several hundred years afterwards it was commonplace to describe the shape of the nose as portending the size of the penis.

Such beliefs remained strong well into the seventeenth century, despite the efforts of anatomists such as Reinier de Graaf to expose them as erroneous. In his work *The Generative Organs of Men*, de Graaf insists that the naso-genital size correspondence is not so, writing: 'In dissecting cadavers, anatomists not infrequently observe the opposite', adding, for clarification of his viewpoint, 'Even if this were so ... sexual capability does not depend on a huge penis.' As well as proclaiming genital size, or status, the shape of an individual's nose was said to convey a sense of their virility. Yet not all physiognomists agreed on which shapes said what. Some subscribed to the notion that the more elephantine the nasal appendage, the stronger the supposed sexual vigour. According to others, it was a snub nose that was the true hallmark of a lustful man.

It's not just men, though, who had their noses sized up, sexually speaking. Women did too. Moreover, correlations between the nose and the genitals were not confined to the west. *Siang Mien*, the Chinese art of reading faces, describes how the nose of a woman or a man can be used as a measure of a person's vitality and sexual powers, of a person's ability to love. The nose, it says is 'the centre of life'. Fascinatingly, it was also believed that the state of a woman's nose could be read as a sign of sexual arousal. According to the ancient Chinese sex manual, *Secret Instructions Concerning the Jade Chamber*, the second of five signs of sexual desire in women is said to be 'breasts hard and nose perspiring'. The manual helpfully adds that a woman's dilated nose and mouth 'means that she wants you to insert your penis'.

The ancient Chinese science of reflexology also teaches that the genitals correspond to the nose and a person's upper lip. And this, it is said, explains why kissing and sniffing are a natural part of sexual foreplay and pleasure. More explanation of this connection is given in Tantric texts, which state that a woman's upper lip is one of her most erogenous zones because of a subtle nerve channel connecting it with the clitoris. This nerve, called the 'Wisdom Conch-like Nerve', is said to be curved like a shell as it anchors to the clitoris, channelling orgasmic energy. This is why sucking and kissing a woman's upper lip is often enough to bring her to orgasm.

Western ideas about the perceived female naso-genital alliance also held that evidence of sexual activity in women was written on their nose. However, while Chinese sex manuals saw this system as a way of making sure that a woman was fully aroused, western men touted the condition of the female nose as a test for virginity. The thirteenth-century writer on physiognomy Michael Scotus alarmingly claimed to be able to tell the sexual status of a woman suspected of moral turpitude by fingering her nasal cartilage. Some doctors today claim to be able to tell from changes in the shape of a woman's nose whether she is pregnant or not.

The idea that the nose and the genitals are connected is also expressed in ancient western theories about the development of the embryo in the womb. By this reckoning, solar system planets held sway over the development of an individual's features, with each planet ascribed a function in the foetus' formation. Mars ruled the third month of development in the womb, and the formation of the head, while the sun influenced the fourth month and the creation of the heart. Not surprisingly, perhaps, the planet Venus, traditionally viewed as the purveyor of venery, pleasure and sexual delight, was thought to bestow concupiscence and desire on the developing infant during its fifth month in the womb. The popular late Middle Age treatise *Women's Secrets* relates how, 'In the fifth month Venus by its perfect power perfects certain of the exterior members and forms certain others: the ears, the nose, the mouth, the penis in males, and the pudenda, that is the vulva, breasts and other members in females. It also causes the separation of the hands and feet and fingers.' Following Venus was Mercury, reigning over the voice, eyebrows and eyes, and making hair and nails grow.

Not surprisingly, perhaps, literature and language does not escape the yoking of nose with genitals. Resemblances between the phallus and the nose were often alluded to in Roman literature. What's more, similarities between a woman's genitalia and her nasal attributes were expressed remarkably succinctly in Latin sexual vocabulary. *Nasus*, the Latin for nose, was also used as a term for the clitoris – the sexual slang of its day. As images in the book *Femalia*, by Joani Blank, show, the crown of a woman's clitoris does sometimes look a little like a nose – a snub nose, that is. The linguistic pairing of the nose and the clitoris is found in other cultures. The Mehinaku tribe of Brazil refer to a woman's clitoris as the nose of her vagina (*itsi kiri*). A woman's clitoris, or vaginal nose, say the Mehinaku, moves about 'searching for its food' – a man's penis – in the manner of a predator sniffing out its prey. Other parts of female genitalia are also equated with facial features, such as the forehead and lips, and the entire vagina is symbolically identified as a mouth.

For the Mehinaku, sex itself is seen as a kind of eating, an idea that is also reflected in their language, whereby the verb to eat also means to have sex. Hence the genitals of one sex are the food of another. Mehinaku myth and ritual also suggest an equivalence between the penis and the nose. Other cultures' rituals underline such associations. For example, an archaic way of mocking a man who is unable to become erect enough for sexual intercourse – who has lost his male sexual power – is for a woman to make a hole in the impotent man's nose and place a cowrie shell there (a symbol of the vagina and female sexual power).

As above, so below

Why the multiple associations between a person's nose and their sexual organs? Can looking at the nose actually be a viable avenue to viewing the vagina? The idea that the nose and the genitalia may be connected in some way has an illustrious history in medicine. Hippocratic doctrine taught that the nose could be used as a diagnostic tool for ailments occurring elsewhere in the body, especially the reproductive organs. The nostrils, in particular, were viewed as important indicators of health. For men, naturally damp nostrils and watery, plentiful sperm were read as revealing a healthy constitution. Nasal discharge, it was reported, could be dried up with a dose of sexual intercourse. Elsewhere, though, religious scribe Celsus (150 CE) advised men to 'abstain from warmth and women' at the first sign of a cold or catarrh, as acts of venery would only inflame and irritate the nose.

Interestingly, Hippocratic medicine held that the affinities between the nose and the genitals were more pronounced in women than they were in men. This enhanced female naso-genital alliance stemmed, it is thought, from the Hippocratic belief that a sexually mature woman's body contained a tube or route (a *hodos*, the Greek for 'way') which linked the nostrils and mouth (orifices of the head) with the genital orifice, the vagina. As the Hippocratic men of medicine saw it, both ends of this tube, or uninterrupted vagina, had a mouth (*stoma*), and so the two were analogous. Remnants of their anatomical reasoning remain in medical terminology and language today. Both the head and the genitals have a neck (cervix), mouth (the mouth of the womb or uterus) and lips (labiae). This idea of the vagina as a second mouth is found in other cultures, such as the Mehinaku, as we've seen. It's also pertinent to recall that reflexology states there is a connection between the mouth and the genitals, and, surprisingly, western medicine seems to suggest there is too, as women are advised to relax their mouths at the final moment of giving birth, because this helps the vagina release the baby. This idea of the vagina as woman's second mouth also helps to explain the saying '*Ella habla por en medio en las piernas*' – 'She speaks from between her legs'.

According to Hippocrates' *hodos* reasoning, the orifices at either end of the tube (nose, mouth and genitals) were used in various ways. One end could be used to detect problems at the opposite end, or either end could be read as a sign of the condition of the internal tube itself. Either end could also be used as the site for the administration of suitable therapy – be it 'from the top' (*anô*) or 'from the bottom' (*katô*) of the tube. Many naso-genital diagnoses and associations were made. 'Dry and blocked, not upright' nostrils were an indication that the mouth of the womb was closed and tilted. Naturally damp nostrils were linked with watery, plentiful *sperma muliebris* (female sperm), and were seen as a sign of a healthy constitution.

Menstruation was one of the most important conditions read by the *hodos* theory. For example, a pain in the throat pointed to the start of the menstrual period. Nosebleeds too were linked to the onset of puberty and menstruation, or could be connected to childbirth. And with a direct route envisaged from vagina to nostrils, nasal blood flow was viewed as evidence of diverted menstruation in those women whose menstrual bleeding was deemed not heavy or frequent enough. According to the medical maxims of the *Hippocratic Aphorisms*: 'If the menses are deficient, it is a good thing when blood flows from the nostrils.'

Hippocrates' ideas of a connection between female genitalia and a woman's nose were enduring. More than a thousand years after their conception they still formed the basis of treatments for female conditions. This is illustrated clearly in the *Trotula*, the most influential compendium on women's medicine in medieval Europe. For instance, the *Trotula*'s advice 'On the Regimen for a Woman Giving Birth' suggests: 'when the time of birth arrives ... let sneezing be induced with the nose and mouth constricted, so that the greatest part of her strength and spirit tends towards the womb ... Likewise, let troches [lozenges] be made from galbanum with asafoetida and myrrh or rue, and let a fumigation be made to the nose. Above all, let her be aware of the cold, and let there not be any aromatic fumigation to the nose. But this can be applied more safely to the orifice of the womb ...'

Rather alarmingly, vaginal or uterine fumigation was common in medieval times. This consisted of a woman sitting on a perforated seat above scented, smoking fumigation pots and stools (see Figure 6.1). Paucity or lack of menstrual blood is one of the conditions that was treated in this way, with the *Trotula* prescribing:

> Take ginger, laurel leaves and savin. Pound them and place them together in a plain pot on live coals, and let the woman sit on a perforated seat, and let her receive the smoke through the lower members, and thus the menses will return. Let this be done three or four times or even more often. But for the woman who frequently takes applications of this kind, it is necessary that she anoint her vagina inside with cold unguents lest she become excessively heated.

The *hodos* theory is perhaps responsible for many of the notions surrounding women's health. Take the 'wandering womb' idea. A woman's womb was seen as capable of wandering along her *hodos*, be it up or down. However, this womb-wandering was seen as causing

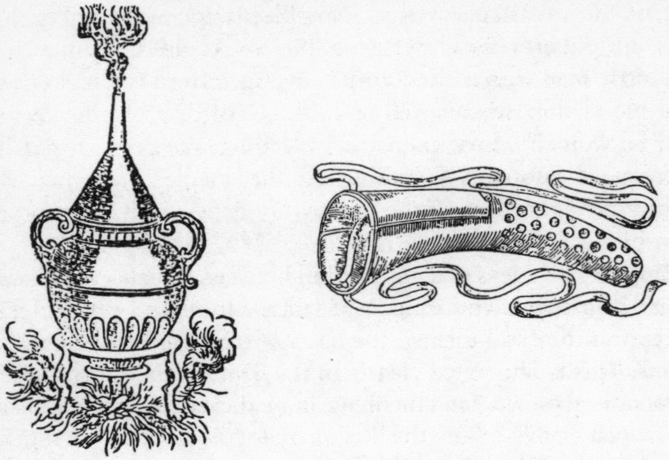

Figure 6.1 Renaissance instruments for vaginal fumigation: The patient sat over a small burner and received either attractive or repellent aromas into her vagina. The perforated instrument on the right is designed to hold the vagina open – the better to receive the healing vapours.

medical problems, such as womb suffocation, or, as it was later known, hysteria. Womb suffocation, it was understood, was a disorder that occurred when the womb moved upwards towards the stomach, chest, heart or throat. Symptoms of womb suffocation, the *Trotula* says, include 'loss of appetite from an overwhelming frigidity of the heart ... Sometimes ... she loses the function of the voice, the nose is distorted, the lips are contracted and she grits her teeth ...'

Remedies for wombs that had wandered too far upwards typically involved applying aromatic potions, which would coax the womb to return to its correct position. According to the *Trotula*, 'the womb follows sweet-smelling substances and flees foul-smelling ones'. Hence the treatments for a raised womb (uterine suffocation) could involve anointing the vagina inside and out with oils with pleasantly scented odours, such as iris, chamomile, musk or nard oil, or smelling the rank aromas of 'castoreum, pitch, burnt wool, burnt linen cloth and burnt leather'. Cupping glasses could also be applied to the groin and pubic areas, or sternatives (substances that induce sneezing) were sniffed.

According to Hippocratic thinking, a woman's genitals-to-head *hodos* also seemed to allow for the free flow of semen backwards and forwards from vagina to brain. This belief may explain why one ancient test for whether a marriage had been consummated or not was for the bride's neck to be measured before and after the wedding night. An increase in size showed a successful union. A similar neck test was also used to trap adulterers. This semen theory probably underpins the belief that indulgence in venery – the pursuit of sexual gratification – can affect an individual's voice. Indeed, Greek and Roman writers believed that it was also possible to tell when a girl had lost her virginity because her voice became deeper. Medieval and Renaissance writers gleefully retold the story of how Diogenes Laertius of Democritus recognises that Hippocrates' daughter has been deflowered during the night from a change in the girl's voice. Perhaps they were having a dig at Hippocrates.

The connection between voice and venery was also thought to affect men. For instance, seventeenth-century authors recorded how voice trainers infibulated a man's penis – enclosing it in bands and fetters – in a bid to protect the singer's glory. Meanwhile, this idea of the voice being affected by sexual activity has persisted into the twentieth century. In 1913, the *New York Medical Journal* published the paper 'Connections of the sexual apparatus with the ear, nose and throat'. In it, the author writes: 'After a night consecrated to Venus, patients which have had any nasal, aural or laryngological abnormality invariably find this condition exaggerated.' On a more serious note, a recent study highlighted the fact that 30 per cent of women with vocal cord dysfunction suffered sexual abuse during childhood.

Scents and sensuality

Significantly for this view of the vagina, it is not just physical similarities and supposed physiology that have pulled the nose and genitalia together. It's the function of the nose too – the sense of smell. Smell has consistently been perceived as the sexual sense, the most intimate sense, the animal sense. It is, according to Rousseau, 'the sense of memory and desire'. The recognition of smell as a powerful sexual stimulus is reflected throughout history – celebrated as an aphrodisiac in perfumes and poetry, yet often maligned as a bad influence by philosophers and governments. Civet, the honey-like marking sexual secretion of the urogenital sacs of the African civet cat, was one of the most sought after aphrodisiac scents. According to the medieval writer Petrus Castellus: 'Civet will cause a woman so much desire for coitus that she will almost continually wish to make love with her husband. And in particular, if a man wishes to go with a woman, if he shall place on his penis this same civet and unexpectedly use it, he will arouse in her the greatest of pleasure.'

Musk too has been viewed as a potent 'provoker of venery' throughout history. In the nineteenth century, French novelist Emile Zola writes this of musk and women: 'With the aid of a piece of musk she abandons herself to forbidden delights. She is in the habit of surreptitiously sniffing it. She drugs herself with it until orgiastic convulsions overwhelm her.' One seventeenth-century writer warns of the dangers of using musk too liberally, writing of a couple who doused their genitalia in musk only to find that, like dogs, they could not disengage from each other after.

Poetry frequently and beautifully twins scents and sensuality. Within poetry's verses, naso-genital associations and allusions, which perhaps could not be spoken of straightforwardly, were free to be eulogised. Such poems read as spellbinding and mesmerising evocations of desire, steeped as they are in smells redolent of lust, love and genitalia. For example, the soon-to-be married couple in 'The Song of Solomon' detail their delight in the power and richness of the odours of each other, writing of mountains of myrrh and hills of incense. Aroused by her bridegroom's passionate portrayal of the bountiful scents of her still-locked 'garden' (vagina), the bride calls on the north and south wind:

> Blow upon my garden, let its fragrance be wafted abroad
> Let my beloved come to his garden, and eat its choicest fruit.

The ecstasy of a woman's revealed perfume is a theme that seventeenth-century English poet Robert Herrick returned to again and again, in both 'Upon Julia Unlacing Herself', and 'Love Perfumes all Parts', in which he rhapsodises:

If I kiss Anthea's breast
There I smell the Phoenix nest:
If I her lip, the most sincere
Altar of incense, I smell there
Hands, and thighs, and legs, are all
Richly aromatical
Goddess Isis can't transfer
Musks and Ambers more from her:
Nor can Juno sweeter be,
When she lies with Jove, than she.

For various reasons, however, the pairing of the sense of smell with sexuality has not always been considered in a positive light. Early philosophers, noting the predilection of animals to go nose to genitalia prior to copulation, chose to rank smell as one of the lower senses. To them, it was an animal sense, incapable of raising humans to elevated heights of creativity, like the senses of sight and sound could and did in art and music. The philosophers of the Middle Ages regarded smell as a vulgar sense, and one that in no way promoted human intellect. Astonishingly, both ancient and modern governments, perhaps recognising that you don't control a people unless you control their sexuality, have deemed perfumes dangerous and intoxicating enough to be banned or have their usage restricted. In 188 BCE, Romans were forbidden to wear all but the most modest amount of perfumery in social ceremonies.

Sixteen hundred years later, the English parliament felt the need to pass an act in 1770 protecting men from 'perfumed women', for fear that scented 'witchcraft' might lure unsuspecting men into marriage. And by the eighteenth and nineteenth centuries, the use of musk, amber and civet was discouraged, for fear of its detrimental and 'decaying effects'. One result of this anti-perfume attitude was that in 1855, Queen Victoria caused a furore during a royal visit to Paris. The problem? The British monarch was wearing perfume with a hint of musk – a scent that at that time was deemed more appropriate to a *salon mondaine* than the fashion-conscious French court.

Downplayed by philosophers, branded the animal sense and associate of sex, and bedevilled by its ephemeral nature, perhaps it's not surprising that the sense of smell remained a poor cousin of science for many centuries. Indeed, even today, smell remains the least researched and funded of humankind's five recognised senses. It wasn't until the end of the nineteenth century that hints that Hippocrates' hunch about a naso-genital alliance might be based in physical reality began to emerge. Charles Darwin, marvelling at the variety of facial and genital features in the animal kingdom, brought attention to them and to the extraordinarily similar naso/genital arrangement of the male mandrill. This Old World monkey's nose of vibrant vermilion red echoes its fire-engine-red penile shaft and anus, while its brilliant cobalt-blue paranasal ridges mirror its pale blue scrotum. The startling effect of this as above, so below colour scheme is topped off by the apparent mimicking of the mandrill's yellow/orange facial beard with pubic hair of a similar hue. Writing about the mandrill, Darwin said: 'No case interested and perplexed me so much as the brightly-coloured hinder ends and adjoining parts of certain monkeys . . . It seems to me . . . probable that the bright colours, whether on the face or hinder end, or, as in the mandrill, on both, serve as a sexual ornament and attraction.'

Other Old World monkeys display naso-genital links, and for some this association is underlined by changes in reproductive status mirroring those seen in the genitals and nose or face. Take female Japanese macaques. The faces of these female primates turn an even brighter pinky-red as their sexual perineal skin swells and blooms during their five-month-long mating period. Male Japanese macaques sport red sexual skin on their face as well as their scrotum and perineum, and out of the mating season, the loss of sexual skin colour is accompanied by their testicles retracting and ejaculation ceasing. In a similar vein, the flamboyant naso-genital blues and reds of the male mandrill become muted if the male is subordinate or solitary, or peripheral to a social group. And as his naso-genital colours fade, his testicles shrink too. Not surprisingly, such colour-challenged males do not enjoy as much mating and reproductive success as their more brilliantly hued brothers. It's also now appreciated that the growth of the extraordinarily long, fleshy and distinctly phallic nose of the male proboscis monkey (*Nasalis larvatus*) is delayed if there is an absence of females in the social group. Peculiarly, some birds, as well as primates, exhibit naso-genital features connected with reproduction. This is the case for the male pelican, whose beak becomes swollen with a large bump during the mating season, despite the fact that this mars his field of vision and interferes with the catching of fish.

The nose has a clitoris?

Following hot on the heels of Darwin's observations of comparable external naso-genital characteristics came the surprising realisation that the internal structures of the human nose and genitalia are actually strikingly similar. In 1884, American surgeon John N. Mackenzie pointed out that the respiratory and olfactory mucosae, which cover the conchae in the nose and, in the case of the olfactory mucosa, line the narrow olfactory slits, were composed of erectile tissue analogous to the *corpora cavernosa* tissue of the clitoris and penis. That is, the nose has a clitoris too. And, just like their genitalic counterparts, the blood vessels of these nasal tissues fill with blood, or vasodilate, in response to sexual excitement. So not only did the human nose resemble the genitalia, it also responded in a similar erectile manner too.

Nasal erections are, in fact, the reason behind the nasal stuffiness, congestion or rhinitis that is experienced by many individuals following orgasm, sexual stimulation or intercourse. The idea that sex goes to the nose is, not surprisingly, recognised by those individuals who rely on their nose for their livelihood. Perfume testers, wine tasters and tea blenders are all aware of the condition known as 'honeymoon rhinitis' – a hypersensitised nose post-sexual activity. For me, the idea of nasal erections has resonance, having experienced personally such extreme nasal arousal post-orgasm. The feeling was of my nose being vibrant, literally quivering, suffused with sensation, and intensely aware of the sexual aromas surrounding me. One more sniff of the sexual landscape I was nestled in, and I felt I would surely dissolve in eternal orgasm. Sadly, I didn't, but the memory remains deliciously strong.

The enhanced blood flow to the nose, which is responsible for resulting in nasal membrane engorgement, also accounts for a rise in temperature of the nasal mucosa. Experiments looking at nasal mucosa immediately before and immediately after sexual intercourse show a mean rise in temperature of 1.5°C. Cold temperatures, too, have an effect on the nose, constricting nasal structures as they do clitoral or penile erectile tissue. The rapid dilation of the erectile tissue of the nose is what is believed to be behind the sudden, and often paroxysmal, sneezing that can accompany sexual desire, genital erection, intercourse and orgasm. In his 1875 text *Observations Rares de Médecine*, Stalpart de Wiel mentions 'individuals in whom the act of coitus was often preceded by sneezing'.

John Mackenzie wrote in 1884 'of a man of sanguine temperament, who every time he caressed his wife sneezed three or four times', while another researcher in 1913 noted the case of a man 'who frequently sneezed at the sight of a comely maiden'. Following one friend's confession of a similar naso-genital phenomenon brought on by sexually arousing thoughts alone, I now view his every sneeze with a wry, quizzical smile. Not just sneezing, but wheezing too, is tied in to sexual situations. The asthmatic breathing 'associated with stoppage of the nostrils' suffered by one Victorian woman was apparently alleviated when she did not engage in sex every night with her husband. Today sexual abuse is recognised as a stressor in cases of paroxysmal sneezing.

The emergence of naso-sexual medicine

The recognition at the end of the nineteenth century that there was a physiological relationship between the human nose and genitalia ushered in a new field of medicine – naso-sexual medicine. Over a period of approximately twenty-five years, a multitude of papers, books, lectures and dissertations were devoted to poring over the possible connections between the nasal passages and the sexual organs. During its heyday, naso-sexual medicine influenced many, including Sigmund Freud, to explore further the connections between the nose, olfaction, genitalia and sexuality. In 1912, at the tail end of the naso-sexual renaissance, E. Seifert proposed that there was a 'reflex neurosis' operating between an individual's genitalia and their nose, and that it was this reflex that was the key to understanding all aspects of human health and fulfilment.

Naso-sexual medicine also resulted in some curious remedies for gynaecological problems. At the end of the nineteenth century, Wilhelm Fliess, one of Sigmund Freud's closest collaborators, sought to pinpoint the precise areas of a woman's nose that were linked with her genitalia. His identification of these 'genital zones' or spots (*Genitalstellen*) on the olfactory mucosa of the nose – which had a tendency to bleed at various times associated with the menstrual cycle and pregnancy – then led to them being used as therapy sites for various gynaecological disorders. The treatments which proponents of nasal genital zones advocated included cauterisation, or the infinitely more pleasurable approach of applying cocaine nasally. During the heyday of naso-sexual medicine, if you were suffering from labour pains, or just plain dysmenorrhoea (painful periods), the doctor could, and did, prescribe a dab of cocaine up the nose for you. Fliess also suggested that several cases of apparently spontaneous abortion were, in fact, triggered accidentally, by intranasal surgical procedures.

Fliess, Mackenzie and other researchers in the field of naso-sexual science were also intrigued by the apparent effect of the menstrual cycle and of pregnancy on the female nose. Female nasal mucosa, it was noted, swelled and reddened, became more sensitive and congested, and subsequently bled, with a periodicity seemingly in concert with that of the 29.5–day human female menstrual cycle. Indeed, the occurrence of nosebleeds (epistaxis) during menstruation was referred to as vicarious menstruation – menstrual bleeding from an alternative orifice. It was also pointed out that, as many pregnancies progressed, an increasing proportion of women presented with either blocked noses or sporadic nasal bleeding.

However, it wasn't until the late 1930s that a scientific rationale for such rhythmic nasal events was realised. The nasal and genital skin of female rhesus monkeys provided the key. Hector Mortimer, a Canadian otolaryngologist, observed that the striking reddening and swelling of the sexual skin that these monkeys sport coincided exactly with the reddening of their nasal mucosa. For these primates, and some others (but by no means all), the sexual swellings of their anogenital region reach peak tumescence immediately prior to ovulation, as the circulating blood levels of the hormone oestrogen come to a head too. Blood oestrogen levels, it was finally appreciated, had an effect on both a female's genitalia and her nose. The thinkers of old were correct in assuming a connection, or route, between the nose and the genitalia. Perhaps hormones are the mysterious *hodos* envisaged by Hippocrates.

It's now accepted that the human nose, and nasal membranes, are stimulated by circulating levels of hormones. Vasomotor rhinitis (inflammation of the nasal membranes) is a common occurrence in both pregnancy and puberty, both times in life when blood oestrogen levels soar. Increases in blood oestrogen levels during pregnancy have also been shown to correlate closely with nasal congestion. It's also interesting to note that around ovulation, many women report a heightened sense of awareness, coupled with (or probably as a result of) an increased sensitivity to odours – again, a result of the effects of circulating hormones on their nasal mucosa. This lower female threshold to aromas around the time of ovulation has also been documented in the laboratory.

The hormonal connection between the nose and the genitals is also underlined by a number of medical conditions. Chronic underdevelopment of the nasal membranes (atrophic rhinitis) is often linked with irregular or non-existent periods (amenorrhea), while Kallman's syndrome is associated with no sense of smell (anosmia) and undeveloped gonads: in women the ovaries contain only immature egg follicles, while men present small testes, do not produce sperm and a prostate cannot be felt. Losing one's sense of smell also has a negative effect on sexuality, with over a quarter of anosmia sufferers becoming sexually dysfunctional. The sense of smell, it seems, is integral to both human sexual development and adult sexuality.

Would like to meet . . .

Human anatomy and physiology highlight how the nose and the genitalia are related, with hormones the messenger molecules shuttling information to and fro via the blood. But why this intimate connection? Why should the nose and the sense of smell be so tied up with human sexual anatomy? The answer lies many millions of years back in time. At its most fundamental level, the sense of smell is the ability of an organism to respond to chemical cues in its environment. At heart, therefore, smell is chemosensory, a chemical sense. It requires the presence of molecules, particulate matter, in the air or water, to effect sensation.

Smell is also an original sense. Communicating via chemicals is as old as life itself, and is an attribute of all organisms on earth, from the smallest to the largest. Even the simplest and most ancient unicellular creatures, which have neither a nervous system nor specialised sensory apparatus, possess the ability (courtesy of chemo-receptors) to respond to chemical cues (chemo-signals) in their environment. Using chemical communication – smell – they find food, or avoid danger, be it toxic substances or predators. And when sexual, rather than asexual, reproduction first arose (an event believed to have begun about a billion years ago), the chemical sense of smell was the only system in place to enable procreation to occur. This, then, is the core reason why smell has a very powerful and central role to play in sexual reproduction. Other senses may since have been co-opted to the job, but smell remains a prime mover.

Sexual reproduction, it is surmised, has a watery origin. Before humankind's ancestors were multiplying on land, they were doing it at sea. But sex at sea, as highlighted earlier, is a risky business for those ocean-dwellers that do not possess internal genitalia. For both sexes, spawning, using the surrogate womb of the vast sea, is fraught with added dangers. Release your gametes at the wrong time or in the wrong place and your shot at procreating stands to be scuppered as your eggs or sperm are washed away before encountering anyone else. Timing – being able to co-ordinate sexual reproduction – is all, and the key to acquiring such rhythm is being able to sense and respond to the presence of others around you. Are they members of the same species, are they of the opposite sex, and are they sexually ripe? Answer yes to all three, and in the absence of immediate danger, and the result could well be the mutual orgasmic rhythmic contractile expulsion of gametes into the surrounding waters. Curiously, many chemicals that cause such explosive and ejaculatory reactions in ancient creatures, such as the sea squirt, are those that humans utilise today, perhaps with a slight spin, or different emphasis, but with the same end result in mind. Human gonadotrophin (ovary- or testis-stimulating) hormones also effect the release of a sea squirt's gametes. Some things just don't change. If it works well once, Mother Nature will use it again.

Over a hundred years ago, German biologist and philosopher Ernst Haeckel envisaged olfaction as a primordial attractive force in the copulatory union of female and male gametes. His theory of erotic chemotropism viewed gonadal cells as possessing a primitive consciousness (*Seelenthätigkeit*), and seeking each other out via a type of primitive smelling. To Haeckel the attraction one organism has for another of the opposite sex was a conscious reaction to the prompting of its gonads. In light of Haeckel's intriguing surmisings, it's now realised that once released, even gametes themselves work to meet their other half. Both the female and male gametes of the aquatic fungus *Allomyces macrogynus* release chemicals which enable their mutual orientation towards each other. The female gametes secrete a compound dubbed sirenin, which acts as a sperm attractant, causing an influx of calcium ions into the cytoplasm of any nearby sperm, and a subsequent change in their swimming pattern and a shift in movement toward the source of the chemical – the female gamete. The male gametes too produce an attractant, named parisin, which the eggs sniff out and then swim towards. Such simple chemo-sensory systems are believed to be the ancestors of life's more specialised communication systems of hormones (messenger molecules which are released internally within a given organism) and pheromones (communication chemicals released by an organism into their immediate environment).

It's important to remember, though, that mammals are far from being simple unicellular organisms. Rather, we are highly evolved creatures, comprised of multiple specialised organs, glands and complex communication systems. In mammals, the nose is the primary chemo-sensory organ, receiving olfactory information and relaying it directly and rapidly to the brain. The conventional view of human chemo-sensory sensitivity is that in comparison to the supersniffing abilities of other mammals, such as bloodhounds, humans just don't make the grade. This, though, is a misrepresentation. Okay, humans are not up to the smell-detecting standards of bloodhounds, but our olfactory sensitivity is not something to be sniffed at. Humans can recognise at least 100,000 different odours.

Humans are also incredibly smelly creatures as a result of numerous secreting scent glands scattered across our skin surface (see Table 6.1). Indeed, among primates, humans seem to be the species most richly endowed with scent-producing glands, smell structures which start firing on all cylinders at puberty – in concert with our reproductive

Table 6.1 Major Scent Gland Regions of the Body

Major anatomical sites	**Gland type**	
	Sebaceous	Apocrine
Scalp	*	*
Face	*	*
Eyelids	*	*
Ear canal	*	*
Vestibulum nasi (nasal vestibule)	*	*
Upper lip	*	
Lining of mouth	*	
Axillae (armpits)		*
Nipples and areolae	*	
Midline of chest	*	
Umbilical region of abdomen		*
Mons pubis		*
Labia majora	*	*
Labia minora	*	
Prepuce/glans penis	*	
Scrotum	*	
Circumanal/anogenital/perineum		*

Human sebaceous glands produce sebum – a thick, oily, unpigmented secretion. Their function is thought to be linked to sexual reproduction as the glands only begin to secrete once puberty is reached. Genital skin has the highest density – with up to 900 sebaceous glands packed into every square centimetre of skin. Human apocrine glands produce a viscid, oily substance which has a surprising range of colours. It can be milky pale grey, clear white, reddish, yellowish or even black. Like sebaceous glands, apocrine glands only start to function at puberty, suggesting that they too have a reproductive role. Women have far more apocrine glands than men. Adapted from Stoddart, D. Michael, *The Scented Ape: the Biology and Culture of Human Odour*, London: Cambridge University Press, 1990.

organs. And smell is a sense we can't avoid. We can close our eyes, cover our ears, but we can't stop smelling. Each inhalation brings an enforced inspiration of aromas. The scent of fear, the smell of food, the odour of arousal; humans, like other mammals, recognise these fragrances and learn to follow their noses. Considering this, it's not too far-fetched to imagine that chemo-sensation could very well be an important factor in communicating human sexual and social information, just as it is in simple organisms.

Girls are made of sugar and spice?

I have two favourite smells. The savoury aroma of my mum's slow-cooked meat and potato pie; and the heady, rich scent of my fertile cunt. Familial love and sexual love, described by mere chemicals. My much-loved vaginal perfume is the deepest, truest smell of me. It's the scent of my fertility, my sexual ripeness and pleasure. It's mercurial too, starting on day four or so of my menstrual cycle. From then until I've ovulated, I am intensely aware of this rich, sweet, deep, creamy and aromatic vaginal incense. Post-ovulation it's somehow fruitier. Although rarely openly discussed, the sexually pleasing and powerful scent that a woman's vagina and its secretions exudes is no secret. This intimate and erotic smell and taste is a sensual joy that different cultures have lauded and lusted after for centuries.

History relates how courtesans in medieval Europe used their sexual secretions as perfume, anointing themselves behind their ears and around their necks, in order to attract customers. It's also said that women in southern Spain would rub a small dab of their vaginal juices behind their ears and into their temples. Mixed in with the delicate essence of themselves were other fragrances, such as jasmine, neroli, myrrh, ylang ylang or frangipani. This particular tradition is understood to have been the secret of Taoist mistresses in ancient China before it was passed on to the Moors and from them to the Spanish. Meanwhile Napoleon is famously meant to have requested that Josephine 'not wash' before he arrived home, while Henry III reportedly remained in love with Mary of Cleves all his life after smelling the scent of her undergarments.

The classical Indian sexological text the *Ananga Ranga* is one surviving document which depicts in glorious detail the sensorial appeal of the vagina. Women, it says, fall into one of four classes, and it then goes on to praise women in terms of their genital scent, taste and style. First, the vagina of the *padmini* (Sanskrit for lotus-woman) is said to resemble the opening lotus bud, and enjoy feeling the rays of the sun and the touch of strong hands. Her sexual secretions (*Kama-salila*) are perfumed like the lily that has newly burst. The *chitrini* (the art-woman) can be recognised by her soft, raised and round *mons veneris* and sweet honey-smelling vagina. Delightfully, her genital fluids are said to taste of honey too. They are also exceptionally hot, and so abundant that they make copious sounds. Then there's the vagina of the *shakhini* (the fairy- or conch-woman), which is, apparently, always moist and loves being kissed or licked. Her genital juice tastes piquant or salty. Finally, the fourth order of woman is the *hastini* (elephant-woman), who takes great pleasure from much clitoral stimulation. Her sexual secretions have the savour of 'musth' – the musky juice which flows from an elephant's temples signalling their sexual excitement.

The strength of the association between female genitalia and their smell is underlined, dramatically, by language. 'Pillow of Musk' and 'Open Peony Blossom' are two Chinese ways of saying vagina, while in eighteenth-century England, honeypot, rose or moss rose were all used to describe the sexual heart of a woman. Honey's vaginal reputation is tenacious. It is not only the *Ananga Ranga* that talks of sweet honey-smelling vaginas; others say all women's vaginal juices taste of honey during certain days of the menstrual cycle. It's surely no coincidence that honey is a core component of many marriage ceremonies, such as the Hindu custom of daubing the bride-to-be's vagina with honey at the marriage feast, or that newly-weds enjoy a honeymoon. Honey also enjoys a reputation as an aphrodisiac, and, of course, we call our loved ones honey.

The myrtle is another deeply perfumed plant that history records as redolent of female genitalia. The 'fruit of the myrtle' is a term that over the years has been used to describe both the clitoris and the labia minora, while a woman's outer lips (labia majora) were, according to the first-century Greek physician Rufus of Ephesus, the lips of the myrtle. Myrtle, with its pink or white flowers and aromatic blue-black berries, is also the sacred plant of Aphrodite, the Greek goddess of love. Legend recalls that when Aphrodite emerged from the waves riding on a sea-shell, only to have her nakedness leered at by lewd satyrs, she chose to cover her genitalia with branches of the fragrant myrtle bush, which grows best near the seashore. It is said that the Greeks identified this plant more than any other with all things that smelt beautiful, and, indeed, the Greek name for the myrtle (*murto*) derives from the same root as that for perfume. And not surprisingly, considering its link to Aphrodite, the myrtle is also considered to be a powerful aphrodisiac. For example, Dioscorides, in his pharmacology compendium *De Materia Medica*, describes myrtle oil as refreshing, aphrodisiac and antiseptic when taken in tea.

'Streaming with the essence of the lily'

How would you describe the heady scent of female genitalia? Is it the scent of the lily or lotus, of sweet aromatic honey? Or is it the 'musks and ambers' that poet Robert Herrick says his lover smells of? One of the most beautiful descriptions of a woman's secret scent comes, I feel, from Pierre Louÿs, who writes of how he feels he is 'streaming with the essence of the lily' as he lies with his cheek on the belly of a young woman. This phrase evokes such potency and pleasure, it's stunning. Louÿs was not alone in dreaming of the vagina as a lily. Lilies or lotuses (the lotus flower is a type of water-lily) are a common symbol of the vagina or *yoni*, in particular in eastern cultures. For example, the Sanskrit word for lotus is *padma*, which is also a word for the *yoni*. Chinese sexological texts refer to the vagina as a Golden Lotus, while the Latin name for the lotus is *nymphaea*, a term applied to a woman's inner labia too.

Some curious and unexpected connections between the lotus and female genitalia are suggested elsewhere. In Greek mythology, the lotus is represented as a fruit that induces a dreamy languor and forgetfulness in those that eat it. Lotus-eaters lie around languidly all day, partaking of the legendary fruit. Precisely what this fruit is is never spelt out, although if it is code for the vagina, then it gives a whole new meaning to the term lotus-eating. Peculiarly, though, lotus-sniffing was one of the pastimes of ancient Egypt. Numerous illustrations show both women and men plunging their noses into the scented heart of the blue lily or lotus (see Figure 6.2). The significance of this act, which appears to be part of ancient Egyptian pleasure rituals, had puzzled historians for years. Recently scientists came up with an intriguing suggestion: astonishingly, sniffing blue lilies acted as an aphrodisiac. This particular lotus has a pharmacological quality akin to that of the prescription medication Viagra. Both contain a chemical, the former natural and the latter not, which results in increased blood flow to the genitals. It seems that the scent of the lotus – whether describing the actual flower or female genitalia – really is a potent aphrodisiac, and lotus and vagina actually are connected via smell. This property of the lotus is also perhaps why the lotus is a sacred flower for Indian, Persian, Egyptian and Japanese cultures.

If I were forced to pick a third favourite smell, I would have to

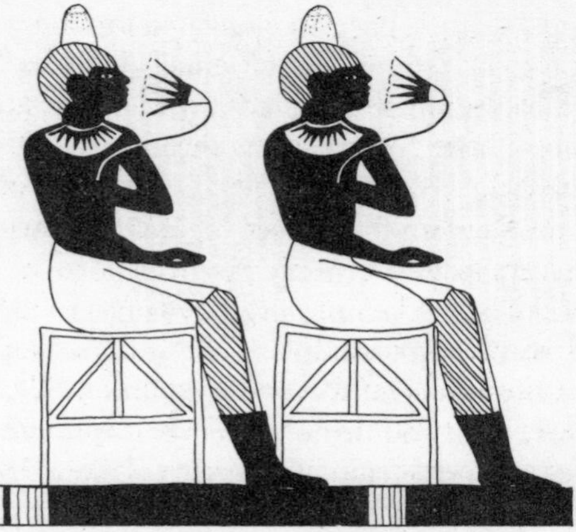

Figure 6.2 From a painting found at the tomb of Nakht, in Thebes, depicting a feast (eighteenth dynasty). The guests wear cones of myrrh attached to their wigs and sniff the aphrodisiacal scent of blue lotuses.

plump for vanilla. In terms of fragrance, vanilla belongs to what is called the ambrosia or musk-like category of scents (the seven classes of odours are detailed below). Not surprisingly, perhaps, the perfumes typically used to describe the vagina fall within this particular category. In fact, it could be said that ambrosial scents are, in essence, the intimate scents of a woman: musk, lily, amber and vanilla, all creamy, luxurious and sensual fragrances. More specifically, ambrosial scents are said to have their roots in amber, the resinous product of the intestinal tract of the sperm whale. Fragrant and attractive, the Greeks referred to amber as *elektron* – a substance that when rubbed releases charged particles. For the Greeks, ambrosial scents were regarded as both the elixir of life and nourishment for the gods.

The smell of vanilla is certainly an ambrosial aroma. It's also a smell that is commonly used to describe the scent of female genitalia, and this aroma association is again underpinned by language. A vanilla is actually a tropical climbing orchid with fragrant greenish-yellow flowers and long fleshy pods containing seeds or beans. It is these vanilla beans and pods that are used as flavouring for foods. The Latin American orchid was given the name *vainilla* by Spanish settlers because its pods – which have an elongated outline with a slit at the top – were said to be reminiscent of female genitalia (no mention is made of whether the smell triggered any memories too). *Vainilla* is the Spanish diminutive for vagina or sheath. Hence, vanilla literally means 'little vagina'.

The taxonomic system that places vaginal fragrances together was devised by the eighteenth-century Swedish botanist Carl Linnæus. Linnæus chose to group odours into seven classes in terms of their hedonic, that is, their pleasurable, qualities. These classes are *Fragrantes* (fragrant, such as saffron and wild lime); *Hircinos* (goaty, the smells of cheese, meat and urine); *Ambrosiacos* (ambrosial or musk-like, as we've seen); *Tetros* (foul; this includes the walnut, also known as Jupiter's Nut or glans of Jove); *Nauseosos* (nauseating, like the foul-smelling resinous gum asafoetida); *Aromaticos* (aromatic, the spicy notes such as citron, anise, cinnamon and clove) and *Alliaceous* (like garlic, which is a type of lily).

Linnaeus wasn't shy about talking about smell. He held that the fragrance of the may flower – the blossom of the may tree or hawthorn – recalled that of female genitalia. This is an association that has survived since medieval times, when may blossom was picked on a May morning and worn by revellers dancing around the maypole on a day dedicated to sexual pleasure. Linnaeus also saw several varieties of rose as reminiscent of female genitalia, and indeed, pink and red roses were common vaginal symbols in the west. Strangely and sadly, though, the plant that Linnaeus chose to bear a directly vaginal name, *Chenopodium vulvaria* (also known as stinking goosefoot), is reported to smell fish-like. Peculiarly piscine is not the scent of a healthy, clean vagina; rather this is the signature note of a bacterial vaginal imbalance, just as the reek of rank cheese is that of a bacterial penile imbalance.

The deeply conservative Linnaeus is also famous for describing plants in terms of their vaginal and penile attributes, their pistils and stamens respectively, as well as referring to their reproduction systems as their marital tendencies. In this vein, he divided the plant world into different classes according to the type of marriage each plant contracted – be it monandrian (one husband, penis or stamen), diandrian (two husbands, penises or stamens) or more, or whether the marriage was public or clandestine. His wife he referred to as 'my monandrian lily', lily having been spun to imply virginal in the west in contrast to its role as a vaginal symbol in the east.

Spice boxes

So why do women smell the way they do? There are two answers to this question. The first centres on the literal reasons for this – the composition of a woman's genital juices and where these secretions come from. The second concerns the effect that a woman's scent has on other individuals, that is, the vital message it conveys. First off, what's in the vaginal mix? A woman's sexual aroma is a complex cocktail of vaginal secretions, exuding throughout female genitalia. Cervix, uterus, Fallopian tubes, vaginal walls, prostate, all these and more add to a female's bountiful fluids. Deliciously, the French refer to this confection of aromas as a woman's *cassolette* – her cooking pot of fragrances.

Female genitalia also incorporate specialised mucus-secreting glandular structures. These include Bartholin's glands (also called major vestibular glands), which are set deep in the lower half of the labia majora, close to the vestibular bulbs and bulbocavernosal muscle. These glands secrete fluid through an excretory duct, 1.5 to 2 cm long, which opens either side of the lower edge of the vaginal opening or vestibule area (at five and seven o'clock). Dotted around the vagina's vestibule are minor vestibular glands of varying numbers. The average is between two and ten, although some women have more than a hundred, and some have none at all. These minor glands also exude fluid. Apocrine glands, scattered around the genitals, also add to the aroma medley.

A woman's inner lips, her labia minora, provide a rich addition to her perfume. Despite not having any hair follicles, the inner labia contain large numbers of sebaceous glands (the small skin glands that emit lubricative and protective sebum on to hair follicles and surrounding skin). These labial sebaceous glands secrete a white oily substance, similar to that produced by a man's preputial skin. This genital secretion fascinated me as a child, although I didn't know, and didn't ask, what it was. For some reason, dark-haired women possess more of these inner labial glandular structures than their blonde sisters do. The labia majora (outer lips) are also rich in sebaceous glands, adding another note to a woman's sexual scent. And if allowed to flourish in all its springy lush splendour, a woman's pubic hair – the triangular crowning glory of her genitalia – then sets off a woman's vaginal perfume perfectly, and piquantly. As nineteenth-century French poet Charles Baudelaire put it:

> Languorous, black, luxuriant locks
> Live pomander, incense burner
> Wafts her wild, musky fragrance

A woman's Bartholin's glands are reputed to be a key source of her signature sexual scent, although there is, as yet, scant evidence in support of this. What is known about this genital fluid is that it is clear, mucoid, alkaline, under ovarian hormonal control, and increases during sexual arousal. These mucus-secreting glands are present in other female mammals. In the platypus, the ducts open at the base of the monotreme's clitoris. In female opossums, the secretions flow into the canal of the urogenital sinus, while in female spotted hyaenas, with their queenly elongated clitoris, complete with urethra running through it, the extremely well-developed Bartholin's glands open into the urethra close to the tip of the clitoris. The equivalent male mammalian structures are called Cowper's, or bulbourethral, glands.

Many female mammals also produce clitoral gland secretions. In the rat, the main excretory duct of the clitoral gland courses along the surface of the clitoris, emptying on the side of the urethral opening, thus communicating with both the urethra and the vagina. Studies show that the odour of these clitoral/urethral secretions is highly attractive to male rats. The clitoral glands are, in fact, homologous to the male's penile preputial glands, which appear as paired structures on either side of the penis. Many mammals' preputial glands are known to be of prime importance in producing secretory and olfactory products. For example, the preputial pouch of male Himalayan deers is the source of the red, jelly-like secretion that is musk.

In comparison, though, to what is known about male accessory glands, very little is known about the female's. This paltry state of affairs is highlighted both by the scientific community's ignorance regarding the existence and function of the female prostate, and by the recent revelation that women have more genital glands than previously thought. In 1991, scientists discovered a completely new type of female genital gland, and intriguingly, it has so far defied all attempts at classification. These anogenital or vulval glands extend deep into the dermis (the inner layer of the skin), twice as deeply as eccrine or apocrine glands, and cannot be categorised as eccrine, apocrine or mammary glands. Ultrastructurally they are unique, as is their vulval secretion product. Although tentatively described as sweat glands, their function remains unknown. Their discoverers call them remarkable, suggesting they may have some sexual function, possibly of an olfactory nature. Their morphology is similar to that of mammary glands, and, indeed, occasionally the glands reach such a complexity that they appear lobe-like. Even more strangely, the existence of this type of vulval gland is suggested to be at the root of a strange and rare medical condition whereby women develop lactating mammary glands in their vulval skin. This peculiar and puzzling genital condition may well account for cases in the past where women were labelled as witches, and killed, as a result of marks akin to nipples on their external genitalia. It's certainly the case that most of the so-called witch marks or devil's teats that were found on middle-aged or elderly women during medieval Europe's witch hunts were noted as being on their vulval skin. 'Mary had teats in her secret parts and they are not like haemorrhoids,' reads one witch-finder's report.

Flagging up fertility

Female genitalia undoubtedly smell memorable and have the requisite odour-producing plumbing in place to give off sexual scent signals, but do they actually do this? After all, merely possessing the hardware is no proof of use. Moreover, is there an effect on other individuals as a result of them smelling *parfum femalia*? An increasing body of evidence suggests that the intimate scent of a female does stimulate such a response, sometimes with startlingly dramatic results. It has long been noted that in the mammal kingdom going nose to genitalia is a typical prelude to sexual activity. In his notebooks, not intended for publication, Charles Darwin wrote: 'We need not feel so much surprise at male animals smelling vaginae of females – when it is recollected that smell of one's own pud. [pudendum] not disagree.'

Tellingly, the majority of male primates pay particular attention to the smell and taste of female genitalia – frequently sniffing, licking and touching the vagina for a number of days each month. For some primates this investigatory behaviour only occurs during oestrus, while others, in particular spider monkeys, sniff female genitalia repeatedly at all phases of the menstrual cycle. In some primate species mutual genital licking or nuzzling is common too. A more detailed vaginal inspection is part of the sexual ritual of mangabeys, macaques, baboons, gorillas, orang-utans and chimpanzees. This involves one or more fingers being used to poke inside the vagina too. The probing digits are then sniffed or licked. Many other male mammals, including red deer, moose and caribou, pay particular attention to licking the female's vulva, as do some species of insect. Oral sex is also a central feature of the sex life of a species of bat, the Gray-Headed Flying Fox, with the male deeply tonguing the female's genitalia for long periods of time. Unfortunately, whether or not it is scented stimuli and information that the male bat is seeking, or something else altogether, is still unclear.

Some studies do point to female genital secretions signalling the status of a female's sexual ripeness. Research with male rhesus monkeys suggests that the sexual status of the female (is she ovulating or not?) is recognisable from her vaginal aroma, and that the time of ovulation is associated with the maximum frequency of male ejaculation. Mice, as well as monkeys, produce vaginal secretions that play an important role in male mating behaviour. Mice studies, though, reveal an extra twist. Female genital oestrous odour only stimulates male mice to approach and mate if they are sexually experienced. Virgin, sexually naïve male mice appear not to hear the olfactory call. Clitoral gland secretions are the calling card of female rats too. These rodent scent glands produce an array of attractant aromas – one of which (6,11–dihydrodibenz-b,e-oxepin-11–one) preferentially attracts males. Amazingly, the scent of a fecund female rat is enough to give a male rat an erection – no physical stimulus is necessary.

The allure of broccoli

The Syrian golden hamster possesses one of the most researched vaginal secretions, and one that is both alluring and arousing to the opposite sex. The night before oestrus, the female hamster marks the perimeter of her territory with her copious, watery vaginal secretions, effectively laying down a genital trail that lures the male to her underground lair. The major attractant molecule in her genital fluid is believed to be dimethyl disulfide, a chemical that smells a little like broccoli and is extremely common in nature – it acts as a nipple attachment molecule in pup rats, as well as being a principle malodorant in human tooth disease. But there's more to come in hamster vaginal mucus. The later stages of golden hamster courtship and copulation are induced by a protein, dubbed aphrodisin, which the male laps up as he licks the female's genitals prior to intercourse. Interestingly, physical contact with aphrodisin is essential in eliciting the male's mounting and pelvic thrusting response.

Unlike golden hamsters, precisely what it is about primate vaginal secretions that signals a woman's reproductive status is still uncertain. Research has highlighted how the chemical composition of vaginal mucus fluctuates throughout the menstrual cycle. Of particular interest are levels of fatty acids, which are produced by the action of essential vaginal bacteria. In rhesus monkeys, levels of these volatile short-chain fatty acids nearly double in concentration prior to ovulation. The same range of molecules plus some other sister compounds are also present cyclically in human vaginal secretions, and have been found to peak in concentration in the period prior to ovulation.

On average a woman's cocktail of genital mucus contains the following concentrations of fatty acids or copulins per ml of secretion:

10.0 μg of acetic
7.0 μg of propionic
0.5 μg of iso-butyric
6.5 μg n-butyric
2.0 μg of iso-valeric
0.5 μg iso-caproic

However, levels vary markedly from woman to woman. One study found that while 63.5 per cent of women had all these fatty acids present in their vaginal secretions, 2.5 per cent had no detectable fatty acids at all, and 34 per cent possessed only acetic acid. Importantly, research also revealed that women who take oral hormonal contraceptives have far lower levels of vaginal fatty acids and do not show the expected increase in concentration mid-cycle. This is not surprising, as levels of vaginal fatty acids are under the influence of internally produced (endogenous) oestrogen. Taking the pill, with its synthetic oestrogenic component, will disturb a woman's natural hormonal equilibrium, and hence a woman on the pill will smell slightly different.

Research investigating how the smell of a woman's vagina is perceived by men has thrown up some contrary results. Of particular interest is the vagina's aroma around ovulation. One study synthesised primate vaginal fatty acids, creating copulin mixtures that mimicked vaginal secretions at various stages of the menstrual cycle. Most men exposed to them said they found them to be unpleasant, perhaps a surprising result, although it has to be recognised that in matters of smell and sex, context, including chemical context, is all. Yet, although the male sniffers appeared to turn up their noses at the copulin concoctions, when they were asked to sniff the synthetic copulins while looking at photographs of women, images they previously rated as ordinary were suddenly reported as being attractive.

It seems the effect of inhaling copulins made their sexual judgement go to pot. What's more, the copulin smells mimicking ovulation made their testosterone levels rocket, suggesting that the chemo-signals a woman gives off may play a role in regulating testicular function. This research tallies with other studies showing that even though most men say they are not aware when a woman is ovulating, their bodies know, as they respond physiologically with increased testosterone levels.

Other, more recent work reveals that men are able to distinguish when their partners are ovulating from smell alone. What is also significant is that these ovulation or fertility aromas were rated more attractive than others. Importantly, there were two major differences in this study. First of all, the odours analysed were naturally produced, and secondly, the women secreting them were involved in long-term relationships with the men smelling them. In this scenario, naturally produced odours emitted around ovulation were rated by this group of men as more pleasant than at any other time of the menstrual cycle. They were also perceived as tending to stimulate and linger for longer, and at the same time produced a desire for more chemo-sensory stimulation. I would suggest that this points to men being able to distinguish, albeit unconsciously, when a woman is ovulating, and to this ovulation aroma being attractive.

A final test of the pulling power of a woman's fertile vaginal perfume is, of course, whether it increases sexual activity or not. With rhesus monkeys, the answer is emphatically yes. Application of a copulin mixture to females unleashed hugely increased levels of male sexual behaviour. However, the results for humans were more equivocal. Women who rubbed synthetic copulin confections into their skin did not report any significant changes in sexual activity with their partner. In fairness to humans, though, this result probably says far more about the complex emotional and sexual lives we lead than our capacity to be influenced by a purportedly aphrodisiacal smear. It may also say something about synthetic copulins.

The odour avenue

Before looking at the reasons why the smell of her genitalia should flag up a female's fertility, what about other genital aromas? For it's not just vaginal secretions that are important in signalling a mammalian female's reproductive status – that is, gametes ready to be released or not, or pregnancy underway. Mammals are rich repositories of odours, with humans no exception, and a whole host of other bodily fluids – including urine, saliva, sweat, tears and more – have been found to exert erotogenic effects in different species. Urine, the original odour avenue, is of immense importance. Composed of a welter of compounds churned out by the kidneys, urine is also perfumed as it makes its way out of the body by all it passes by – in particular accessory glands such as the prostate.

The power of urine to convey information about the status of an individual is astounding. Health, stress levels, reproductive and social status, metabolic idiosyncracies – all can be read from a simple sample of urine. Human urine tends to be dismissed as an excretory waste product – something to be washed away as quickly as possible – rather than an important genital fluid, but female urine is potent, as anyone who has sat waiting for a pregnancy test result can confirm. It stands shoulder-to-shoulder with vaginal secretions in conveying a woman's fertile status, a fact that simple ovulatory kits exploit (other ovulation detection devices resemble wrist-watches and measure the changing acidity of sweat, as determined by a woman's fluctuating hormone levels).

Urine's fluctuating and sometimes intoxicating scent has a sexual potency too – a fact that has not been overlooked by all. The erotic portent of female urine is part of the vaginal qualities prized in Marquesan society. To this end, certain edible fruit, anthropologists report, are not given to girls because they disrupt the pleasant aroma. In India, the smell of a young bride's urine was used in a wedding ritual designed to capture her bridegroom's heart. This practice, known only to women, involved wicks being made out of rags wet with the bride's urine, which the unsuspecting bridegroom was then asked to smell. Magic traditions also suggest that one way for a woman to keep her man in thrall to her is to urinate in his coffee. I haven't tried this one yet, but it has been recommended to me.

Considering the rich potential of urine to signal reproductive status, do females use their urine in this way? The habit of male mammals to use urine or accessory gland fluids to mark their environment is well known, but what about females? Disappointingly, relatively little has been written about how female mammals void urine and their own brand of marking fluids in order to communicate information about themselves, although this is common too. Yet, as more research is undertaken looking at this aspect of female mammalian sexual behaviour, the importance of females using the aromas of their body fluids to advertise their sexual and social status is becoming increasingly evident. The list of female spray-and-displayers includes tigers, monkeys, pigs, pandas, horses and more.

Female pigs (*Sus scrofa*) urinate frequently when in oestrous in order to let surrounding males get the message that they are now fertile. When a male picks up a sow's fecundity flag, he follows its scent to her, but first finds her urine, sniffs or licks it and then urinates too – on top of her marking. Thus begins pig copulation. Female horses and deer also urinate as a sexual gesture. The effect of their oestrous urine on males is striking – the male's head is thrown back, his upper lip curls, and the pressure resulting from this contraction of the lip-raising muscles results in increased exposure to the female's urine. This facial expression is known as the *flehmen*, the lip-curling or flared face, and is seen in other mammals too (the word *flehmen* derives from a German word for coaxing or cajoling).

In the case of horses, the oestrous smell excites stallions to approach the mare, and engage in licking and tactile stimulation of her. The vivifying power of female urine on males is demonstrated more precisely by the effect of female house mouse urine, which stimulates a rapid rise in circulating levels of luteinising hormone (LH) in males. Such effects are seen in primates too. Male lemurs experiencing the effects of seasonality (fewer hours of sunlight during the day) have lower testosterone levels, and are less socially active and less likely to mate. Smelling female lemur urine, though, is enough to raise their testosterone levels and reanimate them socially and sexually.

Female Asian elephants are one of the mammals whose use of urinary signals has been studied in some detail. The oestrous cycle of female elephants is long – between sixteen and eighteen weeks – yet their fertile period is short, believed to be several days, though it may be only a few hours. Flagging up female elephant fertility effectively is therefore critical in determining successful sexual reproduction. Urine solves the timing issue. When female Asian elephants are feeling fecund they signal this to the males by releasing a particular chemical – identified as (Z)-7-dodecenyl acetate – in their urine. This functions as both a sexual attractant and a reproductive-timing signal.

Where this chemical message originates from, though, is uncertain. The urogenital tract of female elephants, which is extremely long and winding (measuring between 120 and 358 cm from vulva to ovary), is packed with extensive mucus-producing glands, which may be the molecule's source. Alternatively, the copious amounts of urine which flush from the kidneys down the elephant's urethra-cum-vagina may be the culprit. It's also suggested that vaginal and/or anogenital secretions help to advertise the female elephant's fecundity. Around ovulation, females smear the hairy end of their tail with vaginal secretions and then fling the tail in the air – raising it like a flag and spreading their sexual signals further. I like this inventive approach to shouting, 'Come here, I'm ready.'

An adapted clitoris?

Some women occasionally envy men for their possession of a tool that enables them to piss while standing up. Women's genitalia, unfortunately, aren't quite so effective at this task. However, one primate female has an extra trick up her sleeve. This primate is the female spider monkey, who, if you remember, has the longest clitoris of any primate. Some say this pendulous erectile organ resembles a penis. However, unlike a penis, it has a broad, shallow groove along its perineal surface along which urine flows (after it is voided at the base of the clitoris). The epithelial lining of this groove is also unique, appearing smooth and more like a mucous membrane. Females like to travel widely through the high canopy of remnant forests in Brazil, and as they do so they mark tree branches with their urine – their calling card – and call out to prospective mates. This tactic of distributing urine and finding potential suitors seems to work very well for the female spider monkey. They are incredibly sexually active primates, choosing a variety of partners, and it's suggested that their ability to distribute their urine via their clitoris plays a part in this.

The idea that female genitals are designed, in part, to distribute urine is not unusual and is used to explain some penile designs. The male goat, for instance, everts its prepuce to form a pendulous tube fringed with hairs – all the better for spraying urine far and wide. Whether other female primates utilise their external genitalia in this way is unknown. In the New World primate family, there are four groups where clitoral enlargement occurs – *Ateles*, *Brachyteles*, *Lagothrix* and *Cebus*. The clitoris of *Cebus capucinus* measures 18 mm, while that of *Ateles belzebuth* extends away from the body for 47 mm (no internal measurements are known). The reasons behind these alterations in genital design remain to be determined – it may be with extended urine dispersal, or possibly extra sexual pleasure in mind, or both.

The inner labia of women also pose something of a design puzzle. One suggestion is that their secretions contribute to a woman's olfactory bouquet, in particular when sexual arousal results in their surface area swelling markedly. However, the fluted nature of a woman's inner labia also sings to me of a design with fluids in mind – be it for urine, prostatic or other vaginal secretions. I don't believe I am the first to have thought this. For a long period of time, from at least the first century to the sixteenth, these vaginal inner lips were, as we've seen, commonly known as *nymphae* (singular, *nympha*), a word meaning 'water goddesses' in Greek.

And finally, a brief word on a musky genital fluid that is a bit of a mystery. Basmati rice, the night-blooming bassia flower, mung beans and female tigers may not appear at first glance to have much in common, but they do. Connecting these four disparate items is 2–acetyl-1–pyrroline (2AP), a seemingly innocuous molecule. The smell, though, of 2AP, is exquisite and not easily forgotten. It is the heady and particular aroma of basmati, the fragrance of a special strain of beautifully smelling mung beans, as well as the scent of the *Bassia latifolia* flower and the smell of a tigress' billet-doux. (Curiously, mung beans also contain a compound which is found in rat vaginal secretions and acts as a sexual attractant.) Tigresses, as well as tigers, frequently mark their territories, jetting an aromatic milky, lipid-rich fluid upwards and backwards away from their bodies. The smell of this fluid is so strong that the Sanskrit word for tiger is *vyagra*, a name derived from a verb root meaning 'to smell' (whether Pfizer, maker of the pharmaceutical Viagra which increases blood flow to the genitals, were aware of this remains unknown).

However, tigress marking spray is something of an enigma. Fatty acids, amines and aldehydes have all been identified in the fluid, and it is known that 2AP imparts its wondrous aroma, but its source and nature remain elusive. Although ejected under some pressure through the urinary channel, and possessing some urinary characteristics, this fluid is not urine. Neither is it an anal sac secretion. Its purpose is also unclear, although the frequency with which it is ejected and the marking strategies employed point to its role as a sexual signaller or territory marker. Do female tigers have an unknown accessory gland that is responsible for producing the fluids ejected in such a dramatic fashion? The image of tigresses ejecting an unknown milky, fragrant fluid pulls my mind immediately to that of a woman spurting opalescent prostatic fluid. Having inhaled deeply the exotic and highly erotic musky aroma of freshly ejaculated female prostatic fluid, I'm willing to place a bet that one function of this female genital secretion is of an olfactory and sexual nature. Perhaps tigresses have prostates too.

Speaking to the sisters

While the smell of female genitalia undoubtedly has an effect on the male of the species, the effects of eau-de-femalia do not stop there.

Information about a female's reproductive status is of vital interest to members of her own sex, as well as the opposite. In fact, females in many mammalian species use olfactory signals from other females in order to help co-ordinate reproduction within a supportive social or physical environment. This is presumably because giving birth and rearing offspring in the secure company of friends, and at the best time of the year, is far more conducive to ensuring a species' survival than going it alone in a cold and dangerous place. Importantly, the first step towards co-ordinating the birth of offspring within a community is to synchronise a female's cyclic ovulation rhythms. That is, female scents force other females in a group to experience their oestrous or menstrual cycles together (menstruation occurs in Old World monkeys and apes, with some prosimians and New World primates also showing some blood loss).

A wealth of evidence highlights this amazing ovulation synchrony phenomenon, and how various genital fluids have an effect. For example, vaginal secretions are understood to mediate the menstrual synchrony shown in the reproductive lives of Old World primates such as crab-eating monkeys, chimpanzees and baboons. In the Holstein dairy cow, a mixture of urine and cervical mucus was found to exert cycle-shifting effects. The most detailed research to date has focused on the role of urine in entraining the oestrous rhythms of rodents, in particular those of rats and golden hamsters. Such work has shown that when females communicate their ovarian rhythms to other females the olfactory message they broadcast, and the effect it has, depends on the point they are at in their oestrous cycle – urine has the olfactory power to both phase-delay the cycle and phase-advance it, a system that allows for synchrony to arise more quickly. For female rats, pre-ovulatory urine odours shortened cycle lengths, while ovulatory urine lengthened them. On average, only three cycles are required for rat synchrony to develop (the rat's oestrous cycle is 4–6 days long).

Menstrual synchrony is also a common phenomenon in human females. However, although commented on for centuries, and demonstrated in women in 1971 in a classic experiment by psychology professor Martha McClintock, the scientific jury remained out until 1998 as to whether menstrual synchrony was truly an example of humans communicating their reproductive status by smell. It was further work by McClintock that gave the unequivocal answer at the turn of the century – yes, human females do communicate such genital information courtesy of their body odours. The ability of women to synchronise their ovulation rhythms and achieve a menstrual quorum was demonstrated in a study where the underarm sweat of human females at differing stages of their menstrual cycles was daubed on the upper lips of other women, and the effects on their menstrual cycles noted (underarm sweat was substituted for urine or vaginal secretions presumably to save the women's sensibilities).

The results were striking. Underarm secretions from the women's follicular phase (in the 12–14 days prior to ovulation) shortened the women's menstrual cycles (-1.7±0.9 days), whereas armpit sweat from the luteal phase (the days preceding ovulation and prior to the onset of menstruation) lengthened the menstrual cycle (1.4±05 days). Compounds in the axillary secretions, although perceived as odourless by the receiving women, advanced or delayed their menstrual cycle length. The net result of this silent female chemical communication – menstrual synchrony.

Two separate points of interest have come out of this and other menstrual synchrony studies. First of all, ovarian synchrony is far more likely to occur if the women concerned are good friends with each other. Simply sharing the same physical environment is not necessarily enough to trigger entrainment. This can be understood in terms of what friendship signifies – safety – and when it comes to getting the timing right, with regard to reproduction, safety signals 'go'. Being in the company of enemies, on the other hand, or simply someone you're unsure of, spells out potential danger, saying 'beware, perhaps it's not a good idea to synchronise with these female foes, and subject your offspring to them and their kind'.

The second point of note from synchrony studies was that the females of some species appear to dominate ovarian synchrony groups – forcing other females to follow in their hormonal wake, as it were. Such an entrainer is known as a *zeitgeber*. The effect of such hormonally dominant females on the ovulatory status of their social sisters has been noted in several primate species, including marmosets and rhesus and talapoin monkeys, as well as in mice and hamsters, and the silver-backed jackal. In some mammalian species, such as the dwarf mongoose, only the dominant females in a group have reproductive cycles. Moreover, in some societies of species, one female will achieve complete ovulation suppression or quiescence of her sisters. For instance, the smell of a fecund queen bee is so potent that it simply stops other female bees' ovaries from developing.

The somewhat disturbing message from these synchrony studies is that feeling subordinate, like a second-class citizen, as a result of being put upon, stressed, unhappy in your environment or cowed by your social group, can delay or halt ovulation. Such ovulation suppression triggers, and not just those arising from female cohorts, are believed to underlie many cases of human female infertility in the twenty-first century's generation of overworked, underpaid and unappreciated women. Stress-related infertility is reckoned to be responsible for 80 per cent of cases of female infertility.

The scent of a man

Considering the potent effect that the smell of a woman can have on a man, perhaps it will be heartening for men to hear that males hold sway too with their personal fragrances. The best studied male fluid, in this respect, is urine, in particular the urine of the male house mouse. Significantly, olfactory signals from the male mouse have an important role to play in regulating all three of a female mouse's major reproductive events – puberty, oestrous and pregnancy. For example, if a male mouse is introduced into a group of female mice, the majority of the females will be in oestrous three days later – pushed and pulled into ovarian synchrony by the scent of the male. His fragrance will also have an affect on pre-pubertal females. Two compounds in male mouse urine, iso-butyl amine and isoamylamine, are known to accelerate puberty. The olfactory effect of a male mouse on pregnant mice is even more dramatic. One whiff of the urine of a strange male mouse is enough to cause any recently pregnant mice to abort their developing foetuses. Incredibly, even extremely small amounts of urine evoke uterine growth in young female mice. Male smell-mediated effects are also seen in other rodent species.

Female rodents are far from alone in reacting genitally to the smell of the opposite sex. For as many women know, we are not immune to the scented charms of a man – be it his urine, breath, semen or sweat. Research shows that women who spent at least two nights in the company of men over a period of forty days had a significantly higher rate of ovulation than those sleeping alone. Other studies have revealed that women who are in the company of men three or more times a week tend to have shorter menstrual cycles than those who spend less time with men.

In a more detailed study of this effect on cycle length, male armpit sweat was dabbed on to the upper lips of women and the effects on their menstrual cycles monitored. The results were startling, and compare neatly with the female menstrual synchronisation study. The smell of a man appears to regulate and optimise ovarian function, as measured by the length of the menstrual cycle. Those women who had begun the experiment with irregular menstrual cycles – i.e., those whose cycle length was either longer or shorter than 29.5 days – found that their rhythms came closer to, or tied in to, this 29.5-day cycle length.

The effect of the smell of a man on a woman's ovulatory rhythm is important from a reproductive perspective, because female fertility is closely tied in with cycle length. Optimal fertility is associated with a menstrual cycle length of 29.5±3 days, while infertile women tend to have either short cycle lengths (less than or equal to 26 days) or long ones (more than or equal to 33 days). These irregular cycle lengths are far more likely to be anovulatory (that is, eggs are not released). The idea that women are far more likely to ovulate when they are around men, and intimate with them, rather than if they are not, makes perfect common sense. If there's no man around, why bother to ovulate and potentially waste an egg? Saving it for a more suitable date seems eminently sensible.

In an amazing coincidence, if it is that, 29.5 days, a woman's optimal fertility cycle length, is the moon's periodicity too – the time it takes the moon to shift from new to full and back again. Even more curiously, women tend to bleed in concert with the full moon and ovulate with the new when enjoying the company of men. In contrast, celibacy, or being predominantly in the company of women, leaves menstruation tending to coincide with the new moon, and ovulation, if it occurs at all, with the full. Science has not yet been able to explain why the moon's periodicity matches a woman's reproductive periodicity precisely, or the links to ovulating and bleeding at the new and full phases of the moon. It is possible, however, that there is a biological connection, as many species use the phases of the moon to co-ordinate their reproductive cycles for optimum fertility. It is also now recognised that the uterine lining of a woman's womb fluctuates in its receptiveness to implantation, although it remains to be seen whether it is most receptive at new moon. Curiously, in gardening lore, the advice over centuries has been to sow seed when the moon is new.

Fascinating rhythms

There's one final way that a male can influence the functioning of a female's ovaries – and that is using his phallus to full effect. It is a fascinating fact that the physical stimulation of copulation can bring about ovulation. For many species this idea is nothing new. A variety of females, including insects and ticks and many mammals such as cats, rabbits, ferrets and mink, are reflex, or mating-induced, ovulators. These females do not ovulate unless they receive sufficient sexual stimuli – a mechanism which is a sensible way of conserving metabolic energy, with their energy channelled into growth and survival rather than unproductive oestrous cycles. So-called spontaneous ovulators, on the other hand, release their gametes apparently in response to regular and cyclic fluctuations in circulating hormone levels. Humans, rhesus monkeys, sheep, pigs, cows and rodents, among others, are spontaneous ovulators.

Ovulation is, however, still a bit of a mystery to scientists, in particular spontaneous ovulation. Why does each ovarian cycle affect only some eggs and not others? Moreover, the actual spark for ovulation – the event that forces a developing ovarian follicle to rupture and extrude, gently, its eggy contents – is still unclear. It is known that there is a build-up of pressure inside the developing ovarian follicle, and that hormones play a critical role in triggering the egg extrusion – specifically a simultaneous surge of luteinising hormone (LH) and follicle-stimulating hormone (FSH) with the LH surge then triggering a cascade of enzymes, which catalytically break down the collagen casing of developed ovarian follicles. However a piece of the puzzle that is spontaneous ovulation is still missing.

Significantly, spontaneous ovulation is not as regular or rhythmic as previously supposed. Many women have irregular cycle lengths, and as noted, these are often anovulatory. Unfortunately, it's hard to say exactly how common anovulation is in women. Anovulatory cycles tend to go unnoticed because ovulation itself typically goes unnoticed by women (although some women, including myself, feel the deep, tight tension squeeze of *mittelschmerz* from an ovary). And as it's hard to say how many women's menstrual cycles are anovulatory, it's also difficult to say with any confidence how common ovulatory cycles are. Do women and other spontaneous ovulators release an egg every month? Very possibly not.

As a sidenote for any women listening out for *mittelschmerz*. First you need to locate your ovaries. The best way to do this is to place both hands palms down on your stomach, with the thumbs lying in a horizontal line and the thumb tips touching at a point directly over your belly button. The idea now is to make a downwards-pointing triangle with your hands – your thumbs form the top side of the inverted triangle, and where your index fingers come together is the lower apex. Finally, the points where the tips of your little fingers lie represent the position of your ovaries – under the skin, left and right. Knowing this makes it easier to spot *mittelschmerz*.

Whether a woman has sex or not is a factor in whether she ovulates or not, and it seems that the more sex, the greater the likelihood of ovulating. Intriguingly, studies show that women experiencing regular sexual activity with men ovulated in over 90 per cent of their cycles, and had regular ovarian rhythms of around 29.5 days, whereas women who abstained from, or participated in only sporadic sexual activity, did not ovulate in over 50 per cent of their cycles. This physical phenomenon is also seen in other species that are classified as spontaneous ovulators. Copulation or stimuli mimicking copulation, such as vaginal or clitoral stimulation (in the case of a cow), has been found to cause ovulation to occur earlier than it would otherwise have done in sheep, swine, mice and rats amongst others. Many unexpected human pregnancies are thought to flow from the erroneous belief that it's impossible to conceive a child late in a woman's cycle. As these parents know, sexual intercourse can all too easily stimulate ovulation and result in conception.

There are a number of ways by which the physical stimulation of sexual intercourse could exert an influence on the likelihood of ovulation occurring (see Figure 6.3). In many, perhaps most, mammals, it's thought that the surge of luteinising hormone (LH)

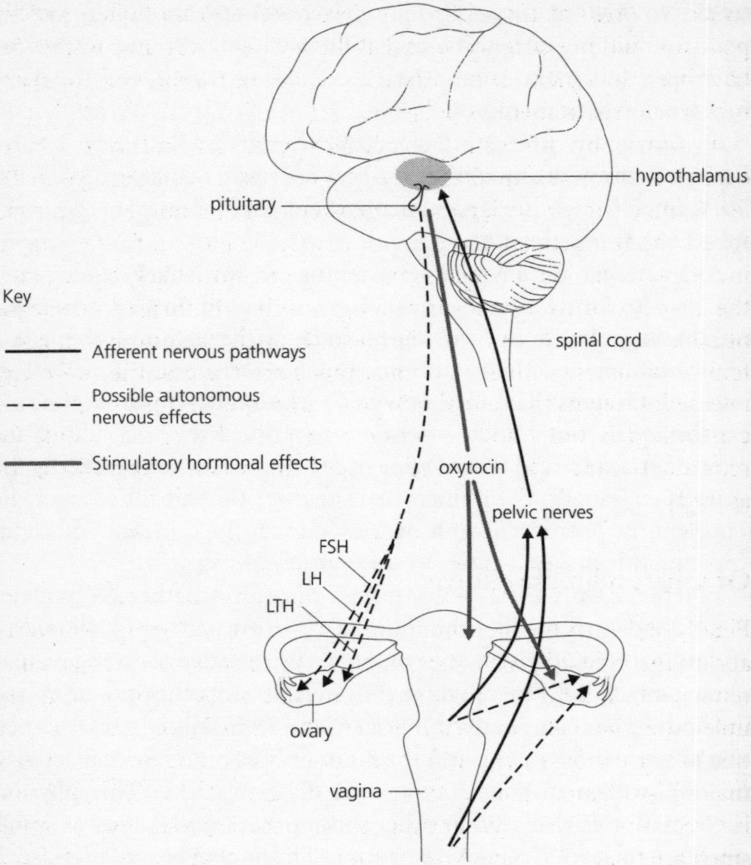

Figure 6.3 The various pathways via which stimulation from sex can induce ovulation in mammals. Sexual stimulation either induces an egg to be released, or induces this event to occur earlier than it would have otherwise: LH luteinising hormone, FH follicle-stimulating hormone and LTH luteotropic hormone (adapted from Jöchle 1975 and Eberhard 1996).

associated with copulation and vaginal/cervical stimulation is a major factor in triggering gamete release. It's also possible that sex may have a more direct influence on the exact moment of ovulation, by inducing contractions of the ovary. Gamete release then occurs when the tension produced by contractions of the whole ovary overwhelms the tensile strength of the wall of the developed ovarian follicle and the pent-up fluid pressure within the follicle. These ovarian contractions have been documented in both reflex ovulators (in this case, cats) and in women (spontaneous ovulators).

If a male, by dint of his sexual technique, can induce a female's ovaries to contract, then this, perhaps coupled with the rise in LH levels, may trigger ovulation. Studies looking at a number of species reveal the importance of copulation style, length and frequency in inducing ovulation. Female prairie voles are more likely to ovulate if the male performs significantly higher numbers of thrusts. The degree of male stimulation can also significantly affect the number of eggs a female ovulates; with female rats, the more thrusts, the more eggs released. It seems that a male's sexual technique, if it is up to scratch, can influence both how a female transports his sperm inside her reproductive tract (as we've seen earlier), and whether she will ovulate as well.

Of mice and mate choice

Finally, a return to the nose. One of the most stunning discoveries about the role of smell centres on a phenomenon that was first reported in mice. Mice possess the enviable ability to be able to size up a potential mate on the strength of their smell alone. They can do this because mouse urine differs in odour depending on what type of major histocompatibility complex (MHC) genes the rodent has (*histos* is Greek for 'tissue'). What's more, the partners that mice select by smell are those that have MHC genes (alleles) that are quite different from their own. That is, mice sniff out and choose to mate with MHC-dissimilar partners. Why?

The answer lies in what the MHC is used for. MHC genes code for proteins in the immune system – the means by which an organism recognises, at a cellular level, whether something is dangerous or not. The more diverse an organism's MHC mix, the more able and flexible an individual's immune system will be, and the better their chances of recognising and dealing with potentially dangerous situations, such as infections. By following their noses, mice choose genetically complementary partners – mates they are more likely to produce healthy, viable offspring with – the strength in diversity approach.

Although mice use the odour of the opposite sex to sniff out a complementary MHC, the effects of a mouse's MHC are not just nasally directed. Studies show that, incredibly, the genitalia of female mice are able to recognise which sperm are more compatible with her than others on the basis of the MHC. Complementary sperm – those with a more dissimilar MHC – are transported more quickly within her reproductive tract than those sperm with similar MHC genes (as we saw earlier). Both a female mouse's nose and her genitalia work in harmony to sniff out Mr Right.

Other species, as well as mice, possess this remarkable ability to choose a mate guided by the MHC or something similar. Moreover, while the MHC plays an important role in immune function in vertebrates, invertebrates, bacteria and plants all have their own chemosensory mate attraction and screening systems in place. The genitals of the female fruitfly distinguish and act on differences in the genetic make-up of fruitfly sperm, sorting and selecting which sperm to use to fertilise her eggs. Flowering plants have an elaborate recognition system in place, that will abort the interaction of stigma (female cell) with pollen (male cell) if the pollen is too closely related to the female cell. Even broccoli has fifty different types of genes in order to avoid getting it together with a too-similar strain of broccoli.

Follow your nose

But what about human mate choice? Is the human nose sensitive enough to read another person's MHC and act on that information? The smell of a sibling, offspring or the opposite sex – these are all odours that women and men can pick out. However, human olfactory sensitivity is far more subtle and extraordinary. Just as mice are able to recognise human MHC types from urine odour alone, human noses can distinguish between mice that are genetically identical, differing only in a single MHC gene position; and just as mice are able to sniff out a well-matched suitor, so too can humans. Human body odours are also influenced by a person's genetic make-up, and women, it appears, are capable of smelling differences as small as one gene. Significantly, perhaps, in all aspects of olfactory capacity, women are superior to men – they can sniff out a smell at a lower threshold and the range of aroma sensations appreciated by women is wider and deeper.

In one MHC study, women were asked to smell T-shirts worn by men for two nights in a row, and then rate the smells in terms of attractiveness to them. The aromas the women found most attractive were, it turned out, those that were most dissimilar to them, in terms of their MHC genes. A separate male sweaty T-shirt sniffing study asked women to rate different male aromas on the basis of which odours they would prefer to be around the whole time. This time women chose the scents of men who had more MHC genes (alleles) in common with them, specifically alleles that the women had inherited from their fathers. It seems women are able to distinguish the fragrance of familiarity, safety and stability (their father's aroma) from unknown male sweat, as well as the heady prospect of novelty, variety and diversity (an MHC stranger).

Further evidence for the effect of human MHC genes on mate choice has come from the Hutterites, a North American religious community who work in communal farms, marry within their own community and shun contraception and divorce. They marry for love, and for life. An analysis of the Hutterite individual's MHC genes and the marriages – mate choices – within this community revealed that these people tend to avoid (statistically significantly) tying the knot with partners who have similar MHC genes. However, data on the Hutterite community also have some stark implications for how too-similar MHCs may affect a couple's fertility (this effect may work at more than one stage of human sexual reproduction). As well as being associated with more miscarriages, Hutterite couples who share a higher proportion of their MHC genes tend to have longer intervals between successive births. As contraception is not used, it's suggested that the longer birth intervals of these couples may result from the loss of embryos early in gestation, even before pregnancy is consciously recognised.

It's also now recognised that couples who suffer from recurrent spontaneous abortions often have a higher proportion of their MHC in common, in comparison to control couples in many different populations. The newborn babies of these couples often weigh less at birth, a factor which is implicated in health problems in later life. One theory is that MHC-correlated spontaneous abortions can be seen as a woman's reproductive organs unconsciously deciding not to go ahead with this pregnancy as the embryo's genetic make-up signals danger to her, in the same way that a person's body chooses to reject a transplanted organ. It's also thought that *in vitro* fertilisation attempts are more likely to fail with MHC-similar couples.

The idea that a person's smell is intimately related to their genetic individuality and their potential as a parent has resonance in the beliefs of different cultures. Odour is the source of personal identity for the Ongee people of the Andaman Islands. The Ongee, and the Japanese, refer to themselves by putting their forefinger on the tip of their nose, while the Temiar people of the Malaysian peninsula equate an individual's odour with their personal life-force. In the west in times past, the body and breath odours of a virile man were referred to as his *aura seminalis*, and were believed to emanate from his semen. One Mexican belief, which some still hold today, is that the fragrance of a man's breath is more important than his sperm in determining whether he will conceive a child with a woman. This last idea is given weight not by just MHC research but also by studies that show that for women, how a man smells is one of the most important factors in choosing whether to be sexual with him or not.

Research also suggests that unpleasant body odour (for whatever reason) is the most potent sensory inhibitor of sexual arousal. Moreover, it's recognised that for both women and men how a person smells is key not only to whether a relationship starts, but also to whether it continues or not. It seems it's impossible for people to maintain an intimate relationship with each other if they don't like each other's smell. This idea of having to like someone's smell in order to like them is expressed in some languages, such as German, where saying you don't like someone translates as: '*Ich kann ihn nicht riechen*' – 'I can't [bear to] smell him.'

While it is certainly true that women can screen men for their genetic complementarity on the basis of their breath, worryingly, studies show that there is one group of women who cannot rely on their sense of smell to do this effectively – women who are taking hormonal contraceptives. The pill appears to interfere with the sexual selection chemistry between a woman and a man, effectively sabotaging what nature has spent millions of years setting up. The result – women on the pill are more likely to plump for a man with MHC genes similar to their own, rather than favouring the fertility-enhancing smell of a man with a dissimilar MHC profile. It is not yet known whether pill-matched couples are more predisposed to infertility and miscarriages, or whether the children of such couples could be more likely to suffer health problems. Such studies remain to be carried out. However, considering the recognised importance in terms of fertility and health of finding a man with a complementary MHC, the effects of hormonal contraceptives on a woman's sense of smell are disturbing.

There is one major argument against the importance of human body odour in signalling a person's potential as a fertile mate. It is that humans, unlike other species, choose to douse themselves in perfumes. Surely this fragrance-cloaking habit, which is a long one, stretching back thousands of years, scuppers any possible human reliance on olfactory signals? However, research investigating connections between human MHC genes and smell has recently thrown up a quirky and somewhat unexpected result. It seems that when women and men spray on their perfume of choice they are, albeit unwittingly, amplifying, rather than masking, their individual MHC-driven body odour.

Astonishingly, when asked to choose their preferred fragrances from a range of common perfume ingredients, women and men with similar MHCs chose similar aromas. It appears that perfumes truly do unconsciously reveal what consciously humans may try to hide. As the biblical love poem 'The Song of Songs' says, 'Your name is like those oils poured.' These findings explain for me why I and my two sisters have, as adults, plumped independently for the same perfume as our favourite signature fragrance – we're advertising very similar genetic wares. Perhaps, they also clarify the appeal to me at seventeen of the smell of vanilla as a perfume, and why my young niece's favourite scent is the same as mine was at a similar age.

The evidence to date suggests the human nose, courtesy of its sense of smell, is an invaluable body structure in the search to find a genetically complementary mate and ensure both successful sexual reproduction and the survival of the species. The importance of a female being able to sniff Mr Right (for her) may help in explaining why women score higher than men in sensitivity to odours, regardless of age group. It seems that the old adage to 'follow your nose' is sound advice. But smell does not act alone in the search for the best father for a woman's offspring; a woman's nose acts in glorious concert with her genitalia, sampling and screening Mr Right Sperm. A woman's nose sniffs him out and her vagina tries him out for size. Nose and genitalia working together give the best possible chance for female reproductive success. It's not surprising, then, that the naso-genital relationship is inscribed indelibly in human consciousness.

7

THE FUNCTION OF THE ORGASM

Pleasure or pain? Ecstasy or agony? Gianlorenzo Bernini depicted the moment as one of voluptuous rapture. St Teresa swoons backwards, lost in the moment, surrendering to her sacred vision. She moans, her lips parted, her face suffused with sensation, her eyes closed. The folds of her clothing stream and flow from her body, fluid as water, caressing her contours, as above golden rays of light surge down from heaven, and the angel of her lord prepares to pierce his flame-tipped spear through her heart, again and again. 'The Ecstasy of St Teresa' (see Figure 7.1), Bernini's sculpture of the Spanish saint of Avila in intimate communion with her god, is both glorious and disturbing, supremely capable of inducing shudders in unsuspecting onlookers.

For many, what Bernini's seventeenth-century hands created – an image of religious, saintly ecstasy – verges on the blasphemous. However, to others it is pure splendour – an emblem of eternal orgasm. St Teresa herself described her moments of mystical communion with Christ in terms imbued with intense passion. In her manuscript *Life*, written in 1565, she describes how 'The pain was so great that I screamed aloud; but simultaneously I felt such infinite sweetness that I wished it to last eternally. It was not bodily but psychic pain, although it affected to a certain extent also the body. It was the sweetest caressing of the soul by God.'

Perhaps it is not surprising that St Teresa was lost as to how to describe her intense sensations, and onlookers remain split as to what they see. Descriptions of orgasm often defy exactitude. What, after all, is one expressing? A pinnacle of pleasure and passion, or simply seconds of sweet, streaming, exquisite suffering? Is it a blissful evanescent and ecstatic moment when a person can stand outside one's conscious life and self, or just deliciously pleasant muscular contractions centred on and around a person's genitalia? Orgasm, it seems,

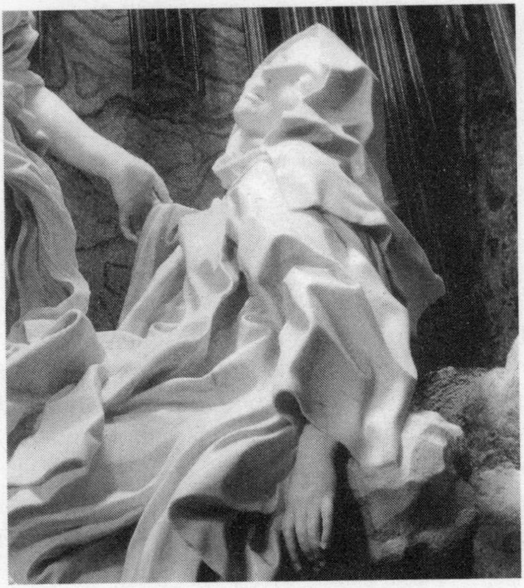

Figure 7.1 Bernini's 'The Ecstasy of St Teresa': is the saint moaning with orgasmic bliss?

is paradoxical. Language tells us the word derives from the Greek *orgasmos*, itself from the term *orgon*, which means to grow ripe, swell or be lustful, words which carry sexual and genital connotations. The Sanskrit *urira* means 'sap' or 'strength' – conveying a sense of sexual energy. However, such words fail somewhat when addressing the complexity and emotion of the experience.

Other English orgasmic expressions – climax, come, spend oneself and the big O – also pale beside the real thing. Latin sexual language utilised metaphors of reaching a goal or arriving (*peruenies*) or accomplishing something (*patratio*) to describe orgasm. French highlights the step to an altered consciousness with *la petite morte*, and expresses the pleasures of orgasm using the verb *jouir* – literally to enjoy or delight in something. However, French perplexes somewhat with the phrase *vider ses burettes* to describe female orgasm. This phrase literally means 'the emptying of her *burettes*', *burettes* being the receptacles for wine and holy water at Mass, but also in Old French a jug or pitcher with a wide mouth. It's also possible that this expression relates to the phenomenon of female ejaculation too. Meanwhile, German adds a bit of fizz with a descriptor of orgasm as *höchste Wallung*, that is, 'maximum bubbling' – a deliciously effervescent portrayal of the pleasure phenomenon.

The difficulty of grasping the heart of orgasm is reflected in the language of other cultures too. Anthropological evidence highlights how, for the Mangaian people, orgasm is *nene*, a word used figuratively to refer to perfection. Synonymous with this is *nanawe*, used for either 'luxuriously comfortable' or 'the pleasantness of a person's talk or of music'. In the Trobiand Islands, the fine line between orgasm and ejaculation is somewhat blurred. *Ipipisi momona* describes the moment of orgasm, but translates literally as 'the sexual fluid squirts/the seminal fluid discharges'. *Ipipisi momona* also refers to nocturnal orgasms, be they female or male, yet the act of ejaculation is described using the word *isulumomoni* – which means 'the sexual fluid boils over'.

Interestingly, the language of the Polynesian people of the Marquesas Islands uses different words to describe different aspects of orgasm, as well as attitudes. First of all they describe orgasm with the word *manini*, meaning literally sweet. However, while *manini* refers mainly to the sensations of pleasure, release and well-being associated with orgasm, Marquesans also describe orgasm in terms of what happens to a person's genitals. This word for orgasm, *hakate'a*, translates literally as 'make semen', i.e. ejaculate, but also possesses overtones of the aspects of *manini*. Neither of these orgasm terms are viewed as being suitable for polite usage – in such circumstances, *pao*, meaning finish, is substituted. This separation into *manini*, *hakate'a* and *pao* is, I feel, similar to English with orgasm, ejaculate and come. Somewhat worryingly, the influence of the sexual views of missionaries on the Marquesan people is evident in their rejigged sexual lexicon. In the southern group of the Marquesas archipelago, both *pe* (rotten) and *hau hau* (bad) are now used to depict orgasm. The phrase *ua pe nei au* translates, disconcertingly, as 'I am rotten now; I have had an orgasm.'

Orgasms for all

The desire to describe, name, quantify and, in doing so, understand orgasm is an age-old itch. Indeed, a multitude of minds – medical, moral, philosophical and just plain curious – have pondered on such questions as 'What is an orgasm?'; 'Why do orgasms exist?'; 'Why do they feel so good?' and, crucially, for an understanding of the vagina, 'What do they say about genitalia?' Ancient western medicine was no exception in this. 'I must now tell why a great pleasure is coupled with the exercise of the generative parts and a raging desire precedes their use,' says Greek physician Galen in *On the Usefulness of the Parts*. Galen, following the lead of Hippocrates, viewed orgasm as a signal of the release of an individual's procreative genital fluids – the seed or semen that they believed both women and men contributed to the conception of a child. That is, orgasm, in their minds, was the means by which genitalia shook forth both sexes' essential generative seed.

Within this two-seed model of conception (as it has come to be known), orgasm could be described as follows. It was associated with a great pleasure that was felt by both sexes and was intimately tied to successful sexual reproduction; both sexes typically emitted genital fluids; the pleasurable sensations felt were a result of both the qualities of the substance emitted, as well as its rapid propulsion; and the woman's womb both secreted her own fluids and then drew up and retained a mixture of her fluids and the male's. This theory viewed both female and male orgasm during sexual intercourse as essential for ensuring successful sexual reproduction. If female orgasm did not occur, a woman would not release her seed, and conception, therefore, could not take place. That is, this view saw both female and male genitalia, and female and male pleasure, having a meaningful role to play in procreation.

Not all early western philosophers of medicine agreed with Galen and Hippocrates' orgasmic views. Aristotle had distinctly different ideas about the nature of both female and male orgasm. Whereas the two-seed theory of conception tied the pleasure of orgasm and the emission of sexual fluids firmly together for both women and men, Aristotle's view of orgasm was completely dissociated from the explosive release of generative seed. Moreover, he underlined this view by refuting that orgasm was a signaller of ejaculation in either sex. For Aristotle, orgasm, or 'the vehemence of pleasure in sexual intercourse', as he put it, was a result of 'a strong friction wherefore if this intercourse is often repeated the pleasure is diminished in the persons concerned'. Orgasm, for him, was not the sensation associated with emission of genital fluids.

In order to back up his 'orgasm separate from seed' theory, Aristotle pointed to his observations that women could conceive without orgasm (although he stressed that this was the exception rather than the rule). And he also highlighted how orgasm was possible for both young boys and old men without the concomitant spurt of ejaculate. Significantly, Aristotle also commented on the changes that occurred in female genitalia during orgasm, noting that as a woman came her cervix acted as a 'cupping vessel', seeming to serve to draw in semen. Aristotle suggested, rather astutely, as we shall see, that 'when this is so there is a readier way for the semen of the male to be drawn into the uterus'. In his view then, female orgasm may not be essential for conception, but it and the changes it wrought in the vagina could certainly improve the chances of conception occurring.

The musings of Aristotle on female and male orgasm were not, however, the ones that gained widespread acceptance in the western world. Rather, it was the Hippocratic idea that female orgasm was crucial for conception that remained in common currency up until and during the eighteenth century. For example, in 1745, French scientist Pierre de Maupertuis still felt confident enough to describe female orgasm in his work *The Earthy Venus* as 'the pleasure which perpetuates mankind, that moment so rich in delight, which brings to life a new being'.

Female orgasm is essential for conception

The theory that female orgasm is essential for conception to occur is, I believe, one of the most influential ideas in the history of the vagina and female sexual pleasure. This is because it had particularly far-reaching consequences for how western women and their genitalia were treated, for, with female orgasm understood as a necessary part of the procreation equation, female sexual pleasure, and how to evoke it, could be viewed in a positive light. Religion could sanction female sexual pleasure and medics could advise on how best to bring about female orgasm because of its intimate connection to creation. The result: female sexual pleasure was deemed acceptable, moral even, by the most important authorities of the day – the church and science.

Fertility advice from physicians emphasised the importance of ensuring that a woman's shudder of orgasm was felt during sexual intercourse. If 'in the very coitional act itself, she notes a certain tremor . . . she is pregnant', Äetius of Amida, physician to the Byzantine emperor Justinian, advised. Moreover, suggesting how best to stimulate a woman to this sexual bliss was also perceived as part of a medic's remit. Soranus' influential second-century medical text, *Gynaecology*, prescribes appropriate foods and massage as the prerequisite preludes to orgasm. He writes of tempting women with meals of aphrodisiacal foods 'to give the inner turbulence an impetus towards coition', and of giving a massage, as it 'naturally aids the distribution of food [and] also helps in the reception and retention of the seed'. Such conception prescriptions were enduring, as the seventeenth-century recommendation of 'sweet embraces with lascivious words mixed with lascivious kisses' shows. History also records the 1740s' story of the young Habsburg princess Maria Theresa, who found herself unable to conceive after her recent marriage. Her physician's advice was: 'I think the vulva of Her Most Holy Majesty should be titillated before intercourse.' This seems to have worked, as Maria Theresa went on to bear more than a dozen children.

The timing – and not just the occurrence – of female orgasm during sexual intercourse was seen as a crucial component of the two-seed theory of successful sexual reproduction. Hippocrates, like his later Greek fellow, Aristotle, noted changes in a woman's genitalia on orgasm. His interpretation was that a woman's womb contracted and closed up after its orgasmic ejaculation, barring entry to any male latecomers, and so the belief that simultaneous orgasm was necessary for conception was born. Rhythm and timing became all important. If a woman came before a man, she could not conceive because her uterus would already be drawn up and closed. If a man orgasmed before a woman, his sperm would douse and extinguish 'both the heat and pleasure for woman'. But if both sexes could come to orgasm together, Hippocrates envisaged, it is as if wine is sprinkled on a naked flame – the flames shoot higher, the heat of the woman's womb blazes most brilliantly, and post-mutual-orgasmic shiver, her womb seals. Success.

Over the centuries many opinions were offered as to what was the best way to ensure a woman came at the same time as a man. Certain times of the day or night were suggested to be better than others, aphrodisiacs could help, as could the right sexual technique. The medieval manuscript *Women's Secrets* advised how 'After the middle of the night or before daybreak the male should begin to excite the woman to coitus. He should speak to her in a jesting manner, kiss and embrace her, and rub her lower parts with his fingers. All this should be done to arouse the woman's appetite for coitus so the male and the female seed will run together in the womb at the same time.' And according to this anonymous male adviser: 'When the woman begins to speak as if she were babbling the male ought to become erect and mix with her.' The final piece of advice? A 'sign of conception is if the man feels his penis drawn and sucked into the closure of the vulva'.

The belief that changes in the structure of female genitalia at orgasm were an integral part of ensuring procreation meant that coital fertility advice was quite far-reaching. The sixteenth-century French surgeon Ambroise Paré counselled on the wisdom of not withdrawing from a woman too soon after her womb had opened from orgasm, 'lest aire strike the open womb', he says, and cool the freshly sown warm seeds, thus harming conception. It seems that sex for women – if a man was aiming to procreate – may well have been more enjoyable than others have presumed: sweet talk and kisses, good food and wine, a sensual massage, mutual orgasm and a long, close embrace afterwards. It sounds good to me.

But sadly for women, the notion that female and mutual orgasm was necessary for conception did not last. Aristotle's beliefs did not disappear entirely and rumours had been circulating the medical world for centuries that female orgasm was not a prognosticator of semination. In the twelfth century, Arabic philosopher and author of a major medical encyclopaedia Averroes reported on the case of a woman who got pregnant from semen floating in her bath water. The death knell sounded in the 1770s when Lazzaro Spallanzani successfully artificially inseminated a water spaniel. Dogs and other animals, at least, the theorists concluded, did not need to enjoy orgasm to conceive. As one doctor commented sagely and succinctly, syringes could not 'communicate or meet with joy'. And what about women and orgasm? Although it took a while longer for the equation of female orgasm with conception to be erased from public consciousness, by the start of the nineteenth century, medical opinion was reaching a consensus. Human female orgasm was not necessary for successful sexual reproduction. What a come-down.

Some entrepreneurial spirits discovered the truth about orgasm and contraception for themselves. Mabel Loomis Todd was one such person. This nineteenth-century American woman, who later became the lover of poet Emily Dickinson's brother, kept a deliciously explicit diary of her sex life, her menstrual cycle, her orgasms (noting them all, including masturbation) and more. May 15, 1879, 'barely eight days over my illness [period]', is the day she chose to put her beliefs about orgasm to the test. 'With me,' she writes, 'the only fruitful time could be at the climax moment of my sensation – that once passed, I believed the womb would close, & no fluid could reach the fruitful point.'

And so she proceeded to test this idea out by having sex with her husband and deliberately coming before he did. As she put it: 'Not at all from uncontrollable passion, but merely from the strongest conviction of the truth of my idea, I allowed myself to receive the precious fluid, at least six or eight moments after my highest point of enjoyment had passed, and when I was perfectly cool & satisfied, getting up immediately, thereafter, and having it all apparently escape.' The result of Mabel's home fecundation experiment – her only child, Millicent.

Orgasms for health – the makings of an orgasm industry

Despite the severing in the eighteenth and nineteenth centuries of a link between female orgasm and conception, one strand of the original two-seed theory remained as part of medical practice. It even flourished as the nineteenth century became the twentieth, evolving into a major part of medical practice. This portion of the two-seed theory was the idea that female orgasm was necessary to maintain a woman's health. As Hippocrates perceived it, orgasm was essential in releasing both sexes' retained seed. However, if this seed was not expelled regularly via orgasm shaking it out, ill health would result from the build-up of seed and subsequent imbalance of bodily fluids. As the medieval manuscript the *Trotula*, in *Treatments for Women*, states: 'Women, when they have immoderate desire to have intercourse and they do not do so, if they do not satiate the desire they incur grave suffering'.

As we shall see, though, this conclusion that female orgasms were necessary in order to maintain physical and mental health had major repercussions for how women, and the diseases attributed to them, were treated by the medical profession.

From Galen's time onwards (129–200 CE), medical texts record, in great detail, how manipulation to orgasm was the standard medical treatment for these non-specific 'women's diseases'. This was because these ailments, which were variously called 'suffocation of the womb'; *praefocatio matricis* ('suffocation of the mother'), and hysteria (literally, womb disease), were believed to stem from the uterus becoming engorged with unexpended seed, and so wandering the body, in search of release. Orgasm was one of the chosen methods of effecting the release, although the prescription for how orgasm was brought about varied. Over the centuries, the methods physicians prescribed to induce orgasm in so-called hysterical women included advocating being 'strongly encountered by their husbands' if they had one. Alternatively, if a woman was single, widowed or confined to a nunnery, the recommendation could be horse-riding, pelvic rocking in swings, chairs or hammocks, or vaginal massage – the latter to be provided by the patient's physician or midwife.

Over the centuries it was practised, vaginal or vulval massage to orgasm became just another skill that male physicians and midwives must perfect for the benefit of their patients. Galen advised how to rub a woman's genitalia until she felt the 'pain and at the same time the pleasure' associated with intercourse – and had emitted a quantity of thick seed. Not surprisingly, different approaches to providing the orgasmic conclusion were suggested. The method Giovanni Matteo Ferrari da Gradi (d. 1472) prescribed was to rub the woman's chest and cover it with large cupping glasses, after which 'the midwife would be instructed to use sweet-smelling oil on her finger and move it well in a circle inside the vulva'. A successful treatment, according to da Gradi, was when the woman experienced '*simul . . . delectatio & dolor*', that is, pleasure and pain at the same time, another description of orgasm that contains echoes of St Teresa's ecstasy.

Many male medics felt it necessary to ask women to help them in their exertions. In his influential early-seventeenth-century medical compendium, Dutch physician Pieter van Foreest recommends to medics confronted with a case of *suffocatio ex semine retento* (suffocation because of retained seed): 'we think it necessary to ask a midwife to assist, so that she can massage the genitalia with one finger inside, using oil of lilies, musk root, crocus, or [something] similar. And in this way the afflicted woman can be aroused to the paroxysm.'

As well as providing descriptions of orgasm, the many discussions of medical vaginal massage provide a rare, intimate and surprising insight into how the vagina was viewed and treated in the last two millennia. Using pleasant or aphrodisiacal aromas seems to have been common, as was applying a particular type of stimulation. In the following case, the recommendation appears to be to stimulate the cervix: 'Let the mydwife anoint her fingers with . . . spike mixed with musk, ambergreese, civet and other sweet powders, and with these let her rub or tickle the top of the neck of the wombe which toucheth the inner orifice.'

Significantly, some accounts touch on what physical effect their actions had on female genitalia, as well as the technique they applied. Äetius of Amida (502–75) describes the moment of orgasmic release as characterised by uterine contractions, muscular spasms throughout the entire body, and the secretion of vaginal fluids. Rhazes, the tenth-century Arabic author of a practical textbook of medicine, details how, when the mouth of the womb is rubbed with a well-oiled finger, there is the sensation 'as if something is pulled up'.

It's important to note, though, that not all doctors were comfortable with providing vulval massage to orgasm for health – from both a moral and practical perspective. The word orgasm is noticeably absent from the majority of descriptions of genital massage, with most orgasm-providing medics preferring to talk about relieving the 'hysterical paroxysms' of women. In 1883, the French physician Auguste Tripier would only admit that what was known as the convulsive crisis of hysteria '*est de même quelquefois que la crise vénérienne*' – 'is sometimes the same as the orgasm'.

One of the few physicians to refer, in print, to the type of relief his profession was routinely providing was Nathaniel Highmore. In his 1660 manuscript *De Passione Hysterica et Affectione Hypochondriaca* he uses the word *orgasmum*, which can only mean one thing in Latin. Highmore also detailed how blood rushed to a woman's genitals during arousal and how the contractions of orgasm seemed to return that blood to the rest of the body. This seventeenth-century doctor

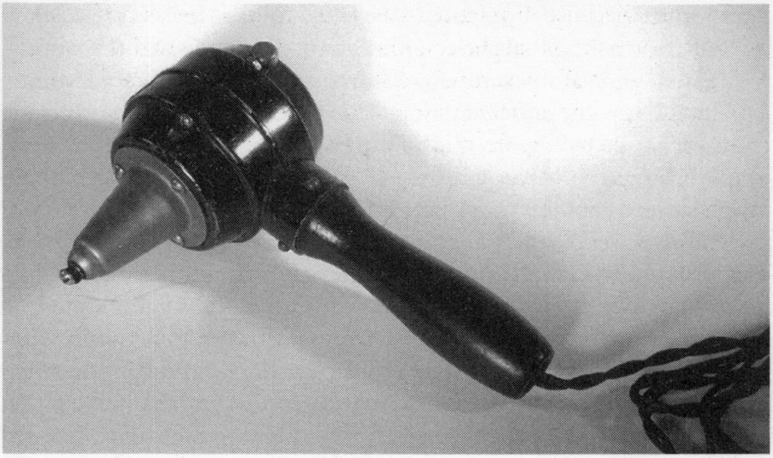

Figure 7.2 The advent of the vibrator: an early twentieth-century vibrator.

was also more direct (and humorous) than most in describing the skill required to effect orgasm via vaginal massage, commenting: 'it is not unlike that game of boys in which they try to rub their stomachs with one hand and pat their heads with the other'. Nearly two and a half centuries later, in 1906, fellow physician Samuel Spencer Wallian was bemoaning not just the expertise called for, but the time taken up too. Manual massage, he complains, 'consumes a painstaking hour to accomplish much less profound results than are easily effected by the *other* in a short five or ten minutes'.

'Aids that every woman appreciates'

The *other* in question was the latest tool of the medical profession – the vibrator. Vibration therapy, as detailed beautifully in Rachel Maines' book *The Technology of Orgasm: 'Hysteria', the Vibrator and Women's Sexual Satisfaction*, was the answer to all tired medics' prayers. Whether steam-powered, water-propelled, foot-operated or, from 1883 onwards, thanks to English doctor and inventor Joseph Mortimer Granville, electromechanical, vibrators provided much-needed relief for physicians and their patients (see Figure 7.2). Female orgasms could now be provided at the flick of a switch. Business, it seemed, boomed. In 1873, it was estimated that in the US 'more than three-fourths of all the practice of the [medical] profession are devoted to the treatment of diseases peculiar to women', with the annual estimated aggregate income which 'physicians must thank frail women for' totalling around $150 million. This is not surprising, considering vulval massage to orgasm was by the end of the nineteenth century a staple medical practice, with some doctors recommending women come in for 'treatments' on a weekly basis. A lucrative outcome indeed.

The difference that the electromechanical vibrator made to the medical profession's treatment of 'hysterical' women was summed up in 1903 in a book by Dr Samuel Howard Monell discussing medical uses of vibration. 'Pelvic massage (in gynaecology),' he wrote, 'has its brilliant advocates and they report wonderful results, but when practitioners must supply the skilled technic with their own fingers the method has no value to the majority.' However, he adds, 'Special applicators (motor driven) give practical value and office convenience to what otherwise is impractical.'

Vibrators took off at home, as well as in the doctor's surgery. In the US in the 1890s, women could purchase a $5 portable vibrator – 'perfect for weekend trips', ran the advertisement – rather than paying at least $2 a pop for a visit to the physician. Delightfully, the vibrator was the fifth household appliance to be electrified, after the sewing machine, fan, kettle and toaster. And as vibrators became available for home use, the ancient art of physician-prescribed vaginal massage to orgasm slowly became defunct. Male medical hands were increasingly freed to perform other healing tasks. Unfortunately, it's not known precisely how many late-nineteenth-century and early-twentieth-century home vibration kits were sold; however, they were certainly popular enough to feature in many mail-order magazines in the US, the UK and Canada up until the 1920s (see Figure 7.3).

The pages of the magazine *Modern Priscilla*, in April 1913, sold vibrators with the promise of 'a machine that gives 30,000 thrilling, invigorating, penetrating, revitalizing vibrations per minute'. Not surprisingly, perhaps, vibrator advertisements (whether directed at doctors or women), did not mention orgasms or sexual pleasure, just the 'health benefits' of vibration. An 1883 text entitled *Health for Women* recommends vibrators as they can treat 'pelvic hyperemia' – congestion of the genitalia. Quite why vibrators fell from medical and public grace and use during the first half of the twentieth century is

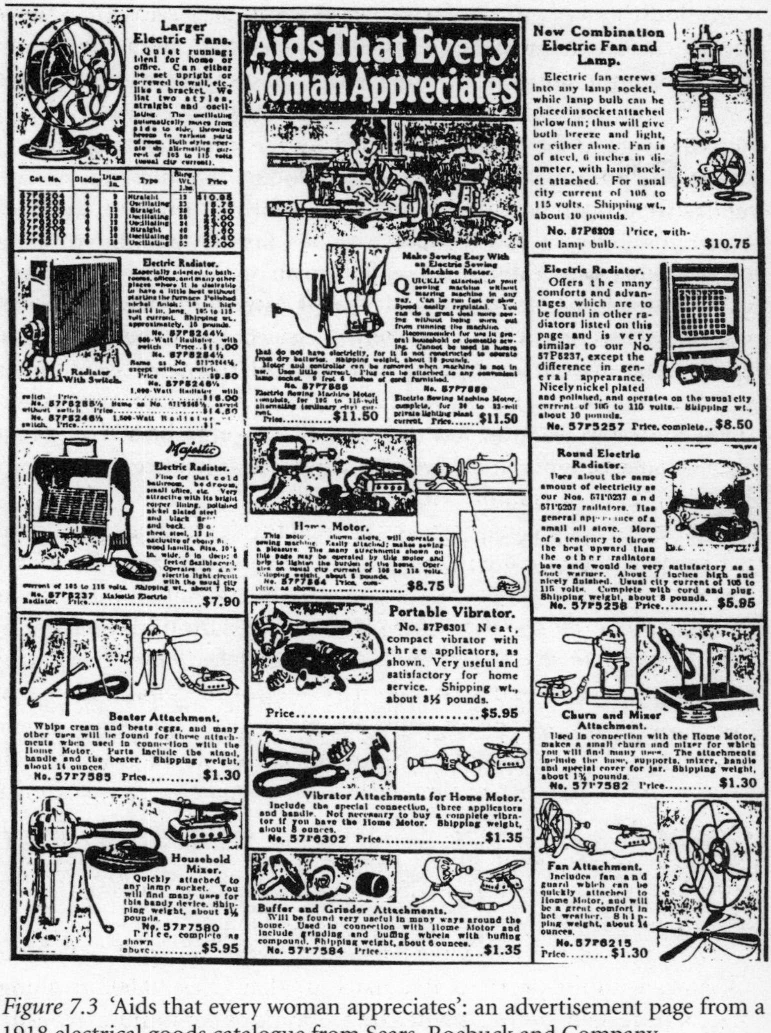

Figure 7.3 'Aids that every woman appreciates': an advertisement page from a 1918 electrical goods catalogue from Sears, Roebuck and Company.

also unclear, although it has been suggested that their exposure in the early erotic films of the 1920s may have changed medical and public opinion as to their 'health' role, and highlighted their sexual one. And sadly, the morals of the day were not in favour of females sexually pleasuring themselves.

Ironically, the orgasm industry in the west was thriving in a time when many medics and men felt confident enough to put forward, and publish, the notion that women were passionless creatures, not much troubled by sexual feelings. While some male doctors were charging women for orgasm provided by them on health grounds, others were promulgating the view that women that did have sexual feelings were mad, bad, dangerous and abnormal. In 1896, Richard von Krafft-Ebing, in *Psychopathia Sexualis*, famously said, 'Woman, however, when physically and mentally normal and properly educated, has but little sensual desire.' He adds that 'if it were otherwise marriage and family life would be empty words', a sentiment that seems to express a fear of what would happen to society if women gave free rein to their sexuality.

The following are just a few comments from other male doctors in this particularly hypocritical period in medicine's history.

> Women have less sexual feeling than men . . . as a rule women have nothing of what is understood as sexual passion. (Charles Taylor, 1882)

> The appearance of the sexual side in the love of a young girl is pathological . . . half of all women are not sexually excitable. (Hermann Fehling,1893)

> Only in very rare circumstances do women experience one tithe the sexual feeling which is familiar to most men. Many of them are entirely frigid. (Nineteenth-century American physican George Napheys)

Meanwhile, writing in 1871, British doctor William Acton did not deny that some women were capable of being aroused; however, he suggested that they were 'sad exceptions', and on a fast track to a 'form of insanity that those who visit lunatic asylums must be fully conversant with'.

Medical massage good, women masturbating bad

Equally, astonishingly and outrageously, while male doctors were manipulating women to orgasm in their surgeries and charging them for it, other male physicians were publishing papers on the problems of females doing it for themselves – manually or mechanically. 'The Neuropsychical Element in Conjugal Aversion', that is, why women say no to sex with their husbands, is the title of an article published in 1892 in the *Journal of Nervous and Mental Disease.* This paper suggested that a common 'source of marital aversion seems to lie in the fact that substitution of mechanical and iniquitous excitations [vibrators and masturbation] affords more satisfaction than the mutual legitimate ones do'.

Other medical journals published articles detailing ways in which male doctors could spot if their female patients were suffering from the 'masturbatory disease'. 'Signs of Masturbation in the Female', by E. H. Smith in *The Pacific Medical Journal* of 1903, is essentially a guide for doctors on how to detect if women have been masturbating. One sign, according to E. H. Smith, was one labium being longer than the other. Other signs of masturbation were that women were more sexually sensitive than they should be. In order to discover whether a woman was more sexually sensitive than she should be, the medical journal advocated sending a 'mild faradic current', i.e. an electric shock, through the urethra.

It seems that western women couldn't win – they were either inferior to men because they were lacking in sexual feeling, or abnormal because they enjoyed and displayed their feelings of sexual pleasure. Many doctors appear to have been very confused. The late-nineteenth-century gynaecologist Otto Adler wrote that up to 40 per cent of women suffered from sexual anaesthesia. However, the women who made up this 'sexually anaesthetic' category included women who said they did masturbate to orgasm; women who said they had strong sexual desires (although they were unable to satisfy them); and a woman who was reported to have had an orgasm as she was being examined by the doctor. Adler's categorisation of what constituted sexual anaesthesia in women seems peculiar indeed, and not particularly robust. Meanwhile the 1899 edition of the reference guide for physicians, the *Merck Manual,* on one page recommended massage as a treatment for hysteria, while on another it suggested sulphuric acid as a remedy for nymphomania. This brings to mind the barbaric idea of pouring carbolic acid on the clitoris as a 'cure' for female masturbation.

This state of confusion in the medical world as to how to understand female orgasm and sexual pleasure is, in part, perhaps explained by the differing messages being received from the authorities of the day. On the one hand, science said female orgasm had no role to play in sexual reproduction, therefore in the eyes of moral and church-going men, sexual pleasure could not be sanctioned in women, as it did not lead directly to procreation. However, on the other hand, science was still teaching (at least up to the end of the nineteenth century) that female orgasm was necessary for health – surely medical ethics demanded doctors do their job? Ultimately, though, just as with the clitoris, the loss of an obvious and immediate role in ensuring successful sexual reproduction meant that it was possible for the medical and scientific community to ignore the troublesome concept of the female orgasm. And in the main, they did, despite having recently routinely provided female orgasms on health grounds.

The history of the west's obsession with orgasms and health would not be complete without the story of Wilhelm Reich (1897–1957), a Viennese doctor and contemporary of Sigmund Freud, who moved to the US in 1939. Orgasm, and how it is linked to health, was Reich's lifetime fascination. In his book *The Function of the Orgasm – sex-economic problems of biological energy*, published in 1927, Reich wrote of his belief that health, in particular psychological health, depends upon what he called 'orgastic potency', that is, the degree to which a person can surrender to and experience orgasm, free of any inhibitions. He suggested that humans store emotions in their muscles, and that during orgasm, the muscular contraction and relaxation of orgasm release these emotions, keeping a person healthy. That is, orgasm regulates the emotional energy of the body and relieves sexual tensions that would otherwise be transformed into neurosis. Orgasm, Reich envisaged,was the free flow of sexual or biological energy (which he called *orgone*) through the body.

The flipside of this, not being able to enjoy full and satisfying orgasms because of psychological or physiological tension blocks in the body, was ill-health. Reich explained and expanded on this in the following way:

> People who are brought up with a negative attitude toward life and sex acquire a pleasure anxiety, which is physiologically anchored in muscle spasms. This neurotic pleasure anxiety is the basis on which life-negating, dictator-producing views of life are reproduced by the people themselves. It is the core of a fear of an independent, freedom-oriented way of life.

Reich's views on the importance of sexual pleasure were not shared by everyone, perhaps because of his controversial exhortations to fuck freely. A propaganda film he made in his youth, *Mysteries of the Organism*, promoting what he called orgasmatherapy, declares:

> The human being averages 4,000 orgasms in a lifetime. Do not turn off this pulsating motor of joy and life force ... The biological charge and discharge produced by the genital embrace causes the orgasmic reflex, supremely pleasurable muscle contractions. Subjection to social disciplines may cause gastric ulcers, respiratory, coronary and vascular diseases. Comrade lovers, for your health's sake: fuck freely.

In a western world which would rather not talk about sex or orgasm, and which only permitted sex within marriage, for procreation purposes, Reich's views were dismissed and ridiculed and more. His books were burnt twice in his life – the first time by the Nazis in Germany in 1933. Later, in the US, his belief that illnesses could be affected by orgasm (*orgone* energy) got him into serious trouble with the drug regulatory authorities there. He remains virtually the only post-war western writer to have their books burned by the American state (1956), and he died in prison a year later, jailed for non-compliance with an injunction that ordered him to refrain perpetually 'from making any statements or representations pertaining to the existence of *orgone* energy'.

It seems ironic that just over fifty years after American doctors were providing orgasms on health grounds, Reich was persecuted for suggesting the same – albeit far more publicly. There is a curious addendum to the Reich story, as there is now some western scientific research that suggests orgasms may well be good for health. Studies looking at men have shown that those who have two or more orgasms a week live longer than those who have one or none, while other studies looking at coronary disease in women and men suggest that a satisfying and orgasmic sex life may contribute to a strong and healthy heart. Is it possible that Reich was right, that the function of the orgasm is ensuring health of body and mind? Unfortunately, the jury is still out on this one. But for what it's worth, I'm happy to put my faith in enjoying an orgasm a day in an attempt to keep the doctor and death at bay.

The elixir of life

Before looking at what science today has to say about female orgasm and its connection with female genitalia, what about outside the Christian western world? How is orgasm understood elsewhere? Moreover, do views of female orgasm differ in cultures where sex is viewed as sacred? Eastern belief systems, such as Taoism, which developed in China, and Tantra, from northern India, also viewed female orgasm as essential for health. First Tantrism. Orgasm in Tantric terms is understood as a resolution of two forces – call them expansion and contraction, or female and male – which results in cosmic harmony. Tantra, which teaches that Buddhahood, some say nirvana, resides in the vagina, places great emphasis on *maithuna* – a Tantric sex rite. During *maithuna*, which is often called *yoni-puja* (worship of the vagina), a man's goal is to feed or fuel himself off the woman's sexual/spiritual energy. In this way, it is said he can revitalise himself and achieve longevity. There's one sticking point though. Having sex is not enough. Successful sexual vampirism is only accomplished by ensuring the woman has an orgasm (and that the man does not ejaculate his semen).

There is also another reason why Tantrism perceives female orgasm to be essential. This stems from the idea that it is orgasm that releases a woman's *rajas* – her vivifying vaginal secretions. Indeed, in some Tantric schools, the main aim of *maithuna* is the production and collection of the woman's *rajas*, which the man will then ingest. Somewhat peculiarly, this can be done by collecting the vaginal juices on a leaf, mixing them with a little water and then drinking the genital cocktail. Or, if a man has truly mastered his Tantric sexual techniques, he can enhance his hormonal system by absorbing the *rajas* directly through his penis – a practice known as *vajroli-mudra*.

Female orgasm is also considered to have benefits for health and a long life within Taoism, which was founded by the sixth-century BCE prophet Lao Tzu. In fact, Taoism teaches that sex is seen as one of the prime ways to come closer to the Tao, that is, ultimate reality, energy, movement and constant change, where the polar opposites of yin (female) and yang (male) are balanced and harmonious, continually uniting and metamorphosing into each other. Indeed, the basic principle of traditional Chinese philosophy says that 'the interaction of the female essence [yin] with the male essence [yang] is the Way of Life [Tao]'. Moreover, as Taoist sexual lore teaches that death is caused by the imbalance of yin and yang, sex is seen as a major force for rebalancing the body and thus cheating death.

For men, the way to garner longevity sexually is by the process of gathering and absorbing essential yin essence (*cai Yin pu Yang*), while withholding their own ejaculation. And just as in Tantric thought, this female elixir (known as *khuai*) is only produced when a woman has an orgasm. However, there is a slight twist. According to the Taoist sex manual *A Popular Exposition of the Methods of Regenerating the Primary Vitalities*, this life-giving essence can be supped from three places: a woman's mouth, her breasts and her vagina – hence it's called The Great Medicine of the Three Peaks. Regarding the vaginal juices, the manual states that it 'is called the Peak of the Purple Agaric, also the Grotto of the White Tiger, or the Mysterious Gateway. Its medicine is called Black Lead, or Moon Flower. It is in the vagina. Usually it does not flow out . . . Only the man who can control his passion and sexual excitement in coitus can obtain this medicine and achieve longevity'.

But what about women? Their orgasms may benefit men, but are orgasms good for female health as well? In Taoist thought, the answer is a resounding and emphatic yes. In fact, in Taoism women seem to have a remarkable win-win situation. Not only are they understood to gain in energy and longevity from their own orgasms, but they can also nourish themselves by gathering a man's essence too (*cai Yang pu Yin*). In contrast, men can only gain from women's orgasms, not their own. Women, it is said, gain longevity via orgasm by allowing their sexual or creative energy (symbolised as the Kundalini serpent) to rise from the vagina, up the spine and to the brain. This type of nourishing whole-body orgasm (where altered levels of consciousness are reached) is understood as a moment of union with the supreme Tao, or universe, and is called an 'orgasm of the valley'. Women are taught that they can help themselves to experience these profound and consciousness-altering orgasms by developing an awareness of and connection with their genital musculature (both vaginal and uterine).

Who has the best orgasm?

Curiously, eastern and western theories of female orgasm have something else in common – other than considering it a health boon. This sharing of ideas surrounds a question that we've all asked ourselves at one time or another – namely, who has the best orgasm, or greatest pleasure during sex? The answer it seems is unanimous – women do. It is a general belief in Greek mythology, Hinduism, Islam, Taoism, Christianity and western medicine that women enjoy greater pleasure during sexual activity. Within Taoist thought, this belief is expressed in the idea of a woman's yin energy being like water, or *k'an*, vast and inexhaustible, and very slow to cool, whereas a man's yang energy is like fire, or *li*, volatile and flaring up quickly, but easily spent and extinguished. Taoism also explains that it is easier for women to draw sexual orgasmic energy up from their genitals as their energy is on balance more yin. That is, as they are more focused inwards, they have a greater ability to be in touch with their internal sensations, hence their greater orgasmic capacity.

The idea that women have greater sexual pleasure is recorded in Greek mythology in the story of Teiresias, a man who was famous for having spent seven years of his life as a woman, during which time he became a celebrated courtesan. Because of his sexual experiences as both a woman and a man, Teiresias was one day called by the Greek god Zeus to settle a dispute between Zeus and his wife, Hera. The married couple were arguing over who enjoyed the greatest pleasure, or the better orgasm (*major voluptas*) during sex. Teiresias' answer was simple:

> If the parts of love-pleasure be counted as ten,
> Thrice three go to women, one only to men.

The tale of Teiresias and his championing of women's greater enjoyment of the pleasures of the flesh is echoed, almost uncannily, in many cultures. Very similar words and numbers are attributed to Ali ibn Abu Taleb, who was the husband of the Muslim prophet Muhammad's daughter, Fatima, and also the founder of the Shiite sect of Islam. According to him: 'Almighty God created sexual desire in ten parts; Then he gave nine parts to women and one to men.'

The legend of Bhangasvana, recorded in the Hindu saga the *Mahabharata*, contains many elements of Teiresias' myth too. Bhangasvana is a powerful king, a tiger among men, but he angers the god Indra, who punishes him by turning him into a woman. As a woman, Bhangasvana cannot rule his kingdom and is forced to live as a hermit. Years later, when Indra forgives the ex-king, the god grants Bhangasvana the choice of becoming a man once more, or remaining as a woman. Bhangasvana's reply? 'The woman has in union with man always the greater joy, that is why ... I choose to be a woman. I feel greater pleasure in love as a woman, that is the truth, best among the gods. I am content with existence as a woman.'

Other Indian stories, including the companion epic the *Ramayana*, convey similar messages – women are capable of enjoying sex more than men, they are more sexual, and are insatiable sexually. One Indian proverb tells how woman's power in eating is twice as great as a man's, her cunning or bashfulness four times as great, her decisions or boldness six times as great, and her impetuosity or delight in love eight times as great. Going back to the third century BCE, the text of the Old Testament both recognises the voluptuousness of the vagina and warns against it with the following lines: 'There are three things that are never sated ... Hell, the mouth of the vulva, and the earth.'

Double pleasure equals double trouble?

Why did all these different civilisations consider women's sexual pleasure or orgasmic capacity to be so much greater than men's? Western medicine, with its emphasis on analysis, made a brave attempt to explain why this should be. In fact, the question appears to have aroused the minds of many men of science, causing great consternation and, perhaps, a little envy and fear. *On Coitus*, a medical treatise written by Constantine the African, an eleventh-century doctor (and possibly the west's first sexologist), suggests that 'Pleasure in intercourse is greater in women than in males, since males derive pleasure only from the expulsion of a superfluity. Women experience twofold pleasure: both by expelling their own sperm and by receiving the male's sperm, from the desire of their fervent vulva.' In other words – women experience double the pleasure as a result of the thrill of both receiving warming male seed and emitting their own.

This idea of women's double pleasure is a frequent theme in western medicine, in particular from advocates of the two-seed theory of orgasm and conception (both women and men ejaculate semen). However, even those medical minds that insisted only men emitted seed during sex stated that women's sexual joy was the greater. According to medieval medic Albertus Magnus, a proponent of the one-seed theory, this greater delight came from 'the touch either of the man's sperm in the womb or of the penis against her sexual part'. Avicenna, on the other hand, upped the stakes and suggested that woman's sexual pleasure was threefold. Women, Avicenna claimed, have 'three delights in intercourse: one from the motion of her own sperm, a second from the motion of the male sperm, and a third from the motion or rubbing that takes place in coitus'.

Sexual vampirism

Sadly for women, the hints of sexual vampirism that are found in the east's beliefs about female orgasm are also present in western ones – with a twist. It was not unusual for male medics to write of how women, via their vaginas, could feed sexually off men. For example, sixteenth-century physician Lemnius, writing of woman's greater sexual excitement, describes not only how 'she draws forth the man's seed and casts her own with it', but also how she 'takes more delight and is more recreated by it'. But in this sex-negative society, where sex was sanctioned only for procreative purposes, men got indignant about being used in this way. It appears that the idea that women have a greater capacity for sexual pleasure seems to have been more threatening than welcoming.

Not surprisingly, perhaps, vampiric associations were made clear. Women, it was said, could use sex to 'suck the vigour of their menfolk, like the vampire'. Today, of course, it is always women that are vamps, never men. And, indeed, the definition of a vamp is a woman who exploits a man. The idea of women as sexually insatiable and vampiric is also very much to the fore in the earlier medieval medical compendium *De Secretis Mulierum* (*Women's Secrets*), which was still popular in the eighteenth century. Written to instruct celibate monks on the facts of life, *Women's Secrets* warns that:

> The more women have sexual intercourse, the stronger they become, because they are made hot by the motion that the man makes during coitus. Further, male sperm is hot because it is of the same nature as air and when it is received by the woman it warms her entire body, so women are strengthened by this heat. On the other hand, men who have sex frequently are weakened by this act because they become exceedingly dried out.

However, *Women's Secrets* is a deeply misogynistic text, with a very strong subtext extolling the evil nature of women. Significantly, it added a very negative flavour to the western medical world's notions of women's greater, boundless sexual pleasure. Woman, the treatise warns, has 'a greater desire for coitus than a man, for something foul is drawn to the good'. Furthermore, it states, 'one should beware of every woman as one would avoid a venomous serpent and a horned devil, for if it were right to say what I know about women, the whole world would be astounded'. Indeed, it is argued that this text on women and the workings of their genitalia directly influenced the *Malleus Maleficarum*, the fifteenth-century inquisitorial treatise on witches, which includes the memorable maligning line: 'All witchcraft comes from carnal lust, which is in women insatiable.'

Defining female orgasm

In the space of two millennia, female orgasm has been perceived in a myriad ways. This planet's greatest pleasure, an essential shake-out of female seed, a source of life-giving energy and a big fat zero – something that simply does not exist. Female orgasm, of course, does exist. And like male orgasm, female orgasm is defined as a perception (the acknowledgement of a sensation transmitted by nerves) accompanied by motor, that is muscular, activity. Brain and body working together beautifully. Without the muscular activity there is no orgasm, and a person must perceive the sensations generated by the muscular activity of the orgasm to experience it too. Another way of putting this is that there has to be tension before there can be release.

Just as many aspects of female sexual anatomy, such as the structure and function of the clitoris or female prostate, remained hidden from view or uncertain until recently, so too has information surrounding female orgasm. More specifically, there is a lack of understanding of the physical characteristics of female orgasm, and the function of the pleasure phenomenon. There are various reasons why a scientific appreciation of female orgasm has been so long in coming. Some of these factors are the same ones that have held back discoveries regarding female genitalia – namely, the reluctance in the west to fund research into projects connected with sex, in particular female sexuality or female genitalia. But one of the other reasons for this state of affairs is less sexist or moralistic. Put plainly, in the past it has been difficult to observe all the physical hallmarks of female orgasm. Nevertheless, while such hallmarks may be harder to view, they are present, and they have been commented on over the centuries. Together they provide a perspective on the vagina that is without equal. Significantly, the view they reveal also says something vital about the function of female genitalia, as well as the function of female orgasm.

More than two millennia ago, Aristotle noted how during female orgasm a woman's cervix acted as a 'cupping vessel', seeming to serve to draw in semen. 'Movements of the matrix' is another description of what physically happened during female orgasm. This cervical/uterine action was also amongst those observed by French physician Felix Roubaud, who published an account of the female sexual response cycle in 1855. Roubaud, like Aristotle, theorised that this cervical response to orgasm sucked up semen, and aided in conception, and in 1876 he published what is thought to be the first scientific account linking female orgasm with powerful pelvic muscle contractions.

Some descriptions of what happens to female genitalia on orgasm came about serendipitously. The following description of how the mouth (the os) of the cervix changes structure and shape during orgasm was made by an American doctor, Joseph Beck, in 1872 as he was treating a female patient. She apparently warned Beck before he touched her that she had a passionate nature and might have an orgasm from the pressure of his fingers. He took the opportunity to provide one of the first detailed reports of the response in female genitalia to arousal and orgasm:

> [Carefully] separating the labia with my left hand, so that the *os uteri* [vaginal opening of the cervix] was brought clearly into view in the sunlight, I now swept my right forefinger quickly three or four times across the space between the cervix and the pubic arch, when almost immediately the orgasm occurred

> ... Instantly the height of the excitement was at hand, the os opened itself to the extent of fully an inch, as nearly as my eye could judge, made five or six successive gasps, as it were, drawing the external os into the cervix each time powerfully, and, it seemed to me, with a regular rhythmical action, at the same time losing its former density and hardness, and becoming quite soft to the touch. All these phenomena occurred within the space of twelve seconds of time certainly, and in an instant all was as before. At the near approach of the orgastic excitement the os and cervix became intensely congested, assuming almost a livid purple color, but upon the cessation of the action, as related, the os suddenly closed, the cervix again hardened itself, the intense congestion was dissipated, the organs concerned resolved themselves into their normal condition.

Some descriptions of how the uterus and cervix respond to orgasm come, strangely enough, from doctors who were treating 'hysterical' women with genital massage. In 1891, a Swedish physician, Lindblom, who at the time was providing 'pelvic massage' on a nearly daily basis, noted how orgasm altered the rhythm of uterus contraction. Others since then have noted the same – how orgasm increases the strength (amplitude) and occurrence (frequency) of uterine muscle contractions.

It's now acknowledged that the muscular organ that is the uterus is actually never at rest. This structure – an upside-down pear or bull's head shape on the outside and an inverted triangle on the inside – exhibits steadily recurring rhythmic contractions and relaxations, with intervals ranging from two to twenty minutes, as Lindblom and others noted. During menstruation these contractions are stronger and more frequent, but can become spasmodic (indeed it's suggested that these spasmodic overactive contractions are the source of cramping period pain). Uterine contractions also increase during REM sleep, as women experience nocturnal erections, that is, increased blood flow to the genitalia.

The reasons why a woman's uterine musculature must pulse so rhythmically throughout her life are unclear. However, the uterus is a highly complex and astounding muscular structure – strong yet sensitive, as befits its remarkable role in reproduction. It has to be capable of supporting life, and have immense muscular force, able to push a bulky child through a confined space. Not surprisingly, uterine muscle is one of the strongest muscles of the body. Perhaps it is because of its important role in reproduction that uterine muscle can never afford to be completely at rest and risk losing its efficacy. It's possible that this is also why a woman's Fallopian tubes continually contract and relax throughout her life (about three contractions per minute), and why a woman's vaginal musculature does too. Spontaneous vaginal contractions originate from the cervical end of the vagina and are reported to occur every eight to ten minutes (in the resting, sexually unstimulated state, and in pregnant and non-pregnant women).

The muscular moment

While a woman's genitalia are never completely quiescent even when unaroused, on orgasm their muscular response is dramatic. Powerful involuntary rhythmic contractions and relaxations shudder throughout this muscular organ, which consists of both smooth and striated muscle. Indeed, it's now appreciated that in women the point of orgasm can be said to be characterised by the rapid forceful and rhythmic muscle contractions of the uterus, cervix, vagina, urethra, prostate and anus (Figure 7.4 shows how these orgasmic contractions affect vaginal and anal pressures). If orgasm occurs, then a woman's pelvic muscles are rippling in concert. Orgasm does not appear to occur without this physical muscular reaction. This, it is suggested, is the physical basis of orgasm. This glorious vibration phenomenon of genital muscle contractions and relaxations is the hallmark of an orgasmic happening.

Scientific studies of female orgasm show that differing numbers of pulsatile pelvic contractions can happen. Some reports mention between five and fifteen contractions at about one-second intervals, others four to eight times at intervals of 0.8 of a second. However, there is no standard, and contractions can be regular or irregular, and both. Curiously, research suggests women can be identified from the characteristic pattern of their pelvic muscle contractions – their frequency, waveform and muscular force. Rhythmic muscle contraction and relaxation can also occur elsewhere in the body, sometimes shuddering up the spine to the head in an orgasm that is reminiscent of the eastern ideas of the Kundalini serpent climbing the spine. And for men too, orgasm is characterised by muscle contractions. Male

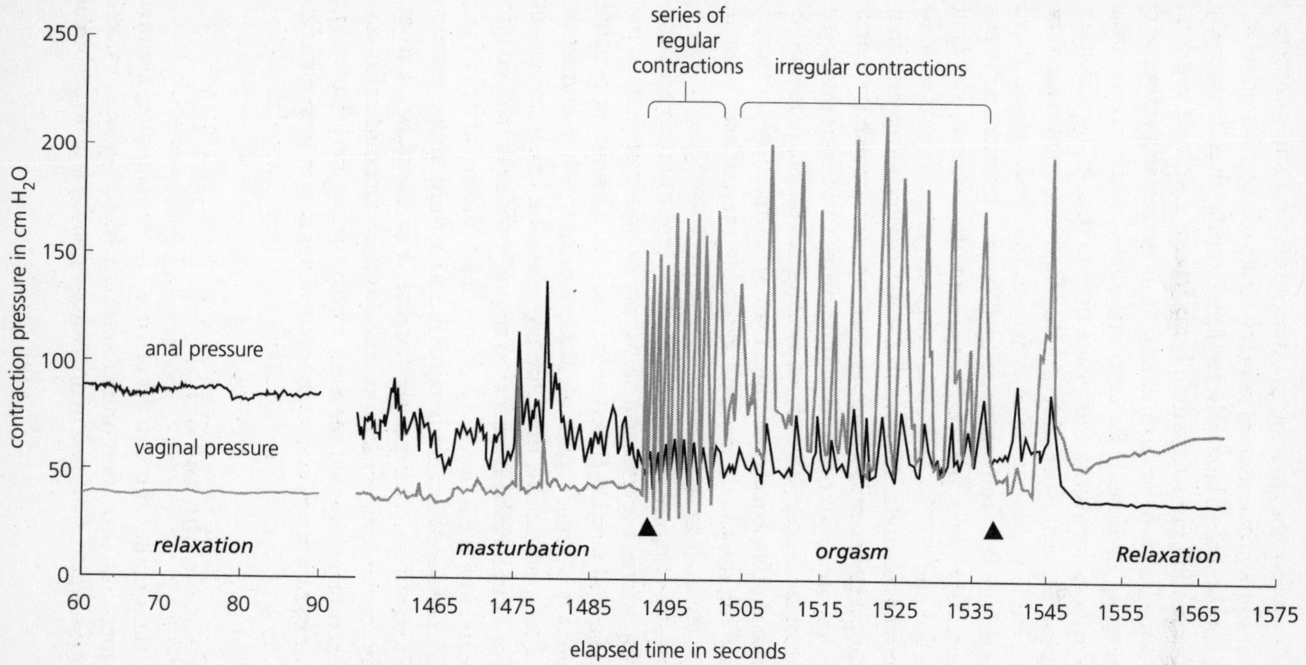

Figure 7.4 Orgasmic contractions: a computer-drawn plot of vaginal and anal pressures recorded during portions of one woman's masturbation sessions. The closed triangles indicate the perceived start and finish of orgasm (adapted from Bohlen, 1982).

contractions involve the urethra, prostate, testes and anal sphincter, with three or four contractions at intervals of 0.8 of a second reported.

Research in the second half of the twentieth century has also thrown up some fascinating facts regarding both female and male orgasm. While the time taken to orgasm differs from person to person, and varies depending on mood, scenario and many other factors, in a laboratory setting the quickest recorded time to orgasm by a woman was just fifteen seconds. It also seems that lengths of orgasm are very variable. In studies, the muscle contractions of female orgasm have been reported to last from thirteen to fifty-one seconds, with the women signalling their own experience of the orgasm as being between seven and 107 seconds. Male orgasm generally lasts around ten to thirteen seconds. Meanwhile, some research suggests that having stronger pelvic muscles appears to enhance the intensity, duration and occurrence of orgasmic contractions. And intriguingly, it seems that orgasms can be truly consciousness-altering, as studies have revealed that electrical recordings (EEGs) of women's brain waves during particularly intense orgasms resemble the patterns seen in people who are in deep meditation.

Orgasms are complex, powerful creatures, and, not surprisingly, they are responsible for triggering a variety of bodily responses, not just muscular and not just aimed at the genitals. It's now appreciated that they elicit strong cardiovascular, respiratory and endocrine (hormonal) responses, and these too are considered as hallmarks of orgasm. For example, the extragenital responses of both women and men typically include a doubling of the heart and respiratory rate, with blood pressure commonly climbing to a third above normal, and pupils dilating. Many people vocalise their shocking, searing, completely overcoming sensations, and 'orgasm faces' are also distinctive. An intense rosy red sex flush across the chest is observed in three-quarters of women, although this is not as common in men (25 per cent).

The story of oh, ohh and ohhh!

Multiple orgasm, the ability to experience one orgasm after another after another, has also come under scrutiny. In the laboratory, the record for the greatest number of orgasms in an hour goes to a woman who, it is said, achieved a spectacular, mind-blowing and eye-watering 134. Not surprisingly, perhaps, how orgasmic a woman is also seems to have a knock-on effect on the time it takes her to come. In a study comparing the time to orgasm of women who are multiply orgasmic with singly orgasmic women, it was observed that, on average, multiply orgasmic women took eight minutes to reach orgasm, whereas singly orgasmic women took twenty-seven minutes. Interestingly, the average time to second orgasm for the multiply orgasmic women was only one to two minutes, as if the first orgasm had primed their bodies. After the second orgasmic event, subsequent orgasms tended to take even less time – thirty-second intervals between orgasms were not uncommon and a few fifteen-second intervals were recorded.

The most immediate difference between the two sexes' orgasms is that women are far more commonly multiorgasmic than men. This is typically because in order to enjoy orgasm after orgasm, men must learn to develop and strengthen their genital musculature, thus enabling them to have greater control over ejaculation. Indeed, if men wish to, they can use their pelvic muscles to stop themselves from ejaculating on orgasm. Men who are capable of separating these two processes report that they are then more likely to enjoy multiple orgasms. Moreover, it should be said that although ejaculation is classically associated as an integral part of male orgasm, strictly speaking this is incorrect. Ejaculation and orgasm are two separate physiological mechanisms. While orgasm is a perception accompanied by motor or muscular activity, ejaculation is just a reflex, a motor pattern that can occur independent of the brain (for example, in a spinal-cord-transected human or animal).

There is some good news for men, though, on the multiple orgasm front. Although male multiple orgasms are typically a result of utilising strong pelvic muscles to stop ejaculation occurring, science has also discovered a small group of men who experience multiple ejaculatory orgasms – that is, they are multiply orgasmic and ejaculate with every orgasm too. These men fall into three groups – some have always enjoyed multiple ejaculatory orgasms, others have taught themselves how to, and for others it has happened serendipitously. In one laboratory study, a thirty-five-year-old man enjoyed six orgasms with six ejaculations, with a period of thirty-six minutes between his first and last orgasm (the first orgasm came eighteen minutes after he started stimulating himself). Despite these heroic efforts, women still come out on top in terms of multiple orgasms. As we've seen, the highest number of female orgasms recorded in a laboratory setting was 134, whereas the top score for men in the same length of time was sixteen. Strangely, the ratio of these figures almost mirrors that given by Teiresias, in his answer regarding who has the greatest pleasure during sex: 'thrice three to women, one only to men'.

An innate capacity?

One of the most startling recent discoveries about the characteristics of orgasm is that these muscle contractions are one of the first sensations humans ever experience. That is, incredibly, both female and male foetuses orgasm in the womb. The following description of female orgasm *in utero* is from the *American Journal of Obstetrics and Gynaecology*, and was reported by two Italian doctors during a routine pre-birth ultrasound scan.

> We recently observed a female fetus at 32 weeks' gestation touching the vulva with the fingers of the right hand. The caressing movements were centred primarily on the region of the clitoris. Movements stopped after 30 to 40 seconds and started again after a few minutes. Furthermore, these slight touches were repeated and were associated with short, rapid movements of pelvis and legs. After another break, in addition to this behaviour, the fetus contracted the muscles of the trunk and limbs, and then clonicotonic movements of the whole body followed. Finally, she relaxed and rested. We observed this behaviour for about 20 minutes. The mother was an active and interested witness, conversing with observers about her child's experience.

The authors concluded their astonishing account of *in utero* female orgasm by saying: 'The current observation seems to show not only that the excitement reflex can be evoked in female fetuses at the third trimester of gestation but also that the orgasmic reflex can be elicited during intrauterine life.' Perhaps it's not surprising to hear that male foetuses too have been found pleasuring themselves in the womb. Indeed, it's not unusual for parents-to-be to see their embryonic son grasping his erect penis *in utero*, while moving his hands in a repetitive masturbatory fashion, for up to fifteen minutes at a time.

How come humans have such an extraordinary capacity for orgasm? One answer is thought to lie with the number of sensory nerve pathways that can play a role in triggering human orgasm and pleasurable sensations. Orgasms don't appear out of nowhere, rather they must be built up to (and curiously and wonderfully, this orgasmic process can be as pleasurable as the orgasm itself). Sexual arousal typically occurs as a result of the activation of various nerves. This nerve stimulation (perhaps from caressing or kissing or more) then causes a further build-up of excitement and arousal until a level is reached that triggers a different, relatively high threshold motor system – and it is then that explosive, rhythmic muscular contractions are felt. Rhythm, the timing of the stimulation, is also a crucial factor in creating orgasm, as rhythm aids in recruiting more and more neural elements to fire together in what will be ultimately orgasmic harmony.

Typically when orgasm occurs, it is a result of one or more of three genital nerves being activated. These are the pudendal, pelvic and hypogastric nerves. These nerves are all genitospinal nerves, meaning they run from the genitalia and then project into a person's spinal cord, with each nerve system having a different level of entry into the spinal cord. This means that in women, if you stroke the clitoris and the sensitive skin (including labia and perineum) surrounding the opening of the vagina, then you're likely to be firing off the pudendal nerve. But if you stimulate the vagina, urethra, prostate and/or the cervix, it's the pelvic nerves that you're affecting. However, there is some overlap, as the hypogastric nerve transmits sensory stimuli from the uterus and cervix, as well as some vaginal sensation. There is also some overlap of the sensory fields of the pelvic and hypogastric nerves in the cervix. In men, the pudendal nerve innervates penile and scrotal skin; the hypogastric nerve transmits sensory stimuli from the testicles and anus; and the pelvic nerve is thought to innervate the prostate.

Variety is the spice of life

Two of the most controversial issues surrounding female orgasm are whether there is more than one type of orgasm, and whether one type of orgasm is better than another. The answer to the latter question is, I suggest, that an orgasm is an orgasm is an orgasm. If it's pleasurable enjoy it. And don't be swayed by the fad of the day. Do it your way, the way that pleasures you the best. But what about the first question? Is there such a thing as a vaginal orgasm, rather than a clitoral or a G-spot orgasm?

The answer, strictly speaking, is yes, but there's more to it than that. Fantastically, in women, because of the different sensory pathways involved in innervating the distinct areas of female genitalia, orgasm can and does come in a glorious variety of ways. Just the cadence of gentle clitoral caressing alone can cause orgasm, but so too can vibratory stimuli focusing primarily on the urethra or prostate (G spot), or singling out the cervix for pulsatile thrusting stimulation, or simply squeezing the vaginal muscles. This appreciation of the nerve pathways underlying orgasm also explains why anal intercourse is an orgasmic activity for women – as the hypogastric nerve also innervates the rectum. And if I was hellbent on classifying, I'd say that the first orgasm was clitoral, the second a G spot, the third cervical, the fourth vaginal and the fifth anal. Importantly, though, when it comes down to it, most women will experience a blend of the above, as in practice it is extremely unlikely that just one nerve pathway will be stimulated. So most orgasms are, in fact, a delicious blend, and what could be wrong with that?

One of the most significant discoveries regarding female orgasm stems from a greater appreciation of the nerve pathways involved in orgasm. While it has been known since the start of the 1990s that the pudendal, pelvic and hypogastric nerves transmit genital sensations, and are therefore key in triggering female and male orgasm, it has only recently been recognised that in the female, another nerve pathway plays an important role. It seems that, pleasingly, for women at least, there are more ways to orgasm than previously supposed.

The first clues that there may be more to understanding how female orgasm can occur came from anecdotal reports in the 1960s and 1970s of women with 'complete' spinal cord injuries (SCI) who nevertheless spoke of experiencing orgasms during their sleep. (Criteria of complete SCI include being unaware of pinpricks or light touch below the level of injury, and also not having any voluntary movement or rectal sensation below this level). Dubbed 'phantom orgasms' by the medical profession, these 'orgasmic' feelings experienced by women with complete SCI were, for the major part, dismissed.

However, evidence pointing to another nerve pathway to orgasm mounted. Other women who were paralysed, with no feeling below the breast, also related how they appeared to have retained some awareness of their internal genitalia, speaking of feeling an 'abdominal glow' during sexual intercourse or of feeling the cramping uterine sensations of menstruation. Reports of such genital sensations posed an intriguing puzzle for the medical community – all known orgasmic and genital sensory pathways involved genitospinal nerves, therefore injuries to the spinal cord would interrupt their input, ultimately denervating a person's genitalia. Without any known nerves innervating their genitalia, how could women with complete SCI perceive and enjoy orgasm? In part because of any physical evidence to the contrary, these reports continued to be dismissed as phantoms or fancies of female imagination.

However, during the 1990s, the anecdotal reports of female orgasm and genital sensations despite a lack of functioning genitospinal nerves were backed up by evidence from scientific studies involving women with complete SCI. These pioneering studies showed that, for these women, despite their injuries, vaginal and cervical stimulation with a genital stimulator elicited both perceptual and autonomic orgasmic responses. That is, the women perceived themselves as experiencing orgasm – indeed, their descriptions of orgasm are indistinguishable from those of able-bodied women. They also expressed physical awareness of the genital stimulator, describing the sensation at the cervix as 'a nice feeling of suction' and as 'deep in the abdomen'. Vaginal stimulation was detailed as 'feeling deep inside'. To add to this, characteristic involuntary responses to orgasm (autonomic responses) were observed too – widening of the pupils, increased heart rate and elevated blood pressure. These women were experiencing orgasm, but how?

The wanderer returns

The answer lies with the vagus nerve, the wandering, seemingly whimsical nerve which, courtesy of its many branches, innervates many of the body's major organs. The vagus, named from the Latin for 'to wander', lives up to its monicker, emerging from the brain stem into the neck and then weaving and wending its way round the body, passing through the chest cavity – heart and lungs – branching out to the pupils of the eye and the salivary glands, connecting with the abdomen, the intestines, the bladder and the adrenal glands, yet – crucially – neatly bypassing the spinal cord. Finally and fortuitously, the circuitous path that the vagus nerve system takes through the body ends with it anchoring itself in the uterus and cervix.

It is because of the vagus' genitalic connection in the uterus and cervix that women with complete SCI can still perceive vaginal and cervical stimulation and enjoy the resulting pleasures of orgasm. It is vagus nerve fibres that are transmitting genital sensations to the brain, and because the vagus bypasses the spinal cord, this system is not affected by spinal cord injuries. (It's estimated that up to 50 per cent of women with spinal cord injuries are able to achieve orgasm.) Whether or not the vagus operates in a similar manner in men is as yet unclear, although there are hints that it may.

As a result of uncovering the role of the vagus nerve in transmitting genitosensory stimulation, and generating female orgasm, some scientists are starting to rethink ideas about genital sensation, orgasm, and the origins of orgasm. The vagus, one of the cranial nerves, is of major significance to species, starting with the most primitive vertebrates, right up to mammals. It is intimately involved in many basic bodily functions – breathing, swallowing, vomiting and digestion. Significantly, it is also, in evolutionary terms, ancient, and has been around since the early primitive vertebrates, such as the lamprey. Taken together, these facts – the vagus' ubiquity, history and present day-genitosensory innervation and orgasm role – suggest that the vagus may represent a primitive system for sensing the genitals and experiencing the muscular contractions and relaxations of orgasm.

Seeing in the dark

We've already seen that the vagina is an incredibly intelligent organ – capable of sorting and selecting sperm with a remarkable specificity. But can you credit that the vagina has extra sensory perception (ESP) too? The discovery of the role of the vagus nerve in human female orgasm suggests that it does. In the studies investigating how women without functioning genitospinal nerves (complete SCI) perceived genital sensations and orgasm, two distinct groups emerged. The first were women who stated that they could consciously feel the genital stimulator in their vagina or against their cervix, and it was this sensation, transmitted by the vagus nerve, that then triggered their orgasms.

However, there was a second group of SCI women who were orgasmic too; and orgasm in these women was more perplexing. These women experienced orgasm with the genital stimulator in their vagina or against their cervix, despite the fact that they did not consciously perceive any physical sensation from the genital stimulator or their genitalia. Somehow, though, their vaginas sensed the applied vibrating genital stimulation (even if they didn't consciously) and responded orgasmically. How can this be so? One suggestion as to how this might occur is that the vagina may be capable of experiencing the phenomenon known as 'blindsight'.

Blindsight is the term traditionally applied to the ability of some people with lesions in the visual cortex to respond appropriately to visual stimuli without having any conscious visual experience. That is, they respond as though they can see, even though they cannot see. And in some of the women with SCI, they respond as though they can feel the genital stimulation, even though they cannot feel it. So is this female orgasmic experience the equivalent in the female genital system of blindsight in the visual system? Moreover, is it the input of the vagus nerves that produces genital blindsight? With research into vaginal blindsight still at a very early stage, perhaps it's not surprising that the jury is still out on these questions. Other questions remain to be answered too. Vaginal blindsight appears to suggest that the female genital orgasmic response is particularly robust. Why should this be so? Is female orgasm or the ability of female genitalia to respond in a characteristic muscular fashion essential for evolution or successful sexual reproduction?

Curiously, the human capacity for orgasm is not limited to arousal stemming from stimulation of genital nerves, be it the pudendal, pelvic, hypogastric or vagus nerves. Orgasm can also be triggered as a result of stimulation of non-genital nerves too. Non-genital orgasms – orgasms resulting from erotic and rhythmic stimulation of the breasts, mouth, knees, ears, shoulder, chin and chest – all these have been recorded in a research setting. Pioneering sex researchers Masters and Johnson observed back-of-the-neck, small-of-the-back, bottom-of-the-foot and palm-of-the-hand orgasms, and chose to view the whole body as a potentially erotic organ. Both women and men with spinal cord injuries anecdotally report that stimulation of the hypersensitive skin zone that develops at or near the level of the injury to the spinal cord is capable of eliciting orgasm.

Laboratory investigations of these orgasmic episodes reveal that orgasm is indeed occurring. In one case, use of a vibrator on a woman's hypersensitive skin zone at her neck and shoulder resulted within several minutes in a characteristic increase in blood pressure, and an orgasm described as a 'tingling and rush'. The woman added how her 'whole body feels like it's in my vagina'. And while such non-genital phenomena demonstrate that orgasms can be produced by sensory stimulation of the rest of the human body, as well as the genitalia, other studies involving women show how, incredibly, imagery alone can be sufficient to trigger orgasm. For this group of women, physical stimulation was not needed to induce orgasm; their minds alone, thanks to fantasy, could take them there – despite being in a laboratory.

Of animals and orgasm

The fact that the phenomenon of female orgasm in humans is so flexible and robust raises the question of whether other females of other species are orgasmic. Although initially disputed and highly controversial, it is now generally accepted that female animals are capable of experiencing orgasm. There is, in fact, a wealth of information showing that many species undergo precisely the same physiological responses that humans do when they come. For example, in both female and male primates, powerful, rapid and rhythmic genital muscular contractions underpin orgasm. Studies show that in many female primates, the signature muscle contractions that shudder through the uterus, vagina and anus during copulation or masturbation typically go hand-in-hand with other physiological responses, such as vaginal engorgement, clitoral erection, tension in the muscles of the body, abrupt heart rate increases and piloerection (hair standing on end). These genital contractions are also associated with behavioural responses, such as copulation calls (rhythmic vocalised expirations), a characteristic 'look back and reach back' at the male reaction, and finally, what is known as the climax, or 'O' face – a distinctive facial expression with the mouth opened in an 'O'.

Amazingly, in female stumptail macaques, detailed measurements of uterine contraction patterns reveal them to begin to change markedly (increasing in intensity and pressure) up to eight to ten seconds before the climax face is shown. These genital contractions then continue to contract and relax for up to fifty seconds. Significantly, the female's climax face occurs when the contractile force of the uterus reaches its peak. This open-mouthed facial expression can then last for up to thirty seconds, disappearing before the macaque's pelvic muscular contractions ebb away to pre-orgasmic levels.

A wealth of other female animals display an orgasmic muscular reflex during and after sexual activity, and also when indulging in non-reproductive sexual activities – be they manipulating their own genitalia or those of fellow females. Following genital and urethral stimulation, female rats display a rhythmic coitus reflex of their pelvic muscles, just like male rats do. Cows respond orgasmically to massage of their clitoris, with muscular contractions of their uterus, cervix and vagina. After only a few minutes' clitoral stimulation, a cow's cervix can be observed gaping open and moving. The domestic cat exhibits an orgasmic genital muscular 'after-reaction', as well as screeching her sensations, while elsewhere in the farmyard, a sow's vagina (with its spiral-shaped cervix) is seen to grasp the male pig's penis during orgasm, as she apparently grinds until she's satisfied. Horse breeders comment on the 'orgasmic' muscular coital reactions of mares.

In fact, it appears impossible to find an internally fertilising female who does not respond to sexual stimulation with characteristic genital muscle contractions. Mice, guinea-pigs, dogs and more have all had their powerful vaginal contractions detailed in the scientific literature. One study looking at female dogs notes, with interest, how the vaginal muscle spasms of the bitch were so strong and violent that they 'could obliterate the urethral lumen of the penis were it not protected by the os penis [the penis bone]'. Indeed, it's suggested that the bones in some males' phalluses, like primates and dogs, are there to prevent penile injury, such as urethral damage, as a result of the female's crushing and potentially pulverising genital contractions. And finally, as previously highlighted, powerful rhythmic movements of the female's pelvic musculature are a key component of sexual activity throughout the insect kingdom too. It seems that genital muscle contractions are a crucial component of female orgasm, and as we'll see, there is a reason for this.

Do animals enjoy orgasm?

But first, a quick comment on animals and orgasm. Do animals enjoy and take pleasure in the vibrations of orgasm? Although many people would perhaps rather presume that other species do not delight in orgasm there is plenty of evidence to suggest that they do. Many mammals show enjoyment of sexual activities, including copulation, same-sex play and masturbation (both in the wild and in captivity). Females not only fondle their external genitalia (as previously detailed), they also find novel ways of stimulating themselves internally. Female chimpanzees and orang-utans insert objects, such as leaf stems and twigs, into their vaginas, moving them repeatedly inside, adding extra lubrication by licking them, and sometimes rocking backwards and forwards on their makeshift sex toy. Female chimpanzees have even been observed carefully biting pieces of plant to the particular length required for insertion and stimulation. In the laboratory, witness the orgasm face of the female stumptail macaque as her genital contractions peak. Or how about the study that revealed how, during thrusting vaginal stimulation, and at the point of orgasm (characterised by peak pelvic contractions), primate females reached back in order to increase the pressure the genital stimulator was applying to their genitalia. It seems they wanted more pleasure.

Astonishingly, female dolphins are equally inventive in their search for internal genital pleasure. Female-female dolphin sex play can include the insertion of one dolphin's fin or tail fluke into the female partner's genital slit. Beak-genital propulsion is another variant on this, whereby one dolphin inserts her snout or beak into the genital slit of another female, simultaneously stimulating her while, swimming, she propels her forwards. Female dolphins have also been observed using their vaginal muscles to carry small rubber balls, which they then rub and squeeze their genitalia against.

The function of the female orgasm

Humans enjoy it, and animals do too. And as we've seen, it's underpinned by characteristic contractions of the genital muscles. But just what is the function of the female orgasm? While female sexual pleasure, be it orgasmic or simply highly stimulating, has in recent centuries been read as having no role to play in sexual reproduction, this, I suggest, is not strictly correct. Significantly, there are a variety of reasons why this is the case. First of all, in the majority of female species, a specific degree of female genital stimulation is essential for successful sexual reproduction to occur. As previously highlighted, the design of female genitalia effectively dictates what a male must do if he is to have a chance of gaining entry to her body, and the opportunity of access to her eggs. Moreover, once inside her, he must then fulfil a whole new heap of genital requirements if the female is to respond in a way that enables his sperm to have the opportunity of having an encounter with one of her eggs. If he does not satisfy these requirements laid down via the design of her vagina, then she has the power to eject, digest or destroy his sperm.

For males, this situation means that if their sexual performance does not come up to scratch – if they do not provide the requisite level of female genital stimulation at the right time and in the right place, both externally and internally – then their opportunity to father offspring will fall by the wayside. They may not get a second chance either, because as most females mate with multiple males, another male will soon take their place. More starkly, if a male never learns the right routine with which to pleasure females of his species then it's very unlikely that he will ever reproduce successfully. In the animal and insect kingdoms, it's never a sensible sexual strategy to enter without permission, dump your sperm quickly and leave. This is why applying the 'correct' level of female genital stimulation, which in some cases may be orgasmic, is essential for successful sexual reproduction.

Some mammals, such as rabbits, cats, ferrets, minks, squirrels and voles, provide a very clear example of the specific degree of female genital stimulation that males must provide if they are to reproduce successfully. These mammals are reflex or mating-induced ovulators – that is, ovulation, the release of an egg, occurs as a reflexive reaction to a requisite level of genital stimulation. In this way, reflexive ovulation is akin to male ejaculation, the reflexive release of semen. In female prairie voles, for example, the likelihood of ovulation is related to the number of vaginal thrusts the female feels (the more she receives, the better the chance of ovulation occurring).

For rabbits, some of the necessary female genital stimuli to trigger ovulation are known. First of all the male rabbit must perform up to seventy rhythmic constant-amplitude, high-frequency extra-vaginal thrusts (too low a frequency and a lack of rhythm does not get results). Vaginal entry is dependent on this particular rhythmic routine, and this stimulation may also begin the cascade of hormonal events necessary to trigger the release of an egg. Once permitted access to a doe's internal genitalia, cervico-vaginal stimulation must then be sufficient to trigger the necessary hormonal conditions for ovulation to occur. Taken as a whole, the specific choreography of rabbit sex shows the importance of the male stimulating the female both internally and externally – providing both foreplay and fucking, if you will.

Why human ovulation is not strictly spontaneous

Many other mammalian species, such as cows, pigs, rats, sheep, mice, hamsters and humans, are termed spontaneous ovulators, that is, they *normally* ovulate in response to cyclical changes in hormone levels. However, the crucial word here is normally. Cows, pigs, rats, sheep, mice, hamsters and humans are also all capable of ovulating reflexively, i.e., in response to a specific degree or type of genital stimulation. Thus sexual choreography in these species is also crucial for males who want to optimise their reproductive success. (Stimulation prompting ovulation in these species is commonly genital, but it can also be olfactory, ocular, acoustic or emotional.) In female cows, ovulation can be brought on by sufficient stimulation of the clitoris, while cervical stimulation hastens the surge of luteinising hormone (LH), which stimulates ovulation.

Studies involving artificial insemination in cattle have also highlighted that genital stimulation can help cows conceive. Put plainly, the effectiveness of artificial insemination in cattle is markedly increased if accompanied by rectal manipulation of the uterus. If a cow does not receive 'enough' genital stimulation then conception rates fall. This same situation occurs with sheep. If animal breeders wish to increase conception rates in ewes significantly, they employ a vasectomised ram to genitally pleasure the female. Simply placing semen in a sheep's vagina is not sufficient to ensure successful sexual reproduction (or a profitable artificial insemination business).

The reproductive need for specific levels of genital stimulation is even clearer with female rats. Here, the number and rhythm of intromissions (the number of times the male's penis is inserted into and enveloped by the vagina, and the timing in between the intromissions) before ejaculation is directly related to whether or not the female becomes pregnant. If the number of intromissions is less than three, then she will not conceive, even though the male deposited his ejaculate (the preferred number of intromissions is between ten and fifteen). Significantly, his failure to father offspring with her is directly related to the level and rhythm of genital stimulation he provided.

Some details of the neuroendocrine mechanisms underlying this rodent situation are understood. It's known that the vaginal stimuli from intromission are picked up in the female rat by the pelvic nerve, and if enough of this particular stimulus is received, it triggers the secretion of the hormone prolactin, which in turn causes ovarian progesterone to be secreted. It is this secretion of progesterone which stimulates uterine growth, preparing it for the implantation of a fertilised egg. Not enough rhythmic vaginal-cervical stimulation equals not enough progesterone secreted equals an unresponsive uterus and the failure of a potential pregnancy. The degree of male stimulation can also significantly affect the number of eggs a female ovulates – the more thrusts female rats receive, the more eggs released.

As previously discussed, women too are not immune to the hastening effects on ovulation of intense genital stimulation and orgasm. However, it remains unclear whether it is the gonadal hormonal surges post-orgasm and genital stimulation that can elicit ovulation, or whether it is orgasmic muscular contractile forces shaking already primed and highly tensile ovaries that can cause ovulation to occur earlier than it would have done. Perhaps both. As the vagus is among the nerves that innervate the ovaries, there is also the possibility that vagally induced orgasm may well have a knock-on effect on the ovaries and egg release. Plus, smooth muscle is a constituent of ovarian tissue, and so compounds that act on smooth muscle may also affect the timing of egg extrusion. The mechanics remain to be determined, although it is clear that orgasm can and does influence the timing of ovulation in women. Curiously, in the 1800s, the moment of ovulation – when the ovarian follicle is at its most swollen and poised to extrude its contents – was known as *l'orgasme de l'ovulation*, a phrase that ties in with the original Greek meaning of orgasm – to grow ripe, or swell. And elsewhere in nineteenth-century medical writings, 'orgasm' implies extreme turgidity or an organ under a great state of pressure.

When the earth moves

As well as affecting the timing of ovulation, the number of eggs released and the viability of uterine implantation, there are other ways in which female genital stimulation and/or orgasm can influence the outcome of sexual intercourse. As we have seen, orgasm and/or genital stimulation has a very striking effect on a female's genital musculature – namely, increasing the intensity and frequency of rhythmic, rippling contractions and relaxations. These characteristic genital muscular vibrations are present in a vast variety of internally fertilising species, perhaps all, from women and chimpanzees, cows and sheep, rats and mice to chickens and dunnocks, bees and beetles. And as previous chapters have demonstrated, sperm transport is primarily a female-dominated affair.

What is significant in terms of sexual reproduction is that it's now increasingly recognised that the contractile forces wielded by a female's genital musculature play a critical role in how she transports sperm through her reproductive system. If the internal vaginal and uterine pressure is just so, and the pelvic muscle contractions are tuned just right, say with contraction waves running from the cervix to the ovary, plus the cervix is poised to dilate at the critical moment, then it is far more likely that any sperm present will be pulled towards a female's ova rather than being ferried away. Some studies, most notably in cows and pigs, have highlighted just how this can work.

Throughout the ovulation cycle of cows and pigs, spontaneous myometrial (uterine muscle) contractions occur. Outside of oestrus, these contractions start at the tubal end of the uterine horns and run towards the cervix – that is, contractions move against any sperm present. However, during oestrus, this pattern of muscle contraction reverses, and contractions start at the cervix and run towards the Fallopian tubes. Any sperm present at this point in the cycle are thus effectively placed on a moving walkway running direct to the female's eggs. Female orgasm during oestrus, courtesy of the increase in strength and frequency of muscle contractions, acts to enhance this directional effect, increasing the likelihood of sperm being retained and conception occurring.

Research in other species also underlines how genital stimulation and/or orgasm affects these sperm-transporting muscle contractions. In the mare, the stimulus of mating results in forceful genital contractions and a strong negative uterine pressure, which results in a forceful 'insuck' of fluid from the vagina into the uterus. In hamsters, what were described as 'dramatic vaginal contractions associated with mating' resulted in the rapid transport (within ninety-one seconds) of sperm into the uterus. In mice, high cervical tension is associated with reduced amounts of semen flowing back out of the vagina. In rats, sperm transport does not take place unless a female receives more than two intromissions.

On the other hand, if not enough stimulation is applied prior to ejaculation, sperm can be summarily digested or ejected. As noted, female damselflies tend to retain the sperm of males who provide more stimulation, and expel the sperm of males who provide less (average forty-one minutes versus seventeen minutes). Significantly, research has shown that stimulation of the sensillae that line the female damselfly's reproductive tract does indeed result in the reflex contraction of the muscles of her sperm storage site. In sheep, stressful, as opposed to pleasant stimuli have been shown to influence sperm transport too, reducing the numbers of sperm reaching the uterus.

Does it work for women too?

And what about women? Studies show that there are two important factors in determining how many of a man's sperm a woman transports and retains. These vital factors are whether or not, and when, the muscular contractions of orgasm occur. Interestingly, research has revealed that if a woman comes any time from one minute before the man to three minutes afterwards, then she will retain more sperm than if she had not come at all, or if she came much earlier or much later than him. This difference is estimated to represent about ten million sperm.

The sperm transport and retention effect is thought to come about because at the onset of female orgasm, muscular contractions cause intrauterine pressure to increase markedly, together with a rise in vaginal pressure. However, immediately post-orgasm, intrauterine pressure drops sharply, creating a pressure gradient between a woman's uterus and her vagina. Hence, if sperm are present in a woman's cervical mucus when she comes, the suction created by this pressure gradient results in the more rapid transport of sperm into her uterus. The cervix and its mucus play an important role in this scenario, as during the build-up to orgasm the cervix dips down further into the vaginal chamber, extruding mucus from its external os. If sex is taking place during a woman's fertile period, this mucus is capable of sequestering sperm in its shimmering folds. Moreover, post-orgasm, the sharp changes in genital pressure result in bodyguard mucus (and its sperm load) being sucked back through the cervical canal and up into the uterus.

The pituitary hormone oxytocin is believed to be at least part of the reason why enough genital stimulation and orgasm results in genital muscle movement and sperm transport. Oxytocin, amongst many other effects, has the ability to stimulate the contraction of smooth muscle. When it comes to female genitalia, this ability is of particular importance, because a female's genitals – including the uterus, cervix, ovaries, vagina and prostate – contain smooth muscle. In women, genital stimulation causes levels of oxytocin to rise, and as arousal increases, so too does muscular tension. Surges of oxytocin are then strongly associated with the strong uterine and vaginal muscular contractions of orgasm, the gaping or dilation of the cervical os, and the widening of a person's pupils. Significantly, the intensity of muscle contractions during human female (and male) orgasm are highly correlated with levels of oxytocin.

In many other mammals too, including cows, rabbits, goats, and ewes, rapid increases in oxytocin are accompanied by forceful uterine or cervical muscle movements. Indeed, oxytocin, from the Greek for 'swift birth', is named after its most dramatic effect on female genitalia – the massively powerful uterine smooth muscle contractions of labour. This striking parturition response to oxytocin is, of course, why pregnant women are often advised to indulge in passionate orgasmic sex. Milk ejection, or letdown, is another of oxytocin's stunning effects. Incredibly, cow's vaginas are so responsive to genital stimulation that blowing air into their vaginas is sufficient to elicit this response, and, fantastically, increase milk yield. Indeed, this technique of blowing into the vagina has been used as an aid to milking for centuries, and still is today.

The choreography of sex

For some species, the movement of a female's vaginal musculature takes on another significant task in sexual reproduction. For these females, controlling the direction of sperm transport is not enough; their muscles are also required to ensure sperm transfer occurs. That is, it is the female's forceful rhythmic muscle vibrations that are responsible for triggering ejaculation of semen. For example, the vaginal muscles of honey bees are believed to be responsible for triggering the male's ejaculation, while the genital musculature of the marsh-dwelling bug is so strong that it effectively sucks sperm from the male's phallus. The idea that it is the contractile force of a female's vagina that provides the necessary physical stimulus for some males to ejaculate is lent weight by artificial insemination techniques. In male boars and dogs, for example, rhythmic pulsation (courtesy of a battery-powered vagina) must be applied to the penis if ejaculation is to occur.

This field of research – understanding how different species' vaginal muscles work during genital stimulation and/or orgasm – is still very much in its infancy, and much more research needs to be done before a clearer picture can emerge of how prevalent this 'ejaculation technique' is. Most of the studies are still confined to insect or mammal species. Yet, in the majority of species, a female's genital musculature is astonishingly steely, capable of providing the necessary phallic squeeze.

When it comes to primates, women are among those that show an ejaculatory muscular wherewithal. If a woman has well-developed vaginal muscles, it is possible, and pleasurable for her, to use them to grip, embrace, squeeze and ultimately cause herself to come, and the man to ejaculate. Movement on the male's part is not essential. It is also the case that the rapid forceful pelvic contractions that occur as a woman orgasms are often the physical (as well as erotic) extra that causes a man to orgasm and ejaculate. This timing – a woman's orgasm triggering a man's ejaculation – sits well with the theory of uterine and vaginal pressure changes and contractions influencing the upsuck of semen.

The idea of a female's orgasmic genital contractions providing the timely trigger for the male is underlined in intimate and surprising detail in a recording of the responses of two stumptail macaques during three consecutive copulations (see Figure 7.5). From the moment when the female presents to the male, to the point where she orgasms seven seconds before him during the first copulation, to the second and third copulations where they orgasm simultaneously, to the post-coital grooming session, an intriguing picture emerges of how synchronised the two stumptail macaques are in their sexual responses to each other. Not only do the climax faces coincide, but the point at which uterine activity increases rapidly and rhythmically in intensity immediately precedes the point of ejaculation each time. Interestingly, in the second and third copulation bouts, the female's 'look back and reach back' action appears to direct or signal the male's thrusting and ejaculatory response. Is she communicating to choreograph mutual orgasm?

In fact, there is a growing body of evidence showing that copulation in primates is characterised by an astonishing level of communication flowing between the female and male – be it facial (head-turning, looking back, climax face), vocal (copulation calls) or physical (reach and clutchback). This communication, it is suggested, plays a role in co-ordinating the male's thrusts and ejaculation with the female's muscular responses and orgasm. Moreover, it is the female who is the prime mover here. It is female rhesus monkeys that reach and clutch back, heralding their orgasm contractions, and seemingly firing off the male's ejaculatory response. Elsewhere, slow-motion films of bonobo sex reveal that the speed and intensity of the male's thrusting is regulated by the female's facial expressions, and/or her vocalisations. Bonobos also communicate sexual information physically. Amazingly, evidence shows that bonobos have developed their own sexual lexicon of hand gestures to negotiate and co-ordinate movements in sexual bouts.

While it is certainly true that today human female orgasm is not essential for conception to occur, I believe that the influence orgasm continues to have on egg extrusion and movement (ovulation and whether implantation occurs), as well as sperm transport and sperm

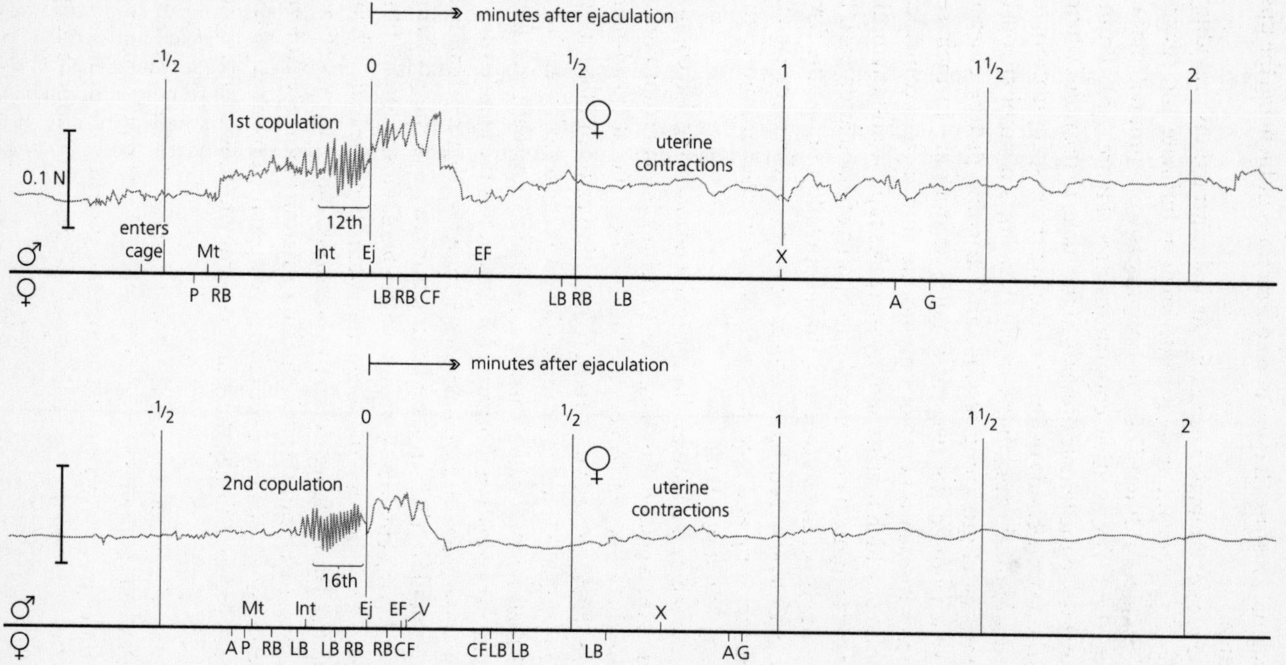
minutes after ejaculation
-1/2
0
1/2
1
1 1/2
2
1st copulation
0.1 N
12th
uterine contractions
enters cage
Mt
Int
Ej
EF
X
P RB
LB RB CF
LB RB
LB
A
G
minutes after ejaculation
2nd copulation
16th
Mt
Int
Ej
EF
V
X
A P
RB
LB
LB RB
RB CF
CF LB LB
LB
A G

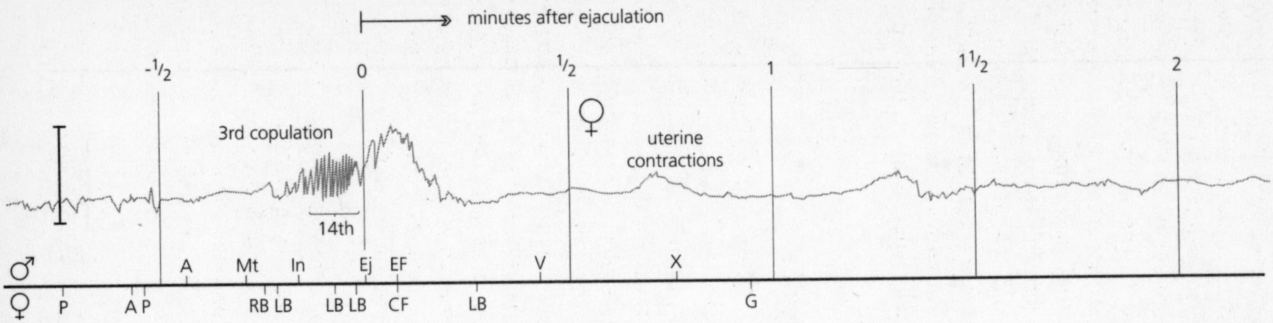

Figure 7.5 Choreographing sex and orgasm: how the uterine contractions and behaviour of a female stumptail macaque compare with those of a male stumptail macaque during three consecutive copulations. Uterine contraction force is measured in Newtons (N) (Adapted from Slob AK, 1986).
Female behaviours include P=present; A=approach; RB=reach back with hand towards male; LB=look back towards male; C=climax face; G=grooming male.
Male behaviours include A=approach; Mt=mount; Int=penile intromission; Th=number of pelvic thrusts; Ej=ejaculation face; V= vocalisation; X=end of penile intromission.

transfer, points to the origin of this pleasurable muscle and nerve phenomenon. I imagine that female orgasm – the rhythmic, forceful, rippling contractions and relaxations of genital muscles – evolved from the female's need to control and co-ordinate the transport of both ova and sperm within her reproductive anatomy. With its accompanying symphony of hormones, the (orgasmic) muscular contractions of female genitalia do indeed manage to orchestrate egg and sperm movement, often with an exquisite amount of precision. Reproductively speaking, it is to every female's advantage to be able to achieve this manipulation of egg and sperm movement inside herself. The result, if a female is allowed free choice of mates and free movement of her genitalia, is conception with the most genetically compatible partner, and hence optimally successful sexual reproduction.

The penis as internal courtship device

This book has looked in large part at the *raison d'ętre* of the vagina – in both sexual pleasure and reproduction. And one particular view explored is why it is essential for internally fertilising females to possess fully functioning, exquisitely sensitive and powerfully muscular genitals. However, this story would not be complete if some further consideration was not given to the penis – most males' vaginal equivalent. If the vagina's primary role is to ensure successful sexual reproduction with the most genetically compatible males, what is the purpose of the penis? Some might say that the penis functions purely as a sperm placement tool, a rigid insertion device shaped to shoot sperm quickly and efficiently into the correct orifice. A quick glance at different species' copulatory routines and the time it takes males to ejaculate reveals that this cannot be the whole tale.

Sex sequences across the animal kingdom are routinely complex and lengthy. Some males spend hours stimulating females, genitally and otherwise, before they even present their phallus to her. Rubbing, caressing, kissing, stroking, vibrating, nuzzling, rocking, even singing and feeding, can form part of a male's essential copulatory courtship. And once genitally surrounded by the female, many other males take far more time than is necessary to give up their gametes if sperm deposition is the only goal of the routine. Spider monkeys stay mounted for up to thirty-five minutes, while sex for greater galagos can last more than two hours. The male marsupial mouse, *Antechinus flavipes*, must thrust inside the female about once every four minutes during the approximately five hours of copulation.

It's not just mammals that delay ejaculation; many other species do to. The male tsetse fly copulates on average for sixty-nine minutes, with sperm transfer only occurring in the last thirty seconds. Many spiders put the majority of their copulatory vigour into foreplay techniques. For example, the Sierra dome spider (*Nereine litigiosa*), will spend between two and six hours using its pedipalps (spider phallus) to stimulate the female genitally. Only after he has done this will he put sperm on the palps and attempt to inseminate her (this can take between 0.5 and 1.4 hours). Post-ejaculation, many species must continue to stimulate the female. Have a thought for the male thick-tailed bushbaby, where intromission (penis insertion) has to be heroically maintained for up to 260 minutes after ejaculation, although it appears that only intermittent bouts of thrusting are called for.

In fact, it is increasingly recognised that the answer to what the phallus is for lies in how a male's phallus can affect the vaginal environment that any sperm land in. As the majority of females enjoy multiple mating habits, the important question for a male is not: Can I place my sperm inside this female? Rather the crucial question is: Can I persuade this female to use my sperm instead of some other male's? Can I convince her, courtesy of the genital stimulation and pleasure my penis can provide, to take my sperm, transport it internally, and use it for fertilisation, rather than dumping it or destroying it? In fact, the primary role of the penis is none other than to act as an internal courtship device – shaped to provide the vagina with the best possible and reproductively successful stimulation. Providing the best, which in all likelihood means the most pleasurable genital stimulation, is, it seems, the way in which a male can persuade a female that he is fit to father some of her offspring.

This idea – that different species' penises are designed to provide maximum vaginal stimulation – is backed up by studies examining penis shape and movement and how this corresponds to vaginal and cervical structures; and by research analysing how increasingly intricate penile designs are correlated with increasingly complex female mating habits. First of all, penis shape and movement, and how it

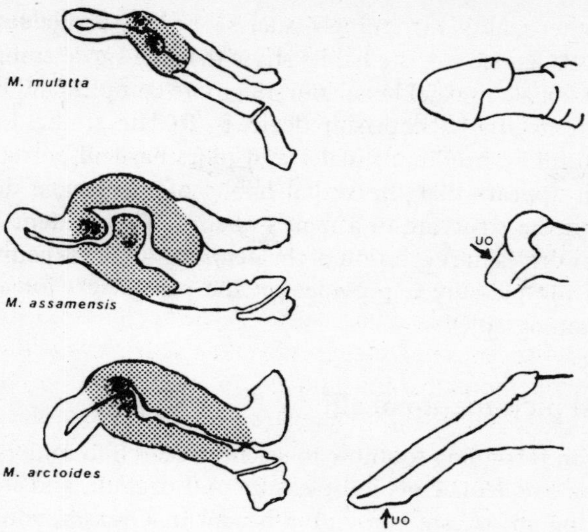

Figure 7.6 Measuring up for optimal stimulation: how the shape of female and male genitalia compare in macaques. The shaded areas of the females' genitalia show the extent of the uterine cervix, uo indicates the urethral opening of the male primate's penis (adapted from Dixson AF, 1998).

complements female genitalia. The curious helical shape of a pig's penis, with its screw-tip ending, appears to fit beautifully with a sow's spiral-shaped cervix. And it seems that this end structure is important in persuading a female pig to retain more sperm. Artificial insemination studies have shown that semen flowback is reduced if an artificial penis with a similar helical tip is used. The tail-like filament at the end of a bull's phallus suggests a similar story. It flips forwards at the point of ejaculation, seemingly designed to do nothing other than stimulate the female. Figure 7.6 shows how the vaginas and cervices of three species of macaques correspond with the males' phalluses.

Whether it is the specifically mushroom-shaped glans; or the frills and lappets surrounding the penile tip; or the elaborate adornments, sculpted lumps, bumps, spines and denticles found on a phallus' surface – all these penile accoutrements are there, it seems, to give the male an additional way of stimulating the female vaginally, in the hope that this stimulation will persuade her to use his sperm rather than another male's. Intriguingly, analyses of how penile design correlates with female mating habits show that the more complex and various a female's sexual behaviour, the more complex and elaborate a male's penis/internal courtship device is. To date, studies looking at bees, butterflies, beetles, primates and more have all borne out this theory. It appears that the sexual habits of the female determine and sculpt the structure of a male's phallus. That is, female sexual behaviour drives the evolution of the penis. And female genital structure and the pleasure it provides set the parameters for a species' sexual choreography.

The best pick-me-up of all?

There is an intriguing footnote to science's search to understand the significance of female genital pleasure and orgasm, and it explains why having an orgasm can cure a headache. Orgasm, you see, is a potent analgesic. That is, female orgasm increases a woman's threshold to pain (the point at which an externally applied increasing pressure becomes painful); in other words, orgasm has a pain-suppressing effect. Critically though, female orgasm does this without affecting a woman's response to tactile or pressure stimulation (it is not an anaesthetic and does not dull sensations). Studies show that women's pain thresholds increase by over 100 per cent as a result of orgasmic vaginal and cervical stimulation.

Research has also revealed that it's not just orgasm that has this effect; vaginal stimulation does too. However, the degree of pain suppression depends on the pleasure experienced – pleasurable vaginocervical stimulation increased women's pain thresholds by 75 per cent. This pain-blocking effect of pleasurable and orgasmic vaginal stimulation is found in other species too, including rats and cats, and these studies have shown the potent analgesic effect to be mediated by two genitospinal nerves – the pelvic and hypogastric nerves. In female rats, the vaginal stimulation of mating produces potent analgesia equivalent to a more than 15 mg/kg dose of morphine sulfate.

Why should vaginal stimulation and orgasm be an analgesic? One answer may lie in the multiple mating habits that the majority of females enjoy. It's suggested that this pain-attenuating mechanism may ensure that repeated copulations do not aggravate, irritate or cause pain to a female's genitalia, which from a reproductive point of view need to be sensitive and highly responsive. Imagine if the intense sensory stimulation of sex commonly resulted in genital hypersensitivity. In this scenario, females and males might never get close enough to each other for long enough to reproduce successfully, which would be disastrous for the survival of a species. In this sense, it is suggested that female sexual pleasure could be a significant adaptive factor in the physiology of reproduction and the evolution of the species.

One of the most common ideas about female genitalia over the last few centuries has been that the vagina has no role to play in sexual pleasure and reproduction other than that of a passive sperm vessel. What this book has hopefully demonstrated is that this notion is incorrect. Female genitalia are highly sensitive and responsive because they have a very significant and powerful role to carry out in both sexual reproduction and pleasure – for both the female and the male.

The pleasure principle

I would like to finish this book with a comment on a person's capacity for genital pleasure and orgasm. Everyone begins their life with an infinite capacity to experience and enjoy pleasure. This is as true of genitally focused pleasure as it is of any other source. Foetuses orgasming in the womb underline this. Significantly, though, it is increasingly recognised that how an individual responds to sexual pleasure (or any kind of pleasure) during their life is a mixture of both the physical processes the body is undergoing, and a completely subjective perception of what those processes represent. That is, a person's perception of sexual pleasure can be as contingent on their past experiences of genital pleasure (or lack of pleasure), and the rules and values their society promotes, as it is on the sea of chemicals that arousal and orgasm send coursing through their bloodstream.

First of all, how experience influences the enjoyment of genital pleasure. A lifetime, or merely a childhood, of being told to ignore genital sensations, or, on the other hand, never having anyone in 'authority' explain that genital pleasure is to be valued, can and does have a blunting effect on how an individual responds to the build-up and release of genital/sexual sensations in their body. For some lucky individuals, these sensations are taught as ones to be valued and are therefore rated as pleasurable; for others, their previous experiences teach them to ignore or suppress these stimuli or label them negatively. How subjective the perception of pleasure can be is illustrated by people's responses to orgasm. Some descriptions of orgasm talk of the sensation as being frightening; others speak of it being the most exciting, fulfilling and enjoyable sensation imaginable. The flood of chemicals may be the same, but the emotional response to that rush differs depending on a person's history.

The brain is, in fact, an amazingly powerful sexual organ, perhaps the most powerful, and is supremely capable of overriding sexual signals, if a person's past has taught them that it may be 'safer' or 'better' to do so. Indeed, studies have shown that the physical effects of female arousal and orgasm can be 'overlooked' or ignored. And ignoring or suppressing feelings of genital arousal is, it's suggested, easier for women to do, as they do not have an obvious visual sign of arousal to underline or emphasise how their body is actually feeling. Men, on the other hand, have in their erect penises a very handy feedback device, reminding them of how they feel, and making it a lot harder to 'ignore' genital sensations.

Secondly, society's role in valuing genital pleasure and orgasm. In the western world and the majority of societies, knowledge about genitalia and sexual pleasure has, until very recently, been shrouded under layers of religious and scientific ideology, much of it misleading or damaging. This is particularly true when it comes to discussions about female genitalia and female sexual pleasure. For these reasons, I don't find it particularly surprising that not all women enjoy their vaginas as much as they could. Anthropological evidence contrasting different cultures' attitudes towards information about sex and genital pleasure have revealed over and over again striking variations in orgasmic response. In societies where little or no sex education is given, and sex is decreed to be for procreation not pleasure, female orgasm and sexual pleasure can be relatively unknown. Yet, in those societies where women and men are taught from an early age to appreciate their own, and each other's, genitalia, as well as the pleasure genitals give, orgasm is achieved virtually universally and without difficulty for both sexes.

In 1948, the anthropologist Margaret Mead, after observing several

Pacific Island societies, made some remarkably astute observations on the cultural factors that affect a woman's capacity to experience sexual pleasure and orgasms (they also apply to men). Mead wrote that in order for a female to find sexual fulfilment:

1. She must live in a culture that recognises female desire as being of value.
2. Her culture must allow her to understand the mechanics of her sexual anatomy.
3. Her culture must teach the various sexual skills that can make women experience orgasm.

Fortunately for women (and men) the three tenets of this vital sex education message are starting to come across in the west, albeit slowly. Unbiased information about female genitalia and their role in sexual pleasure and reproduction is increasingly available, and the vagina is beginning to be viewed as valuable, from both a scientific and a cultural perspective – just as mythology tells us it should be. Unlike the sixteenth-century St Teresa, women can, and do, rejoice in their genitals and the pleasure they bring, as the following twentieth-century description of female orgasm shows: 'Without any effort or trying on my part, my body was moved from within, so to speak, and everything was right. There was rhythmic movement and a feeling of ecstasy at being part of something much greater than myself and finally of reward, of real satisfaction and peace.' Pride, pleasure and the miracle of creation – this view of the vagina is the real story of V.

FURTHER READING

Chapter 1: The Origin of the World

Andersen, Jørgen, *The Witch on the Wall: Medieval Erotic Sculpture in the British Isles*, Copenhagen: Rosenkilde & Bagger, 1977.

Ardener, Shirley, 'A note on gender iconography: the vagina', *The Cultural Construction of Sexuality*, ed. Pat Caplan, London: Tavistock (1987) 113–42.

Bishop, Clifford, *Sex and Spirit*, London: Macmillan Reference Books, 1996.

Camphausen, Rufus C., *The Yoni: Sacred Symbol of Female Creative Power*, Vermont: Inner Traditions, 1996.

Camphausen, Rufus C., *The Encyclopaedia of Sacred Sexuality: From Aphrodisiacs and Ecstasy to Yoni Worship and Zap-Lam Yoga*, Vermont: Inner Traditions, 1999.

Clark, Kenneth, *The Nude*, London: Penguin Books, 1956.

Estés, Clarissa Pinkola, *Women Who Run With the Wolves: Contacting the Power of the Wild Woman*, London: Rider, 1992.

Frank, Anne, *The Diary of a Young Girl: The Definitive Edition*, new translation, ed. Otto H. Frank and Mirjam Pressler, London: Puffin, 1997.

Frymer-Kensky, Tikva, *In the Wake of the Goddesses: Women, Culture and the Biblical Transformation of Pagan Myth*, New York: Fawcett Columbine, 1992.

Gimbutas, Marija, *The Gods and Goddesses of Old Europe – Myths and Cult Images*, London: Thames and Hudson, 1982.

Gimbutas, Marija, *The Living Goddesses*, Los Angeles: University of California Press, 1999.

Gimbutas, Marija, *The Language of the Goddess*, London: Thames and Hudson, 2001.

Halperin, David M., Winkler, John J., Zeitlin, Froma I., *Before Sexuality*, Princeton: Princeton University Press, 1991.

Jöchle, W., 'Biology and pathology of reproduction in Greek mythology', *Contraception*, 4 (1971), 1–13.
Lederer, Wolfgang, *The Fear of Women*, New York: Harcourt, Brace, Jovanovich, 1968.
Lubell, Winifred Milius, *The Metamorphosis of Baubo: Myths of Woman's Sexual Energy*, Nashville: Vanderbilt University Press, 1994.
Marshack, A., 'The Female Image: A "Time-factored" Symbol. A Study in Style and Aspects of Image Use in the Upper Palaeolithic', *Proceedings of the Prehistoric Society*, 57 (1991), 17–31.
Marshack, A., *The Roots of Civilisation*, New York: McGraw-Hill, 1972.
Murray, M. A., 'Female Fertility Figures', *Journal of the Royal Anthropological Institute of Great Britain and Ireland*, 64 (1934), 93–100.
Neumann, Erich, *The Great Mother: An Analysis of the Archetype*, trans. Ralph Mannheim, New Jersey: Princeton University Press, 1963.
Rudgeley, Richard, *Lost Civilisations of the Stone Age*, London: Arrow Books, 1999.
Singer, Kurt, 'Cowrie and Baubo in Early Japan', *Man*, 40 (1940), 50–53.
Stevens, John, *The Cosmic Embrace: An Illustrated Guide to Sacred Sex*, London: Thames and Hudson, 1999.
Stone, Merlin, *When God Was a Woman*, Florida: Harcourt Brace, 1976.
Suggs, R. C., *Marquesan Sexual Behaviour*, New York: Harcourt & Brace, 1966.
Taylor, Timothy, *The Prehistory of Sex: Four Million Years of Human Sexual Culture*, London: Fourth Estate, 1997.
Weir, Anthony, and Jerman, James, *Images of Lust: Sexual Carvings on Medieval Churches*, London: Routledge, 1986.
Yalom, Marilyn, *A History of the Breast*, London: Pandora, 1998.

Chapter 2: Femalia

Adams, J. N., *The Latin Sexual Vocabulary*, London: Duckworth, 1982.
Blank, Joani, *Femalia*, San Francisco: Down There Press, 1993.
Burgen, Stephen, *Your Mother's Tongue: A Book of European Invective*, London: Gollancz, 1996.
Chia, Mantak, and Chia, Maneewan, *Cultivating Female Sexual Energy: Healing Love Through the Tao*, New York: Healing Tao Books, 1986.
de Graaf, Reinier, 'New Treatise Concerning the Generative Organs of Women', 1672, annotated translation by Jocelyn, H B., and Setchell,

B.P., *Journal of Reproduction and Fertility*, Supplement 17, Oxford: Blackwell Scientific Publications, 1972.
Dickinson, Robert Latou, *Human Sex Anatomy*, Baltimore: Williams & Wilkins, 1949.
Dreger, Alice Domurat, *Hermaphrodites and the Medical Invention of Sex*, Cambridge, Mass.: Harvard University Press, 1998.
Eisler, Riane, *The Chalice and the Blade*, California: HarperCollins, 1988.
Ensler, Eve, *The Vagina Monologues*, New York: Villard, 1998.
Fagan, Brian, *From Black Land to Fifth Sun: The Science of Sacred Sites*, Reading, Mass.: Perseus Books, 1998.
Fissell, Mary, 'Gender and Generation: Representing Reproduction in Early Modern England', *Gender and History*, 7 (3) (1995), 433–56.
Laqueur, Thomas, *Making Sex: Body and Gender From the Greeks to Freud*, Cambridge, Mass.: Harvard University Press, 1990.
Lemay, Helen Rodnite, *Women's Secrets: A Translation of Pseudo-Albertus Magnus' De Secretis Mulierum with Commentaries*, New York: State University of New York Press, 1992.
Paros, Lawrence, *The Erotic Tongue: A Sexual Lexicon*, New York: Henry Holt & Company, 1984.
Porter, Roy, and Hall, Lesley, *The Facts of Life: The Creation of Sexual Knowledge in Britain, 1650–1950*, New Haven and London: Yale University Press, 1995.
Schiebinger, Londa, *The Mind Has No Sex? Women in the Origins of Modern Science*, Cambridge, Mass.: Harvard University Press, 1989.
Tannahill, Reay, *Sex in History*, London: Abacus, 1989.

Chapter 3: A Velvet Revolution

Arthur Jr, Benjamin I., Hauschteck-Jungen, Elisabeth, Nothiger, Rolf, Ward, Paul I., 'A female nervous system is necessary for normal sperm storage in *Drosophila melanogaster*: a masculinized system is as good as none', *Proceedings of the Royal Society of London B*, 265 (1998), 1749–53.
Ben-Ari, Elia T., 'Choosy Females', *BioScience*, 50 (2000), 7–12.
Birkhead, T.R., and Møller, A. P., (eds.), *Sperm Competition and Sexual Selection*, London: Academic Press, 1998.
Birkhead, Tim, *Promiscuity: An Evolutionary History of Sperm Competition and Sexual Conflict*, London: Faber and Faber, 2000.

Calsbeek, Ryan, and Sinervo, Bary, 'Uncoupling direct and indirect components of female choice in the wild', *Proceedings of the National Academy of Sciences*, 99 (23) (2000), 14897–902.

Eberhard, William G., *Sexual Selection and Animal Genitalia*, Cambridge, Mass.: Harvard University Press, 1985.

Eberhard, William G., *Female Control: Sexual Selection by Cryptic Female Choice*, New Jersey: Princeton University Press, 1996.

Frank, L.G., Glickman, S.E., Powch, I., 'Sexual dimorphism in the spotted hyaena (*Crocuta crocuta*)', *Journal of Zoology*, 221 (1990), 308–13.

Frank, Laurence G., 'Evolution of genital masculinization: why do female hyaenas have such a large "penis"?', *Trends in Ecology and Evolution*, 12 (1997), 58–62.

Hellrigel, Barbara, and Bernasconi, Giorgina, 'Female-mediated differential sperm storage in a fly with complex spermathecae, *Scatophaga stercoraria*', *Animal Behaviour*, 59 (1999), 311–17.

Hrdy, Sarah Blaffer, *The Woman That Never Evolved*, Cambridge, Mass.: Harvard University Press, 1999.

Hrdy, Sarah Blaffer, *Mother Nature: Natural Selection & the Female of the Species*, London: Chatto & Windus, 1999.

Margulis, Lynn, and Sagan, Dorion, *What is Sex?*, New York: Simon & Schuster Editions, 1997.

Neubaum, Deborah M., and Wolfner, Mariana F., 'Wise, winsome or weird? Mechanisms of sperm storage in female animals', *Current Topics in Developmental Biology*, 41 (1999), 67–97.

Newcomer, Scott, Zeh, David, Zeh, Jeanne, 'Genetic benefits enhance the reproductive success of polyandrous females', *Proceedings of the National Academy of Sciences*, 96 (102) (1999), 36–41.

Pitnick, Scott, Markow, Therese, Spicer, Greg S., 'Evolution of multiple kinds of female sperm-storage organs in *Drosophila*', *Evolution*, 53 (6) (1999), 1804–22.

Pizzari, T., and Birkhead, T. R., 'Female feral fowl eject sperm of subdominant males', *Nature*, 405 (2000), 787–9.

Small, Meredith F., *Female Choices: Sexual Behaviour of Female Primates*, Ithaca: Cornell University Press, 1993.

Tavris, Carol, *The Mismeasure of Woman*, New York: Simon & Schuster, 1992.

Wedekind, Claus, Chapuisat, M., Macas, E., Rulicke, T., 'Non-random fertilization in mice correlates with MHC and something else', *Heredity*, 77 (1995), 400–9.

Chapter 4: Eve's Secrets

Angier, Natalie, *Woman: An Intimate Geography*, London: Virago, 1999.
Bagemihl, Bruce, *Biological Exuberance: Animal Homosexuality and Natural Diversity*, London: Profile Books, 1999.
Chalker, Rebecca, *The Clitoral Truth*, New York: Seven Stories Press, 2000.
Cloudsley, Anne, *Women of Omdurman: Life, Love and the Cult of Virginity*, London: Ethnographica, 1983.
de Waal, Frans, and Lanting, Frans, *Bonobo: The Forgotten Ape*, Berkeley: University of California Press, 1997.
Dixson, Alan F., *Primate Sexuality: Comparative studies of the prosimians, monkeys, apes and human beings*, Oxford: Oxford University Press, 1998.
Fisher, Helen, *Anatomy of Love: A Natural History of Mating, Marriage and Why We Stray*, New York: Ballantine Books, 1992.
Galen, *On the Usefulness of the Parts (De usu partinum)*, Book 14.9, Vol. II, trans. Margaret Tallmadge May, Ithaca, New York: Cornell University Press, 1968.
Lowndes Sevely, Josephine, *Eve's Secrets: A New Theory of Female Sexuality*, New York: Random House, 1987.
Lowry, Thomas Power (ed.) *The Classic Clitoris: Historic Contributions to Scientific Sexuality*, Chicago: Nelson-Hall, 1978.
Moore, Lisa Jean, and Clarke, Adele E., 'Clitoral Conventions and Transgressions: Graphic Representations in Anatomy Texts, *c.* 1900–1991', Feminist Studies, 21 (1995), 255–301.
Moscucci, Ornella, *The Science of Woman: Gynaecology and Gender in England 1800–1929*, Cambridge: University of Cambridge Press, 1990.
O'Connell, Helen, Hutson, John, Anderson, Colin, Plenter, Robert, 'Anatomical relationship between urethra and clitoris', *The Journal of Urology*, 159 (1998), 1892–7.
Pinto-Correia, Clara, *The Ovary of Eve: Egg and Sperm and Preformation*, Chicago: University of Chicago Press, 1997.
Schiebinger, Londa, *Nature's Body: Gender in the Making of Modern Science*, Boston: Beacon Press, 1993.

Sissa, Giulia, *Greek Virginity*, trans. Arthur Goldhammer, Cambridge, Mass.: Harvard University Press, 1990.

Chapter 5: Opening Pandora's Box

Austin, C.R., 'Sperm fertility, viability and persistence in the female tract', *Journal of Reproduction and Fertility*, Supplement 22 (1975), 75–89.

Cabello Santamaria F., and Nesters R., 'Retrograde ejaculation: a new theory of female ejaculation', paper given at the 13th Congress of Sexology, Barcelona, Spain, August 1997.

Carr, Pat, and Gingerich, Willard, 'The Vagina Dentata Motif in Nahuatl and Pueblo Mythic Narratives: A Comparative Study', *Smoothing the Ground, Essays on Native American Oral Literature*, ed. Brian Swann, Los Angeles: University of California Press, 1983.

Douglas, Nik, and Slinger, Penny, *Sexual Secrets: The Alchemy of Ecstasy*, Vermont: Destiny Books, 1979.

Douglass, Marcia, and Douglass, Lisa, *Are We Having Fun Yet?: The Intelligent Woman's Guide to Sex*, New York: Hyperion, 1997.

Faix, A., Lapray, J.F., Courtieu, C., Maubon, A., Lanfrey, Kerry, 'Magnetic Resonance Imaging of Sexual Intercourse: Initial Experience', *Journal of Sex & Marital Therapy*, 27 (2001), 475–82.

Graber, Benjamin (ed.), *Circumvaginal Musculature and Sexual Function*, New York: S. Karger, 1982.

Gräfenberg, Ernest, 'The Role of the Urethra in Female Orgasm', *The International Journal of Sexology*, Vol. III (3) (1950), 145–8.

Gregor, Thomas, *Anxious Pleasures: The Sexual Lives of an Amazonian People*, Chicago: The University of Chicago Press, 1985.

Huffman, J.W., 'The Detailed Anatomy of the Paraurethral Ducts in the Adult Human Female', *American Journal of Obstetrics and Gynecology*, 55 (1948), 86–101.

Ladas, Alice Kahn, Whipple, Beverly, Perry, John D., *The G Spot and Other Discoveries about Human Sexuality*, New York: Bantam Doubleday, 1982.

Morgan, Elaine, *The Descent of Woman: The Classic Study of Evolution*, London: Souvenir Press, 1985.

Overstreet, J. W., and Mahi-Brown, C. A., 'Sperm Processing in the Female Reproductive Tract', *Local Immunity in Reproduction Tract Tissues*, ed. P.D. Griffin and P.M. Johnson, Oxford: Oxford University Press, 1993.

Perry, J.D., and Whipple, B., 'Pelvic muscle strength of female ejaculators: Evidence in support of a new theory of orgasm', *Journal of Sex Research*, 17 (1981), 22–39.

Raitt, Jill, 'The *Vagina Dentata* and the *Immaculatus Uterus Divini Fontis*', *The Journal of the American Academy of Religion*, XLVIII/3 (1980), 415–31.

Ruan, Fang Fu, *Sex in China: Studies in Sexology in Chinese Culture*, New York: Plenum Press, 1991.

Schleiner, Winfried, *Medical Ethics in the Renaissance*, Washington, D.C.: Georgetown University Press, 1995.

Stuart, Elizabeth, and Spencer, Paula, *The V Book: vital facts about the vulva, vestibule, vagina and more*, London: Piatkus, 2002.

Sundahl, Deborah, *Female Ejaculation & the G spot*, Alameda, California: Hunter House Publishers, 2003.

Van Lysebeth, André, *Tantra: The Cult of the Feminine*, Delhi: Motilal Banarsidass, 1995.

Walker, Barbara, *The Woman's Encyclopedia of Myths and Secrets*, San Francisco: Harper San Francisco, 1983.

Zaviacic, Milan, and Whipple, Beverly, 'Update on the Female Prostate and the Phenomenon of Female Ejaculation', *The Journal of Sex Research*, 30 (2) (1993), 148–51.

Zaviacic, Milan, *The Human Female Prostate: From Vestigial Skene's Paraurethral Glands and Ducts to Woman's Functional Prostate*, Bratislava: Slovak Academic Press, 1999.

Zaviacic, Milan, and Ablin, R.J., 'The female prostate and prostate-specific antigen. Immunohistochemical localization, implications of this prostate marker in women and reasons for using the term "prostate" in the human female', *Histology and Histopathology*, 15 (2000), 131–42.

Chapter 6: The Perfumed Garden

Ackerman, Diane, *A Natural History of the Senses*, New York: Random House, 1990.

Barefoot Doctor's *Handbook for Modern Lovers*, London: Piatkus, 2000.

Blakemore, Colin and Jennett, Sheila (eds.), *The Oxford Companion to the Body*, Oxford, Oxford University Press, 2001.

Brahmachary, R.L., 'The expanding world of 2-acetyl-1-pyrrolline', *Current Science*, 71: Issue 4 (1996), 257–8.

Everett, H.C., 'Paroxysmal sneezing following orgasm (answer)', *Journal of the American Medical Association*, 219 (1972), 1350–1.

Fabricant, Noah, 'Sexual functions and the nose', *American Journal of the Medical Sciences*, 239 (1960), 156–60.

Green, Monica H., *The Trotula: A Medieval Compendium of Women's Medicine*, Philadelphia: University of Pennsylvania Press, 2001.

Jacquart, Danielle, and Thomasset, Claude, *Sexuality and Medicine in the Middle Ages*, Princeton: Princeton University Press, 1988.

Jöchle, Wolfgang, 'Current Research in Coitus-induced Ovulation: A Review', *Journal of Reproduction and Fertility*, Supplement 22 (1975), 165–207.

Kannan, S., and Archunan, G. 'Chemistry of clitoral gland secretions of the laboratory rat: Assessment of behavioural response to identified compounds', *Journal of Biosciences*, 26 (2001), 247–52.

King, Helen, *Hippocrates' Woman: Reading the Female Body in Ancient Greece*, London: Routledge, 1998.

Mackenzie, John N., 'Irritation of the sexual apparatus as an etiological factor in the production of nasal disease', *American Journal of the Medical Sciences*, 87 (1884), 360–5.

Milinski, Manfred, and Wedekind, Claus, 'Evidence for MHC-correlated perfume preferences in humans', *Behavioural Ecology*, 12: No. 2 (2001), 140–9.

Ober, Carole, Weitkamp, L.R., Cox, N., Dytch, H., Kostyu, D., Elias, S., 'HLA and human mate choice', *American Journal of Human Genetics*, 61 (3) (1997), 497–504.

Poran, N.S., 'Cyclic Attractivity of Human Female Odours', *Advances In the Biosciences*, 93 (1994), 555–60.

Purves, R., 'Accessory breasts in the labia majora', *British Journal of Surgery*, 15 (1928), 279–81.

Stern, Kathleen, and McClintock, Martha K., 'Regulation of ovulation by human pheromones', *Nature*, 392 (1998), 177–9.

Stoddart, D. Michael, *The Scented Ape: The Biology and Culture of Human Odour*, London: Cambridge University Press, 1990.

van der Putte, S.C.J., 'Anogenital "sweat" glands: Histology and pathology of a gland that may mimic mammary glands', *The American Journal of Dermatopathology*, 13 (6) (1991), 557–67.

Veith, Jane L., Buck, Michael, Getzlaf, Shelly, van Dalfsen, Pamela, Slade, Sue, 'Exposure to men influences the occurrence of ovulation in women', *Physiology and Behaviour*, 31 (1983), 313–5.

Vroon, Piet, with van Amerongen, Anton, and de Vries, Hans, *Smell: The Secret Seducer*, New York: Farrar, Straus and Giroux, 1994.

Wallen, Kim, and Schneider, Jill E. (eds.), *Reproduction in Context: Social and Environmental Influences on Reproduction*, Cambridge, Mass.: Massachusetts Institute of Technology, 2000.

Watson, Lyall, *Jacobson's Organ and the Remarkable Nature of Smell*, London: The Penguin Press, 1999.

Wedekind, Claus, Seebeck, Thomas, Bettens, Florence, Pearce, Alexander J., 'MHC-dependent mate preferences in humans', *Proceedings of the Royal Society of London* Series B, 260 (1995), 245–9.

Chapter 7: The Function of the Orgasm

Allen, M. L., and Lemmon, W. B., 'Orgasm in Female Primates', *American Journal of Primatology*, 1 (1981), 15–34.

Baker, R. Robin, and Bellis, Mark A., 'Human Sperm Competition: ejaculate manipulation by females and a function for the female orgasm', *Animal Behaviour*, 46 (1993), 887–909.

Bohlen, Joseph G., Held, James P., Sanderson, Margaret Olwen, Ahlgren, Andrew, 'The Female Orgasm: Pelvic Contractions', *Archives of Sexual Behaviour*, 11 (5) (1982), 367.

Bullough, Vernon L., and Bullough, Bonnie (eds.), *Human Sexuality: An Encyclopaedia*, New York: Garland Publishing Inc., 1994.

Chia, Mantak, and Arava, Douglas Abrams, *The Multi-Orgasmic Man: how any man can experience multiple orgasms and dramatically enhance his sexual relationship*, San Francisco: Harper San Francisco, 1996.

Eberhard, W., 'Evidence for widespread courtship during copulation in 131 species of insects and spiders, and implications for cryptic female choice', *Evolution*, 48 (1994), 711–33.

Eberhard, W.G., Huber, BA., Rodriguez, R.L., Salas, I., Briceno, R.D., Rodriguez V., 'One size fits all? Relationships between the size and degree of variation in genitalia and other body parts in 20 species of insects and spiders', *Evolution*, 52 (1998), 415–31.

Eisler, Riane, *Sacred Pleasure: Sex, Myth and the Politics of the Body*, San Francisco: HarperCollins, 1995.

INDEX